APPLIED MICROBIOLOGY FOR NURSES

Dinah Gould
and
Christine Brooker

First published 2000 by
MACMILLAN PRESS LTD
Houndmills, Basingstoke, Hampshire RG21 6XS
and London
Companies and representatives
throughout the world

ISBN 0–333–71425–3 paperback

A catalogue record for this book is available
from the British Library.

This book is printed on paper suitable for recycling and
made from fully managed and sustained forest sources.

10 9   8   7   6   5   4   3   2   1
09 08 07 06 05 04 03 02 01 00

Editing and origination by
Aardvark Editorial, Mendham, Suffolk

Printed in Malaysia

APPLIED MICROBIOLOGY FOR NURSES

APPLIED MICROBIOLOGY FOR NURSES

Contents

Contents

APPLIED MICROBIOLOGY FOR NURSES

List of figures

APPLIED MICROBIOLOGY FOR NURSES

List of tables

APPLIED
MICROBIOLOGY
FOR NURSES

Preface

Nurses in every area of practice provide care for patients who are at risk of infection and those who already have an established infection. One in every ten patients admitted to hospital is likely to develop an infection, and patients in a variety of community settings, including their own homes, will have infections. In addition to problems that have been around for decades, and the resurgence of others such as tuberculosis, many 'new' conditions such as BSE and HIV are now known to be caused by infective agents.

A knowledge of how infection occurs, the precautions required to contain it and methods of preventing it occurring in the first place are essential information for every nurse. Experienced practitioners and infection control nurses may have access to a range of advanced texts and journal articles, as well as the latest findings on the World Wide Web. The needs of students and non-specialist nurses getting to grips with the subject, however, have tended to be overlooked.

This book is aimed at exactly this group of readers. It introduces the important concept of applied microbiology with the aid of clinical application boxes, and the core principles of infection control. Chapters 1 to 3 cover basic microbiological information with the emphasis on clinical application and relevance to nurses. The principles of infection prevention, control and treatment are covered in Chapters 4 to 6. Chapters 7 to 13 deal with specific issues, such as urinary and wound infection, and the infection risks posed by blood and body fluids. The concluding chapter looks at epidemiology and some specific diseases, both old and new. Numerous cross-references between chapters help to link microbiological theory with what nurses do and see in practice.

Each chapter is extensively referenced and where appropriate readers are offered suggestions for further reading and other information sources. Many informative illustrations help readers to 'make sense' of new material. Chapter outcomes at the start of each chapter inform the reader about what they should know after reading the chapter, and provide a framework for learning. All chapters conclude with a list of suggested activities linking knowledge to clinical practice, and a revision check list of the key areas. Self-assessment questions for every chapter means that readers can check their knowledge and identify topics needing further work. A comprehensive glossary of the 'language' of microbiology and infection control is provided.

This book will help readers to develop their evidence-based practice and most importantly assist in the continual efforts required to improve the quality of health care.

*APPLIED
MICROBIOLOGY
FOR NURSES*

Foreword

For anyone who would limit what nurses 'need to know' in terms of the life sciences, this book is a perfect antidote. Nurses, as part of a multidisciplinary team, are in the front line of applied microbiology in the form of infection control. In the parlance of Project 2000, the 'knowledgeable doer' is a better doer than the one who simply follows procedures without understanding their significance. The authors have a track record of publication in the life sciences for nurses and I have had the privilege of working with both of them on a number of projects. Being asked to write this foreword, therefore, is both a pleasure and an honour.

It amuses me to think what Florence Nightingale would make of a textbook on microbiology for nurses, because she did not believe that micro-organisms were responsible for the spread of infection. She nursed at a time not far removed from the days when the theory of 'spontaneous generation' of life was still held as an explanation for the appearance of rats in rubbish and mould on food. Most nursing practice relating to infection was based on nothing more than ritual and Pasteur's elegant proof of the existence of airborne micro-organisms is relatively recent. However, I well remember conducting aseptic technique – a fundamental aspect of my practical assessment to register as a nurse – that bore no relation to anything that I had ever learned about micro-organisms in my previous life as a biologist. This text, while restricting itself to those aspects of microbiology that nurses need to know, takes in a wide range of relevant issues such as immunology and the work of the hospital microbiology laboratory. It also devotes chapters to issues specific to nursing such as urinary tract and wound infection.

In the age of clinical governance, where individuals and institutions are required to account for a range of clinical parameters, the work of nursing staff in relation to infection control is likely to come under the spotlight as never before. New policies and practices to reduce infection, on the one hand, and audit outcomes, on the other, will only go so far to address this. Nurses who understand the implications of their practice in terms of the ubiquity and sheer adaptability of micro-organisms and the contribution which malpractices such as the overuse of antibiotics can make to the safety of their patients will formulate and implement the best strategies. Nurses also need to know the dangers of infection to themselves. At one time infection was a serious issue because the means to combat it effectively were not available. The stakes are higher now for all health professionals with the advent of HIV and the more widespread occurrence and increase in strains of hepatitis for which there is no cure. This book is a significant step towards ensuring that nurses are duly prepared, to paraphrase Nightingale, to continue to do neither the patient nor themselves harm.

ROGER WATSON BSc PhD RGN CBiol MIBiol
Professor of Nursing, School of Nursing
University of Hull, England

*APPLIED
MICROBIOLOGY
FOR NURSES*

Acknowledgements

Thanks to Ann Osborne at King's Lynn Health Service Library, Queen Elizabeth Hospital, for her invaluable assistance.

Special thanks to Alex Dallas, veterinary surgeon, for providing information about toxoplasmosis, and advice about bovine tuberculosis, BSE and rabies.

Note from the authors

This book should not be used as a primary source for prescribing, dispensing or administering drugs. While all reasonable care has been undertaken to ensure accuracy, the authors and publishers are not responsible for any damage caused to any person which may occur if a reader prescribes, dispenses or administers drugs on the basis of information given here. Readers are responsible for checking the manufacturer's product information and a National Formulary before calculating doses or administering any drug.

Readers should also be aware that the publication of new research findings and guidelines concerning infection control will continue to affect their evidence-based practice.

1 Micro-organisms and disease

CHAPTER OUTCOMES

After reading this chapter, you should be able to:

- List the main groups of micro-organism causing infection

- Explain the terms infection, colonisation, commensal, pathogen, opportunist and virulence

- Give examples of bacteria of the following morphological types: bacilli, cocci, spirochaetes and vibrios

- Give an example of each of the following and in each case state the nature of the infection caused: Gram-negative bacterium, Gram-positive bacterium, acid-fast bacillus

- Explain how viruses cause disease and give an example

- List the main mechanisms by which micro-organisms are disseminated, and for each route suggested give an example

- State the ways in which micro-organisms gain access to the internal tissues of the host, and give an example for each mechanism suggested

- Describe the main morphological characteristics of bacteria that allow them to behave as pathogens, giving examples

- List the ways in which bacteria multiply, and point out their clinical significance

- Provide examples of a spore-forming bacterium, an aerobe, an anaerobe, a human mycosis and a helminthic (worm) infestation

Introduction to medical microbiology and micro-organisms causing disease

Microbiology is the study of micro-organisms – living organisms that are too small to be examined without a microscope. Organisms with a diameter of 0.1 mm are just visible to the naked eye, but magnification is required to study them in detail. Medical microbiology is the study of micro-organisms that play a role in human infection.

Infection is caused by bacteria, viruses, fungi, protozoa and a few minor groups (mycoplasmas, rickettsiae and chlamydiae). Parasitic worms are multicellular and often clearly visible to the naked eye, but their eggs and larvae are microscopic, so the presence of infection is frequently detected in specimens sent to the microbiology department. In recent years, minute virus-like protein particles called prions have also been implicated in causing infection. An example is the agent causing bovine spongiform encephalopathy (BSE).

Bacteria

Bacteria live everywhere. Most are saprophytes (organisms that live on dead organic material) present in soil and water. They play a vital role degrading complex organic molecules from dead animals and plants into simple organic ones. These molecules are recycled during metabolism by living organisms.

Pathogenic activity

Approximately 50 species of bacteria are pathogenic (able to cause disease). Virulence – the ability to generate infection – is a complex phenomenon related to the physiology of both pathogen and host. Some bacteria are always highly virulent. For example, exposure to *Yersinia pestis* (which causes plague) will almost certainly result in infection. However, some bacteria, particularly those causing infections in hospital, are of low pathogenicity. They cause infection only in people whose immune status is compromised by illness, drugs or the invasive procedures they have undergone (for example surgery, intubation or the insertion of an intravenous line). They do not attack healthy tissues. These bacteria are called opportunists. *Pseudomonas*, *Klebsiella* and *Proteus* are typical opportunists.

Other bacteria live harmlessly in or on one particular part of the body. These make up the normal flora and are called commensals (Table 1.1). They receive shelter and benefit the host by keeping potentially dangerous micro-organisms at bay. If they gain access to a different anatomical location, however, they can generate infection. *Escherichia coli (E. coli)*, normally present in the bowel, can cause urinary tract infection if it gains access to the bladder. This is an example of endogenous (self) infection, occurring when the organisms responsible originate from the same individual. Exogenous (cross) infection occurs when micro-organisms originate from another source: patients, staff or the environment.

Table 1.1   The normal human flora

Anatomical location	Organisms
Skin	*Staphylococcus epidermidis* Micrococci Diphtheroids
Upper respiratory tract	*Streptococcus viridans* Diphtheroids *Neisseria catarrhalis*
Large intestine/bowel	*Bacteroides* spp. *Escherichia coli* *Streptococcus faecalis* *Proteus* Clostridia Lactobacilli
Vagina	Lactobacilli *Staphylococcus epidermidis*

Infection and colonisation

Infection occurs when pathogens gain access to host tissues and elicit a response. Infection in a wound is indicated by the appearance of inflammation and pus. The patient may become pyrexial, and a wound swab will indicate the presence of large numbers of the causative organism.

The response to the pathogens may, however, be slight or absent, a situation described as colonisation. A colonised wound is free from inflammation, a swab indicating scanty bacterial growth. When colonisation occurs, several species of bacteria may be present, often referred to as 'mixed bacterial growth' on laboratory reports. Colonisation is of clinical significance because the organism may multiply in large numbers to form a reservoir. Colonisation is usually the precursor to infection when outbreaks occur (Muder *et al.*, 1991), and even if the original patient escapes the clinical signs and symptoms of disease, cross-infection may still occur.

Clinical Application

Being Alert to the Possibility of Infection

There are many situations in which infection is more difficult to diagnose: the very young, older adults, those with communication problems and people with mental health problems and learning disabilities. The expected signs of infection, for example an elevated temperature, may not be present in older people. Nurses need to be alert to other signs, symptoms and changes in behaviour that may indicate an infection. The list provided offers some examples, but you will be able to think of other examples from your own observations and practice:

- Complaints of feeling generally unwell
- A rash characteristic of the infection
- Chills and shivering
- Changes in vital signs other than temperature
- General aches and pains in the muscles and joints
- A dry mouth with a furred tongue
- Loss of appetite
- Nausea and vomiting
- Diarrhoea
- Headache
- Loss of continence in adults
- 'Accidents' in previously continent toddlers and children
- Behavioural changes in children, becoming fretful and miserable
- Increasing confusion and disorientation in older adults
- Enlarged and tender lymph nodes.

NB. The knowledge that a particular infection, for example chickenpox or gastroenteritis, is present in the population at the time should alert nurses to the possibility of infection.

Describing bacteria

Bacteria can be described in terms of their:

- Morphology (shape)
- Ultrastructure
- Response to dyes used on microscope specimens:- for example, the Gram stain reaction
- Spore formation
- Oxygen requirement.

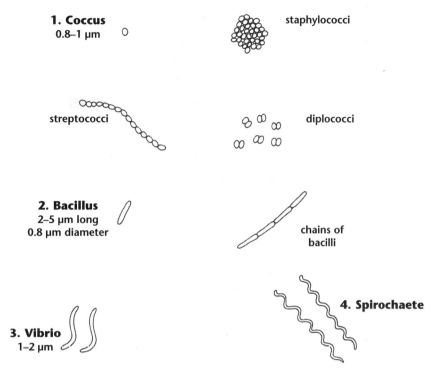

Figure 1.1   Bacterial morphology I

Morphology

Four morphological forms exist (Figure 1.1):

- **Cocci** are round. When they are arranged in pairs, they are known as diplococci. Examples include *Streptococcus pneumoniae* (which causes pneumonia) and *Neisseria gonorrhoeae* (leading to gonorrhoea). Clusters of cocci are termed staphylococci. Examples include *Staphylococcus aureus*, a constituent of the normal skin flora, which is in some members of the population also able to operate as a wound pathogen, and *Staphlyococcus epidermidis*, an opportunist able to cause infection in very sick people, although not in the healthy. Streptococci are round bacteria attached to one another in chains. They cause sore throats and a wide range of other infections encountered in hospital and the community (Cleary *et al.*, 1992).

- **Bacilli** (for example *Pseudomonas*, *Klebsiella*, *Proteus* and *E. coli*) are rod shaped, occurring singly or in chains. They are notorious for their ability to cause infection in hospital. Several bacteria causing food poisoning, including *Shigella* and *Salmonella*, also belong to this group.

- **Vibrios** are curved bacteria. Examples include *Vibrio cholerae* (resulting in cholera) and *Campylobacter* (responsible for food poisoning).

■ **Spirochaetes** are very small, flexible, spirally shaped bacteria. Typical members of the group include *Treponema pallidum* (which causes syphilis), *Leptospira interrogans* (serotype *icterohaemorrhagiae*) (Weil's disease) transmitted to human hosts from infected rats and *Borrelia burgdorferi* (Lyme disease).

All bacteria are unicellular, but their size and shape vary widely (Figure 1.1). Specimens must be 'fixed' (killed) and stained before they can be examined with the light microscope. Advances in electron microscopy have made it possible to study the ultrastructure (fine detail) of cells. The cells are, however, still dead because examination must be performed with the specimens in a vacuum. The image that appears does not represent the dynamic, living state.

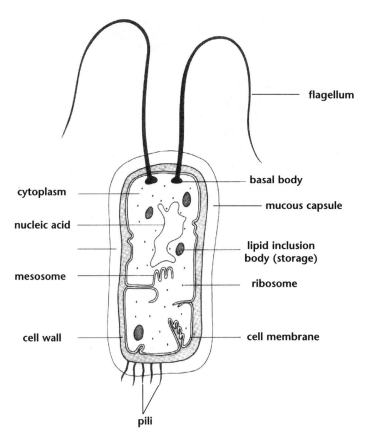

Figure 1.2   The 'typical' bacterial cell

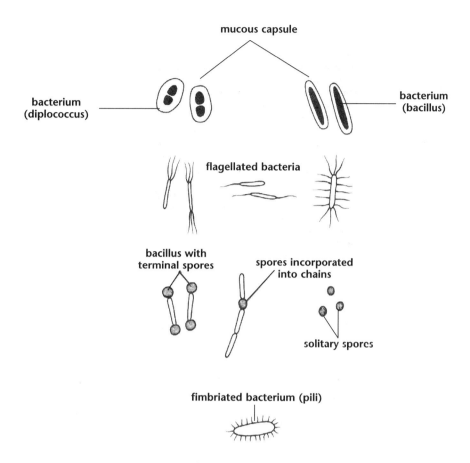

Figure 1.3   Bacterial morphology II

Ultrastructure

The bacterial cell ultrastructure differs from that of multicellular organisms. The cells of multicellular organisms are eukaryotic (that is, they have a true nucleus). Their genetic material is enclosed in a membrane to form this nucleus. Numerous cytoplasmic organelles are also present, a few exceptions being membrane bound. In contrast, bacteria are prokaryotic (lacking in a true nucleus and nuclear membrane). The chromosome containing the genetic material (nucleic acid) lies directly in the cytoplasm, as do all the organelles, including the ribosomes (sites of protein synthesis) and storage granules. The mesosome, an infold of the outer membrane, is the site of respiration, analogous to the eukaryotic mitochondria.

Figure 1.2 depicts a 'typical' bacterial cell, although few species display all the possible features shown. Some species (for example, *N. gonorrhoeae*) possess hair-like processes called pili used to attach the bacterium to a potential host while other, highly motile forms (for example, *Salmonella* and *Proteus*) have one or more flagella (Figure 1.3). However, all bacterial species are surrounded by a rigid mucopeptide cell wall, giving the cell support and protecting its contents. This is absent in eukaryotic cells. Some bacteria have a mucous capsule around the cell wall, reducing the risk of desiccation in dry conditions. Strains of *Klebsiella* equipped with a mucous capsule are particularly likely to contribute to cross-infection and to result in outbreaks of disease because they survive well on dry skin (Casewell and Desai, 1983).

The Gram stain reaction

In the natural condition, bacteria are colourless. The Gram staining reaction is used in the first step of laboratory identification (Table 1.2).

Table 1.2   The Gram stain reaction

- A thin film of the specimen is smeared onto the surface of a glass microscope slide
- The slide is passed through the flame of a Bunsen burner 3–4 times to 'fix' (kill) the micro-organisms
- The slide is covered with purple dye (methyl or crystal violet) for 15 seconds, the excess fluid then being poured away
- The slide is flooded with Gram's iodine for up to 1 minute, after which the iodine is drained
- The slide is flooded with acetone for 2–5 seconds before being washed with water or ethanol to rinse away any dye not taken up by the bacteria
- The bacteria are counterstained by pouring a red dye (carbol fuchsin) onto the slide for 20 seconds
- The slide is blotted dry and is then ready for examination. Gram-positive organisms retain the violet dye and appear deep purple. Gram-negative bacteria stain pink because they lose the violet stain, taking up the red counterstain instead

Examples of typical Gram-positive and Gram-negative bacteria are shown in Table 1.3.

Mycobacterium does not respond well to Gram staining because the thick, waxy cell wall is impermeable to the dyes. It is identified by the acid-fast (Ziehl–Neelsen) staining technique. *Mycobacterium tuberculosis* (tuberculosis) is thus described as being 'acid fast' or as the 'acid-fast bacillus' (AFB).

Table 1.3 · · · **Typical Gram-positive and Gram-negative bacteria**

Gram-positive bacteria	Gram-negative bacteria	
Staphylococcus	Klebsiella	Bacteroides
Streptococcus	Proteus	Vibrio
Bacillus	Escherichia coli	Haemophilus
Clostridium	Acinetobacter	Yersinia
Corynebacterium	Salmonella	Neisseria

The Gram stain reaction is valuable because it distinguishes structural differences between Gram-positive and Gram-negative bacteria and provides an indication of their behaviour. Much of the difference between the two groups is explained by a variation in the chemical composition of the cell wall (see Chapter 4). Gram-positive bacteria tend to be more resistant to desiccation and tolerate dry conditions. Gram-negative species thrive in damp situations and are generally more resistant to antibiotics. Few species of Gram-positive bacteria are flagellated, so they lack motility.

Spore formation

Clostridium and *Bacillus* form spores under adverse conditions. The cell becomes surrounded by a thick, protective capsule, and its metabolism slows. In favourable conditions, the spore germinates, releasing the bacterium. Spores are very resistant to heat and desiccation, remaining viable over long periods. The ability to form spores that will survive in adverse environmental circumstances is restricted to the Gram-positive species. The spores of *Bacillus anthracis* (which gives rise to anthrax) and *Clostridium tetani* (tetanus) survive dormant for years, able to withstand extremes of temperature and exposure to disinfectants that would destroy vegetative cells. Germination occurs when conditions become favourable for growth and reproduction.

Oxygen requirement

Bacteria display a variety of oxygen requirements (Table 1.4):

- They are described as obligate aerobes if their growth demands an environmental oxygen supply
- Those unable to tolerate the presence of oxygen are called obligate anaerobes
- A third group, the facultative aerobes, can grow whether or not oxygen is available.

Table 1.4   Oxygen requirements of some medically important bacteria

Oxygen requirement	Example
Aerobic/facultatively aerobic	*Neisseria meningitidis*
	Neisseria gonorrhoeae
	Salmonella
	Shigella
	Campylobacter
	Klebsiella
	Proteus
	Escherichia coli
Anaerobic	*Bacteroides*
	Treponema pallidum
	Clostridium

The process of infection

Establishing infection

Before infection is possible, a susceptible host must encounter a virulent micro-organism. The pathogen must complete the following stages:

- Gaining access to the host tissues
- Moving to a favourable site
- Multiplying successfully in spite of the defence mechanisms mustered by the host
- Reproducing so that new pathogens can escape to be disseminated, thus completing the life cycle.

Gaining access: portals of entry

Invasion occurs by inhalation or ingestion, via the urogenital tract, by inoculation and by vertical transmission.

- **Inhalation** occurs via the respiratory tract, the nose or mouth being the route taken by colds and influenza viruses and organisms causing tuberculosis, diphtheria and the infections of childhood (measles and mumps). Infectious airborne particles are released as aerosols. Droplet transmission only occurs when an individual with an infectious respiratory condition exhales forcefully, sneezes or coughs. Only the smallest particles (1–5 μm) can reach the lower airways. The length of contact between the source and the potential new case increases the risk of transmission. This is because the longer the period of exposure, the greater the risk of inhalation.

- **Ingestion** via the mouth into the gastrointestinal tract occurs when food or water is contaminated. *Salmonella*, *Shigella*, *Campylobacter*, *Vibrio* and the virus causing poliomyelitis enter by being ingested.

- The **urogenital tract** is the route taken by pathogens causing sexually transmitted infections (*N. gonorrhoeae*, *T. pallidum* and *Trichomonas vaginalis*). Urinary pathogens, principally Gram-negative bacilli, gain access via the urethra.

- The **inoculation** of pathogens via the skin or mucous membranes can occur during surgical incision, accidental injury or injection with a needle (hepatitis B, hepatitis C and human immunodeficiency virus [HIV]), or via the mouth parts of an insect (*Plasmodium* following a mosquito bite).

- **Vertical transmission** occurs via the placenta from the maternal to the fetal circulation (rubella virus and *T. pallidum*) or by contamination as the baby travels down the birth canal at parturition. *N. gonorrhoeae* can be transferred to the eyes of a neonate from an infected mother in this way, resulting in ophthalmia neonatorum. *Chlamydia trachomatis* can cause serious respiratory and eye infections in babies exposed to the organism during birth. Women infected with HIV may transmit the infection to their children via the placenta, in breast milk or at parturition when the infant is exposed to contaminated blood and cervical secretions (Francis, 1994). A baby may develop shingles if its mother had varicella (chickenpox) during pregnancy (Enders *et al.*, 1994).

Virulence

The ability to establish an infection depends on virulence. Several factors contribute, including the size of the inoculating dose and the ability to invade host tissues and damage them.

Size of the inoculating dose

Except in the case of very virulent pathogens a large number of micro-organisms is more likely to overwhelm the host defences, and there is a greater chance that at least some will reach a site suitable for growth and multiplication. Most pathogens invade specific sites. *N. gonorrhoeae* invades the delicate cervical and urethral epithelia but not the tough squamous cells lining the mouth or vagina.

Viruses responsible for colds invade the nasal epithelium and conjunctivae but not the oral mucosa.

Ability to invade host tissues

This depends on the bacterium's morphological characteristics and its production of enzymes and toxins.

Morphological characteristics

Pili on the surface of *N. gonorrhoeae* allow it to attach to epithelial cells on the cervix uteri and urethra. Mutant strains without pili lack virulence. The presence of a protective mucous capsule surrounding the cell wall reduces the risk of desiccation in particular strains of Gram-negative bacteria, so they survive longer on the hands and are more likely to cause cross-infection (Cooke *et al.,* 1981).

Enzyme production

Enzyme production is a property of many bacteria. Staphylococci, streptococci and *Clostridium perfringens* release haemolytic enzymes, which destroy erythrocytes. *Staphylococcus aureus* releases an enzyme called coagulase, which clots plasma, thus protecting the bacteria from phagocytosis (Chapter 2).

Toxins

Toxins are of two types, depending on the mechanism of synthesis and secretion.

1. **Exotoxins** are secreted by Gram-positive bacteria and released outside the cell into the surrounding extracellular fluid, dissolving and being carried throughout the tissues. Exotoxins destroy host cells or inhibit specific metabolic functions. They include some of the most lethal chemicals known. The exotoxin secreted by *Clostridium botulinum* (which causes botulism) interrupts the transmission of nervous impulses, paralysing the victim. *Clostridium tetani* (the causative organism of tetanus) releases an exotoxin that excites neurones in the central nervous system. The muscular spasms of 'lockjaw' result. Exotoxins released by *Staphylococcus aureus* and *Bacillus cereus* result in food poisoning.

2. **Endotoxins** develop as part of the cell wall of Gram-negative bacteria. They include *Salmonella typhi* (which causes typhoid), *Neisseria meningitidis* (meningococcal meningitis) and *Shigella sonnei* (dysentery). The release of endotoxins corresponds with symptoms of fever and malaise experienced by the host.

Ability to damage host tissues

The ability to damage host tissues is closely related to the ability to invade. Damage may be structural (the tissues being physically destroyed) or physiological (normal function becoming disturbed). In most cases, both types occur. *Staphylococcus aureus* destroys tissue because the infection causes abscess formation. Pyrexia occurs simultaneously with this.

Bacterial growth requirements

A knowledge of bacterial growth requirements is essential when attempts are made to grow and identify organisms in the laboratory. Bacteria are unicellular and therefore more susceptible to environmental fluctuations than larger, more complex multicellular organisms. As with higher forms of life, their growth requirements include:

- Water
- An energy source
- A suitable pH
- A suitable temperature
- Protection from ultraviolet rays.

Water

Water accounts for more than 80 per cent of the bacterial cell volume and is essential for the growth and survival of vegetative bacterial cells. Some Gram-positive species (for example, *Bacillus* and *Clostridium*) avoid desiccation by forming resistant spores under adverse conditions.

An energy source

Nourishment is derived from substances available within the environment. Bacteria vary enormously in their ability to utilise different sources of nourishment:

- Phototrophs use carbon dioxide as their sole source of carbon to synthesise all the complex organic molecules they need. Like plants, they obtain their energy from sunlight.

- Chemotrophs obtain energy by oxidising inorganic material.

- Heterotrophs require a supply of organic nutrients such as carbohydrates or amino acids. Most pathogens are heterotrophs. Generally speaking, the more adapted the organism is to a strictly pathogenic existence, the more demanding its growth requirements (for example, *Pseudomonas*, *E. coli* and *Klebsiella*). In contrast, *N. gonorrhoeae* has complex growth requirements and cannot survive long outside the human host. *T. pallidum*, which is even more fastidious, has never been cultured outside living tissues.

Bacteria also vary in their ability to use sources of energy during respiration (see Oxygen requirement, above):

- Obligate aerobes (for example, *M. tuberculosis*) are unable to grow in the absence of oxygen.

■ Facultative aerobes are tolerant of the presence of free atmospheric oxygen in their environment and will grow whether or not it is available. Most human pathogens belong to this group.

■ Obligate anaerobes cannot grow unless all traces of oxygen are removed from their environment. They tend to cause infections deep within the tissues. *Clostridium* spp. cause gangrene and tetanus, infections originating when the bacteria gain access to the deep tissues.

■ Microaerophilic bacteria grow more rapidly in the presence of only traces of free oxygen.

A suitable pH

Bacteria vary widely in their tolerance of acidic or alkaline conditions, ranging from pH 4–9. Human pathogens generally prefer a pH within the range 7.2–7.6, but there are exceptions. Cholera vibrios, for example, thrive best at pH 8. They affect the small intestine, which receives pancreatic fluid at the same pH. Lactobacilli (part of the normal flora) inhabiting the vagina grow best at a pH of about 4.

A suitable temperature

All species have a preferred temperature range, but within this there is an optimum temperature at which they grow best:

■ Mesophilic bacteria thrive within the 25–40 ^{0}C range. Human pathogens fall into this group, thriving optimally at 37 ^{0}C.

■ Psychrophilic bacteria grow best at approximately 20 ^{0}C and slowly at 4 ^{0}C. They influence health not by causing infection, but by their ability to spoil food that has not been properly refrigerated.

■ Thermophilic bacteria, growing at temperatures of 55–90 ^{0}C do not operate as human pathogens.

Protection from ultraviolet rays

Most pathogenic bacteria grow best in darkness and are rapidly destroyed by ultraviolet light, whether it is natural, in sunlight or arising from an artificial source. This is the rationale behind 'airing' clothing in the sun as it dries.

Bacterial reproduction and genetics

Binary fission

Binary fission is a simple, asexual process involving the division of a bacterial cell into two genetically identical daughters. The rate of binary fission depends on the particular species and the environmental circumstances. In ideal conditions (for example, a warm, damp hospital ward), a typical Gram-negative bacillus such as

E. coli will divide about once every 20 minutes. Others, for example *M. tuberculosis*, divide very slowly. The results of laboratory tests for *E. coli* are available within 24 hours, but a firm diagnosis of tuberculosis may not become available for weeks. Treatment for tuberculosis may, however, be started on the basis of clinical findings and other tests, for example skin tests, radiography and the presence of AFBs in a sputum specimen.

Asexual reproduction does not involve the exchange of genetic material so there can be no provision for genetic variation, a disadvantage as the organisms are thus limited in their ability to respond and adapt to environmental pressures.

Sexual reproduction

Sexual reproduction is, however, possible in particular bacteria containing a small amount of extrachromosomal DNA lying within the cytoplasm. This is called a plasmid. It accounts for approximately 1 per cent of the total amount of genetic material present in those cells which contain it. A transfer of genetic material between bacteria is possible according to three mechanisms: conjugation, transduction and transformation.

Conjugation

Conjugation is an important means of genetic exchange, particularly among Gram-negative bacilli. Sex pili coded by the DNA of a donor or 'male' cell attach to the recipient or 'female' cell. Plasmid replication follows, one copy passing to the recipient, the other remaining within the cytoplasm of the donor.

Transduction

Transduction occurs when a bacteriophage (a viral parasite of bacteria) invades a bacterial cell. Phages operate in a manner similar to that of conventional viruses, entering the bacterium and replicating to release a large number of new infective agents, which in turn attack more bacteria. Transduction results when new phages carry extrachromosomal genetic material from the old host to a new one that previously lacked a plasmid.

Transformation

Transformation takes place when a strand of extrachromosomal DNA is absorbed via the cell well into the cytoplasm of a bacterium.

Sexual reproduction in bacteria is of great clinical significance as genes conferring antibiotic-resistance can be exchanged, resulting in the emergence of antibiotic-resistant strains. The widespread, indiscriminate use of antibiotics encourages the survival of bacteria carrying plasmids conferring antibiotic resistance on their hosts.

Escape and dissemination

In many cases, bacteria leave the body via the entry route, but there are exceptions. Those causing gastroenteritis gain access via the mouth and leave in the faeces, thus being said to be disseminated by the faecal-oral route.

Micro-organisms are spread from one individual to the next by direct and indirect contact. Dissemination is also possible via the airborne route, in contaminated food and water, and by insects.

Contact

Contact is the major route of spread in hospital and probably in the community too (Gould, 1991).

In hospital, bacteria are spread chiefly on the hands of staff because patients and equipment are handled so frequently, increasing the number of opportunities for cross-infection. The relationship between handwashing and a reduction in infection rate was first demonstrated by Ignaz Semmelweiss in a series of epidemiological studies in the 1840s (Newsom, 1993). Since this time, controlled trials in hospital have been notable by their absence because withholding hand decontamination would be ethically and aesthetically undesirable (Larson, 1988). There is, however, a wealth of indirect evidence to implicate hands as vectors of cross-infection.

Persuasive evidence is provided by Casewell and Phillips (1977), who demonstrated that the hands of staff in an intensive care unit were contaminated with *Klebsiella* of the same strain as those colonising and infecting the patients. Laboratory studies indicated that the bacteria could remain viable for up to 150 minutes following artificial inoculation onto the hands of volunteers – ample time for cross-infection to occur during normal nursing activities. Clothing, air and ward dust were seldom contaminated with the same strains, confirming earlier views that Gram-negative bacteria are not readily disseminated by the airborne route (Noble *et al.*, 1976). In later studies within the same unit, the rate of cross-infection declined following the introduction of a strict regimen of hand decontamination (Casewell and Phillips, 1977).

In the community, there is evidence that many pathogens traditionally thought to rely on droplet spread are in fact disseminated by contact (Worsley *et al.*, 1994). Laboratory simulations demonstrate that individuals are more likely to develop upper respiratory tract infection after contact with hands and objects (fomites) contaminated with virus than after exposure to virus-laden aerosols (Gwaltney *et al.*, 1978). It has been suggested that coughing and sneezing release infected droplets that settle onto surfaces, including clothes, in the immediate environment. They are then transferred by hands to other objects (crockery, door handles and so on), reaching new victims after their hands have in turn become contaminated. The virus reaches the nose and conjunctivae when the face is touched. Hand hygiene can reduce the incidence of upper respiratory tract infection (Leclair *et al.*, 1987).

Clinical Application

Handwashing

Handwashing is the most effective infection control measure, but it is performed too seldom by hospital staff, often because they are too busy. Hands should be washed even when gloves are worn because virus particles can leak through and contamination can occur as the gloves are removed (Gould, 1994).

Hand hygiene is equally important in the community, where it can be more difficult to achieve. The difficulties arise when a large number of people are seen quickly in clinics and health centres (Gould, 1997).

Similarly, rotavirus, responsible for vomiting and diarrhoea, although released in droplets, appears to be spread by hand contact. In an experimental incidence study conducted in a day nursery, a reduction in the rate of infection was demonstrated when handwashing was promoted among children and the staff attending them (Black *et al.,* 1981). It is worth remembering that handwashing is a simple and cost-effective way to reduce infection (Gould, 1997; May 1998).

Airborne spread

Airborne spread occurs only over short distances for Gram-positive pathogens and for viral infections such as chickenpox. An extensive review of the literature confirms that cross-infection by this route is unusual outside high-risk environments such as theatres and burns units (Ayliffe and Lowbury, 1982). In theatre, skin scales laden with staphylococci gain access to open tissues, often by landing on the drapes from the air. They may originate from either the patient or the attendants. The airborne route is also important in burns units. The skin is the body's chief defence against bacteria, and when it is no longer intact, patients become extremely susceptible to infection.

Contaminated food and water

Contaminated food readily operates as a vehicle for bacteria. Such infection is the result of poor hygiene in homes, restaurants, fast food outlets, shops and factories (North, 1989; Hobbs and Roberts, 1993). In most cases, contamination occurs via the hands. *Salmonella* contaminating the fingers from infected food sources can survive handwashing. Spread is therefore by the faecal-oral route.

Waterborne spread occurs in areas where sanitation is poor. Cholera is endemic throughout much of the developing world, including Asia, but outbreaks rarely occur in the UK. Typhoid is also transmitted via contaminated water. Legionnaires' disease (caused by *Legionella pneumophila*) is disseminated in contaminated aerosols (Woo *et al.,* 1986); outbreaks of this occur in the UK.

Insect vectors

Insect vectors disseminate infection by mechanical and biological transmission. Mechanical transmission occurs when pathogens are transferred from one locality to another via the surface of the insect, often on its feet. Houseflies operate as mechanical vectors for *Shigella* (Cohen *et al.,* 1991). In hospital, flies, Pharaoh's ants and other arthropods may carry pathogenic bacteria present within the clinical environment (Fotedar *et al.,* 1992).

Biological transmission involves a complex interaction between pathogen and vector. *Plasmodium*, the agent responsible for malaria, multiplies within the gut of the mosquito, increasing the number of protozoa available to contribute to an infective dose. Transmission occurs when the insect bites a human host.

Reservoirs of infection

Reservoirs of infection develop when favourable conditions promote the growth and reproduction of a large number of bacteria. Reservoirs may develop on the skin of staff or patients, leading to cross-infection. The contribution of environmental reservoirs to cross-infection depends on their situation. A large reservoir of bacteria in a drain is unlikely to contribute to nosocomial infection (infection acquired in hospital) because there are few opportunities for transfer to susceptible individuals, but if the reservoir involves objects that have the potential for contact with patients or staff, the risks are considerable. Epidemiological studies have contributed enormously to our understanding of infection risks and to the development of infection control guidelines to reduce spread. They provide overwhelming evidence that when patients become infected or colonised, the organisms responsible originate from other people rather than from distant sites in the inanimate environment (Casewell and Phillips, 1977; Mulhall, 1997).

Viruses

Viruses are the smallest micro-organisms known to be infective agents. They vary in size between 10 and 300 nm, being visible only under the electron microscope. Each virus particle consists of a core of nucleic acid – either DNA or RNA but never both (Table 1.5). The nucleic acid is surrounded by a protein coat to protect it from adverse environmental conditions (Figure 1.4). Prions (see above) are less complex structures that consist of proteins but no nucleic acids. 'Enveloped' viruses are surrounded by a lipid and protein capsule with structures permitting them to attach to their hosts. Attachment is always at specific sites on the cell surface for which the virus has particular affinity. For example, the influenza virus attaches itself to mucoprotein receptors. Viruses lacking a capsule are described as 'naked'. Viruses are classified by their shape and by the type of nucleic acid they contain – DNA or RNA.

Table 1.5   Medically significant viruses

Family	Type	Diseases/conditions
DNA viruses		
Papovavirus	Papilloma virus	Warts, tumours
Adenovirus	Adenovirus	Sore throat, conjunctivitis
Herpesvirus	Herpes simplex types 1 and 2	Cold sores, genital infection
	Varicella zoster	Chickenpox, shingles
	Epstein–Barr virus	Glandular fever, Burkitt's lymphoma
	Cytomegalovirus	Cytomegalovirus infection
Poxvirus	Variola	Smallpox
Hepadnavirus	Hepatitis B	Hepatitis B
RNA viruses		
Picornavirus	Enteroviruses	Poliomyelitis, respiratory infection, hepatitis A
	Rhinovirus	Common cold
Togavirus	Flavivirus	Yellow fever, dengue
	Rubella virus	Rubella
Reovirus	Rotavirus	Gastroenteritis
Rhabdovirus	Rabies virus	Rabies
Arenavirus	Lassa virus	Lassa fever
Orthomyxovirus	Influenza virus	Influenza
Paramyxovirus	Parainfluenza virus	Parainfluenza
	Respiratory syncytial virus	Respiratory infection
	Mumps virus	Parotitis
	Measles virus	Measles
Retrovirus	Human immunodeficiency virus	HIV disease
	HTLV-I, HTLV-II	Leukaemia
Filovirus	Ebola virus	Ebola virus disease
	Marburg virus	Marburg virus disease

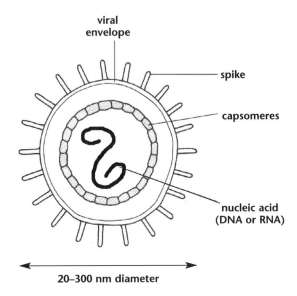

Figure 1.4   The structure of a typical virus

Viruses are responsible for a wide range of human, animal and plant infections. Some, called bacteriophages (phages), attack bacteria. Viruses depend on living organisms to provide a host; they are not capable of growth or reproduction outside living cells. Lacking cellular structure and the characteristics of living organisms, they may occupy the 'grey' zone between animate and inanimate organisms, perhaps resembling life as it first appeared on earth. It is, however, more likely that they represent degeneration into highly successful and sophisticated parasites. Their existence as the earliest form of 'life' in the absence of potential victims is hard to explain.

Life cycle

The virus gains entry by endocytosis (a bulk transport process that transfers material into cells) and is carried into the cytoplasm in a vacuole via the cell membrane (plasma membrane), leaving its protein capsule redundant on the cell's surface (Figure 1.5). Viral nucleic acid is then released to take over the genetic machinery of the host cell. Viral DNA becomes incorporated into the DNA of the host, assuming command of genetic control. The host synthesises viral proteins rather than its own so that new virus particles are generated and eventually released, completing the life cycle. RNA viruses use the enzyme reverse transcriptase to manufacture DNA templates of their own RNA for incorporation into the genome of the host. Some viruses lie dormant within the host cell for long periods of time but can become activated to produce active infections, herpes zoster (shingles) being a good example.

Viruses and malignancy

The earliest relationship between viruses and malignancy was demonstrated in 1908 when it was established that, in chickens, a certain type of leukaemia could be transmitted to previously healthy birds from those with the disease. It is now known that viruses are responsible for malignancies in many animals, and they appear to play a role in the development of some human cancers. There is an established association between the papilloma wart virus and cervical cancer (Barton, 1994) and between the Epstein–Barr virus and Burkitt's lymphoma (Anderson *et al.*, 1976).

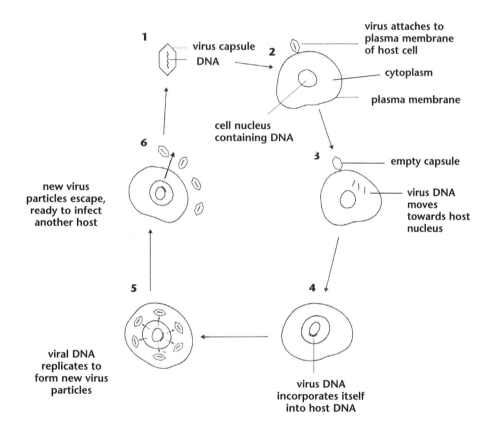

Figure 1.5   The life cycle of a typical virus

Fungi

Fungi are classified independently of plants and animals. Over 300,000 species are known but like bacteria, most are harmless saprophytes. Approximately 200 species cause human disease. In common with other micro-organisms, some fungi (for example, *Candida albicans*) can cause opportunistic infections in people who are immunocompromised. All fungi are eukaryotic, and because of the similarities between fungal and mammalian cells, it has never been easy to develop antifungal agents. The drugs used to treat fungal infections are often highly toxic, and few are available without a prescription (White, 1991). Some fungi, for example yeasts, assume a simple structure and exist as single cells, but complex forms exist with filamentous hyphae branching to form an extensive interwoven mesh called a mycelium (Figure 1.6). These forms are visible to the naked eye, but as microscopic examination is necessary for identification, the diagnosis of fungal infection (mycosis) is made in the microbiology laboratory.

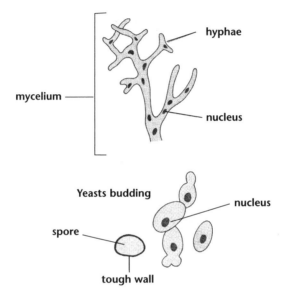

Figure 1.6   Fungal morphology

There are three types of mycosis:

1. **Superficial mycoses** occur when infection is superficial or restricted to the skin and its appendages (hair and nails), for example athlete's foot (*Trichophyton interdigitale*), or mucous membranes, as in the case of vaginal thrush (*Candida albicans*).

2. **Subcutaneous mycoses** (for example, mycetoma) affect the skin, subcutaneous tissues and bone. Slow, localised spread occurs.

3. **Systemic mycoses** (caused by, for example, *Cryptococcus*) develop, and then hyphae penetrate the deeper tissues. In temperate climates, systemic mycoses are uncommon except in the immunocompromised patient.

Table 1.6 gives examples of fungi that may cause human disease.

Table 1.6   Human mycoses

Fungus	Mycosis
Candida albicans	Thrush
Trichophyton interdigitale	Athlete's foot
Cryptococcus neoformans	Meningitis (immunocompromised patients)
Microsporum audouini	Ringworm
Aspergillus fumigatus	Respiratory infection (immunocompromised patients)

Protozoa

Protozoa are unicellular, microscopic animals (Figure 1.7). Most species are harmless, but some operate as human pathogens, especially in hot climates. Others are a threat to the immunocompromised host (Table 1.7). *Plasmodium*, the protozoan responsible for malaria, is discussed in Chapter 14.

Table 1.7   Pathogenic protozoa

Protozoan	Condition
Trichomonas vaginalis	Vaginal infection
Plasmodium spp.	Malaria
Trypanosoma rhodesiense	Sleeping sickness
Leishmania donovani	Kala-azar
Entamoeba histolytica	Amoebic dysentery
Toxoplasma gondii	Latent infection, damage to fetus in utero

Rickettsiae and chlamydiae

These organisms bridge the gap between viruses and bacteria. Like viruses, they are small and rely on their hosts to grow and reproduce, but they are susceptible to antibiotics. Typhus, caused by *Rickettsia prowazeki*, is spread by human head and body lice. *Chlamydia trachomatis*, responsible for non-specific urethritis, is discussed in Chapter 13.

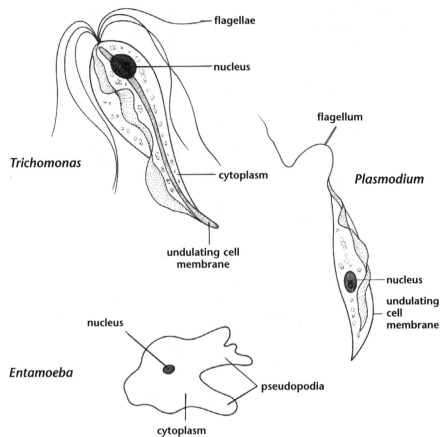

Figure 1.7 Pathogenic protozoa

Mycoplasmas

Mycoplasmas are similar to bacteria but lack cell walls. Without a rigidly supporting outer structure, they change shape readily during growth, often becoming filamentous. The most significant mycoplasma operating as a human pathogen is *Mycoplasma pneumoniae,* which infects the lungs.

Helminths

Numerous species of helminths (worms) give rise to human infestation. Some are large and multicellular, others microscopic (Figure 1.8). There are two main groups: round and flat (Table 1.8). It is impossible to cover all types and with that in mind only the threadworm will be discussed.

(b) A tapeworm

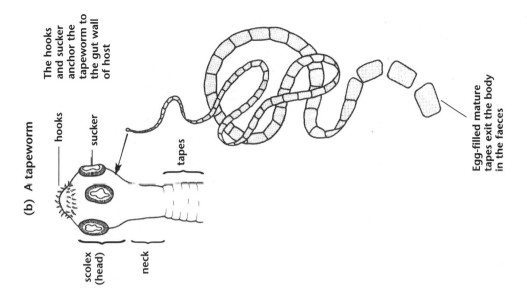

The hooks and sucker anchor the tapeworm to the gut wall of host

hooks

sucker

scolex (head)

neck

tapes

Egg-filled mature tapes exit the body in the faeces

(a) A roundworm (*Ascaris lumbricoides*)

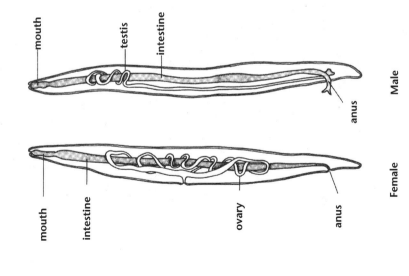

mouth

testis

intestine

anus

Male

mouth

intestine

ovary

anus

Female

Figure 1.8 Helminthic infestation

Clinical Application

Controlling Threadworm Infestation

Control is achieved by:

- All household members taking one of the proprietary antihelminthic agents such as piperazine, which acts by paralysing the worms. It can be purchased without prescription, but instructions (such as taking a second dose 2 weeks later to remove newly hatched worms) must be followed carefully. Newer preparations such as pyrantel embonate or thiabendazole may be prescribed
- Good handwashing and scrubbing of the nails, which should be kept short
- Vacuuming the house (carpets and upholstery) to remove eggs and avoid reinfestation
- Avoiding sharing towels and flannels. Towels, flannels and bed linen should be frequently laundered.

Table 1.8   Medically significant helminths

Helminth	Type
Enterobius vermicularis	Round (threadworm)
Ascaris lumbricoides	Roundworm
Toxocara canis	Dog roundworm
Trichinella spiralis	Pork roundworm
Necator spp.	Round (hookworm)
Taenia saginata	Beef tapeworm
Taenia solium	Pork tapeworm
Schistosoma haematobium	Fluke

Enterobius vermicularis, the threadworm, is probably the most common helminthic parasite in the Western world. It is not carried by cats, dogs or any other domestic animals; humans are the only hosts. The eggs are swallowed, hatch in the small intestine and migrate to the large intestine, where they live. Within 2 weeks, the worms reach maturity, mate and migrate to the rectum, emerging at night to lay their eggs on the perianal skin. The eggs adhere to the skin by a sticky fluid, which causes intense itching. When the victim scratches, a large number of eggs are transferred to the hands and fingernails. These are thence transferred back to the mouth, recommencing the cycle of infection. People of any age can catch threadworms, but children are the most commonly affected. The entire family should be treated, however, as the eggs are easily transferred on to towels, soap and upholstery, and may be ingested with food if it is touched with inadequately washed hands. The eggs can survive in the environment for several weeks. Threadworms are not dangerous but they can be a nuisance, causing discomfort, irritability and sleeplessness.

REVISION CHECKLIST: KEY AREAS

❏ Introduction to medical microbiology and micro-organisms causing disease

❏ Bacteria: Pathogenic activity, Infection and colonisation, Describing bacteria

❏ The process of infection: Establishing infection, Gaining access, Virulence, Bacterial growth requirements, Bacterial reproduction and genetics, Escape and dissemination

❏ Viruses: Life cycle, Viruses and malignancy

❏ Fungi

❏ Protozoa

❏ Rickettsiae and chlamydiae

❏ Mycoplasmas

❏ Helminths

Activities – linking knowledge to clinical practice

1 **Draw** a table to compare and contrast the main groups of micro-organism responsible for human infection.

2 **Identify** five situations in your clinical area that constitute a risk for cross-infection. Document these carefully, giving reasons for the specific hazards you identify, and suggest strategies for prevention.

SELF-ASSESSMENT

1. Helminths are always microscopic.
    True? ☐ False? ☐

2. Most bacteria and fungi are pathogenic.
    True? ☐ False? ☐

3. Which of the following are typical opportunists?
    (a) *Proteus* ☐
    (b) *Candida* ☐
    (c) *Legionella* ☐
    (d) *Staphylococcus aureus* ☐

4. Which of the following are bacilli?
    (a) *Pseudomonas* ☐
    (b) *Staphylococcus epidermidis* ☐
    (c) *Candida albicans* ☐
    (d) *Mycoplasma pneumoniae* ☐
    (e) *Salmonella typhi* ☐

5. Protozoa cause human mycoses.
    True? ☐ False? ☐

6. *Plasmodium* is a protozoan.
    True? ☐ False? ☐

7. Viruses contain either RNA or DNA but never both.   True? ☐ False? ☐

8. Virulence is . . . .

9. Most micro-organisms are disseminated by the airborne route.   True? ☐ False? ☐

10. *Staphylococcus aureus* never forms spores, even under dry conditions.
    True? ☐ False? ☐

References

Anderson M, Klein G, Zeigler JL *et al.* (1976) 'Association of Epstein–Barr viral genomes with American Burkitt lymphoma'. *Nature* **260**: 357–9.

Ayliffe GAJ and Lowbury EJL (1982) 'Airborne infection in hospital'. *Journal of Hospital Infection* **3**: 217–40.

Barton S (1994) 'New therapies for the treatment of genital warts'. *Nursing Times* **90**(20): 38–40.

Black RE, Dykes AC, Kern EA *et al.* (1981) 'Handwashing to prevent diarrhoea in day centres'. *American Journal of Epidemiology* **113**: 445–51.

Casewell M and Desai N (1983) 'Survival of multiply-resistant *Klebsiella aerogenes* and other Gram-negative bacteria on the finger tips'. *Journal of Hospital Infection* **4**: 350–60.

Casewell MW and Phillips I (1977) 'Hands as a route of transmission for *Klebsiella* colonisation and infection in an intensive care ward'. *Journal of Hygiene* **80**: 295–300.

Cleary PP, Kaplan EL and Handley J (1992) 'Clonal basis for resurgence of *Streptococcus pyogenes* disease in the 1980s'. *Lancet* **339**: 518–21.

Cohen D, Green M and Block C (1991) 'Reduction of transmission of shigellosis by control of houseflies (*Musca domestica*)'. *Lancet* **337**: 993–7.

Cooke EM, Edmonson AS and Starkey W (1981) 'The ability of strains of *Klebsiella aerogenes* to survive on the hands'. *Journal of Medical Microbiology* **14**: 443–50.

Enders G, Miller G, Craddock-Watson J *et al.* (1994) 'Consequences of varicella and herpes zoster in pregnancy: a prospective study of 1739 cases'. *Lancet* **343**: 1548–51.

Fotedar R, Banerjee U, Singh S *et al.* (1992) 'The housefly (*Musca domestica*) as a carrier of pathogenic micro-organisms in a hospital environment'. *Journal of Hospital Infection* **20**: 209–15.

Francis B (1994) 'The incidence of HIV/AIDS in children and their care needs'. *Nursing Times* **90**(26): 47–9.

Gould D (1991) 'Nurses' hands as vectors of hospital-acquired infection: a review'. *Journal of Advanced Nursing* **16**: 1216–25.

Gould D (1994) 'Nurses' hand decontamination practice: results of a local study'. *Journal of Hospital Infection* **28**: 15–30.

Gould D (1997) 'Giving infection control a big hand'. *Community Nursing Notes* **15**: 3–6.

Gwaltney JM, Moskalski PB and Hendley JO (1978) 'Hand to hand transmission of rhinovirus colds'. *Annals of Internal Medicine* **88**: 463–7.

Hobbs BC and Roberts D (1993) *Food Poisoning and Food Hygiene* (6th edn). Edward Arnold, London.

Larson E (1988) 'A causal link between handwashing and risk of infection? Examination of the evidence'. *Infection Control and Hospital Epidemiology* **9**: 28–34.

Leclair JM, Freeman J and Sullivan BF (1987) 'Preventing nosocomial respiratory syncitial virus infections through compliance with glove use and gown isolation precautions'. *New England Journal of Medicine* **317**: 329–34.

May H (1998) 'Now wash your hands'. *Nursing Times* **94**(4): 63–6.

Muder RR, Brennan C, Vickers RM *et al.* (1991) 'Methicillin resistant colonisation and infection in a long-term care facility'. *Annals of Internal Medicine* **114**: 107–12.

Mulhall A (1997) 'Epidemiology in infection control'. *Nursing Times* **94**(45): 68.

Newsom SWB (1993) 'Pioneers in infection control: Ignaz Philipp Semmelweiss'. *Journal of Hospital Infection* **23**: 175–87.

Noble SWB, Habbema JDF, Van Furth R *et al.* (1976) 'Quantitative studies of the dispersal of skin bacteria into the air'. *Journal of Microbiology* **9**: 53–61.

North N (1989) 'Food scares: the role of the Department of Health' in Harrison E and Gretton A (eds) *Health Care UK – An Economic, Social and Policy Audit*. Policy Journals, Newbury, pp. 65–77.

White G (1991) 'Management of fungal infections'. *Nursing Standard* **6**(9): 38–40.

Woo AH, Yu VL and Goetz A (1986) 'Potential in-hospital modes of transmission of *Legionella pneumophila'. *American Journal of Medicine* **80**: 567–73.

Worsley M, Ward K, Painer L, Privett S and Roberts J (1994) *Infection Control: A Community Perspective*. Daniels, Cambridge.

Further reading and information sources

Crewe W and Haddock DWR (1985) *Parasites and Human Disease*. Edward Arnold, London.

Kerr J (1998) 'Handwashing'. *Nursing Standard* **12**(51): 35–9.

Postgate J (1992) *Microbes and Man*. Cambridge University Press, Cambridge.

Schaeter M, Medoff G and Schlessinger D (1994) *Mechanisms of Microbial Disease*. Williams & Wilkins, Baltimore.

2 Response of the body to infection

CHAPTER OUTCOMES

After reading this chapter, you should be able to:

- Name the cells of the immune system and list their functions
- Distinguish between innate and acquired immunity
- Describe the role of innate immunity in defending the body against infection
- Describe the role of acquired immunity in defending the body against infection
- Explain the meaning of the following: 'antigen' and 'antibody' (immunoglobulin) and give examples
- List the factors that may influence individual susceptibility to infection
- Discuss the concept of 'herd immunity' and the factors that may affect it
- Explain why hospital inpatients are at particular risk of developing infection

Introduction to the immune response, immunity and immunology

Immunity is a state of resistance to an infectious agent. It depends on the ability of the body to recognise and dispose of foreign micro-organisms and other naturally occurring organic substances, including pollen, dust and cells from other organisms. Immunology is the study of the cells and molecules responsible for recognising and destroying foreign substances.

The immune response involves:

- Detecting foreign substances or their toxins within the body
- Communicating this information to the parts of the system responsible for their neutralisation and destruction
- Recruiting the immune attack
- Suppressing the immune response once the harmful agent has been eliminated.

Types of immunity

There are two types of immunity that interact and are necessary for survival. These are innate (natural) immunity – the same in health for every member of the species – and adaptive, or acquired, immunity, which is subject to individual variation.

Innate immunity – preventing invasion

Innate immunity helps the body to resist invasion. If its mechanisms fail, it attempts to contain the pathogens by limiting their access to the tissues.

Invasion is prevented by the anatomical arrangement of the tissues, the secretion of fluids that wash foreign materials from the body and the presence of normal flora covering the skin and lining the gut. Intact skin and mucous membranes are the body's chief defences against infection. The skin has a low pH because sebaceous secretion is acidic (the 'acid mantle'), supporting a population of commensal bacteria that keep pathogens at bay. Infection supervenes when the skin is broken or becomes excessively moist. Moisture beneath the breasts or between the toes frequently leads to infection, especially if hygiene is poor.

The gastrointestinal system is protected by its powerful acid and alkaline secretions. The pH of gastric acid is too low for most bacteria to survive. Its effectiveness has been demonstrated by an epidemiological investigation revealing that, during an outbreak of dysentery, infection was confined to patients whose natural gastric secretions had been suppressed by taking antacids (Horan, 1984). In the small intestine, the high pH (8–9) destroys most pathogens, although the bacteria responsible for typhoid and cholera survive.

The respiratory system is protected by the coughing and sneezing reflexes. Inside the nose, the turbinate bones increase the surface area of the mucosal surface and cause air to eddy, thus trapping small particles as inspired air travels over them. Lymphoid tissue in the pharyngeal, palatine and lingual tonsils traps any remaining pathogens. The entire respiratory tree, except for the alveoli, is lined with specialised mucus-secreting epithelium. The mucus traps foreign substances and is then carried upwards to the pharynx by the action of the cilia. Smoking paralyses the action of the cilia, eventually destroying them altogether and thus contributing to the development of lower respiratory tract infections in heavy smokers.

The vagina contains lactobacilli. These bacteria metabolise glycogen in cervical secretions, forming lactic acid. The pH of the healthy adult vagina is approximately 4.5, inhibiting the growth of other organisms. Before the menarche and after the menopause, the cervical secretions are scant because oestrogen production is low. The vaginal pH is correspondingly higher, and infection is more common in older women. Women taking antibiotics to treat recurrent infections are at risk of devel-

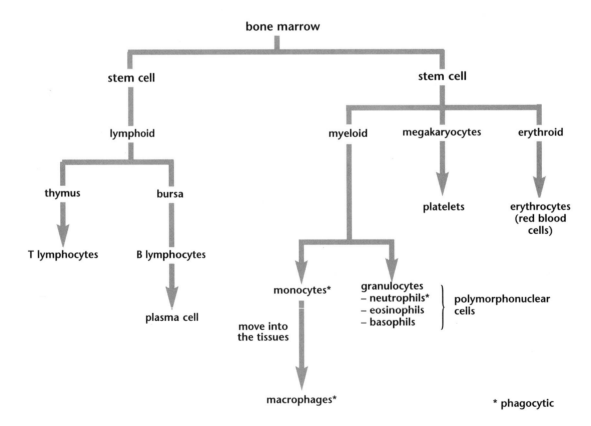

Figure 2.1   Origins of the leucocytes

oping vaginal infections such as candidiasis (thrush) because the normal vaginal flora are suppressed (Sawyer *et al.*, 1994).

The bladder has little protection against pathogens, and urinary infections are common, especially during pregnancy. This is probably because the hormone progesterone has a relaxing effect on the tissues, including the urethral aperture, allowing bacteria to enter the bladder more easily. However, the regular and complete emptying of the bladder tends to militate against infection by flushing micro-organisms out of the bladder and urethra.

Lysozyme, an enzyme secreted by macrophages (leucocytes), is present in many body fluids, including tears and saliva. It destroys bacteria by attacking their cell walls but is inactive against strains protected by a thick extracellular mucus coat (see Chapter 1).

Innate immunity – limiting spread

After invasion, inflammation and the activity of phagocytic cells in the blood and tissues limit the spread of the infection. These form part of the innate immune response because they offer the same protection for everybody, operating in the same way. Their origins and properties are shown in Figures 2.1 and 2.2.

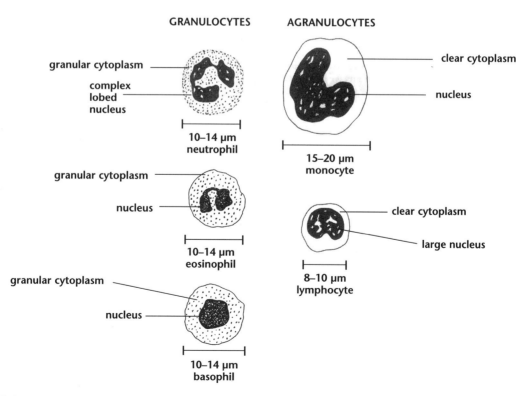

Figure 2.2 Leucocytes

Inflammation and phagocytosis

Inflammation is the response of tissues to trauma, whether injury involves cuts, chemical damage, extremes of temperature or pathogenic invasion (Figure 2.3). The classic hallmarks of inflammation are:

- Erythema (redness)
- Swelling
- Heat
- Pain
- Loss of function (depending on the extent of the injury).

The capillary walls vasodilate in immediate response to injury, becoming more permeable. This action is triggered by the release of prostaglandins from platelets, and other locally acting hormones, particularly bradykinin and histamine. Bradykinin comes from the neutrophils and is responsible for the pain experienced during inflammation. Histamine is produced by the basophils.

Leakage of plasma into the intercellular space accounts for the swelling (oedema) and contributes to the pain of inflammation by exerting pressure on adjacent nerve endings. Increased blood supply explains the erythema and sensation of heat. This increased blood supply is beneficial because it boosts the local availability of neutrophils and macrophages (derived from monocytes) to combat infection, while the greater volume of fluid helps to dilute the toxins.

Neutrophils begin to appear within the damaged area about an hour after the initiation of inflammation, stimulated by the release of leucocyte-releasing factors, which increase the activity of leucopoietic (leucocyte-producing) tissue in the red bone marrow. Neutrophils entering the blood are carried along the edges of the capillaries to the site of injury (mural flow), escaping into the tissues via slits between the capillary cells (diapedesis). Migration to the injured area takes less than 2 minutes and is caused by chemical attraction (positive chemotaxis). As the inflammatory response progresses, macrophages begin to congregate within the damaged area, engulfing debris and spent neutrophils. The phagocytic and cytotoxic activity of both neutrophils and macrophages is similar.

Phagocytosis occurs when a neutrophil or macrophage engulfs a pathogen (Figure 2.4). The first step is opsonisation, the attachment of a ligand (particle or group of molecules) to the surface of the phagocytic cell, stimulating the action of the contractile proteins myosin and actin that are present within the cytoplasm. Endocytosis follows: the pathogen is engulfed, entering a vacuole created by the phagocytic membrane. Lysozomes in the cytoplasm fuse with the vacuole, emptying strongly acidic enzymes (catalase and myeloperoxidase) onto the pathogen and destroying it.

Opsonins are 'chemical tags' – antibodies and complement proteins with receptors enabling them to recognise and attach to receptors on the surface of foreign molecules, labelling them in order to enhance phagocytosis. Further receptors permit the opsonin to link itself in turn to a phagocyte so that it operates as a bridge between the pathogen and the cell that will engulf it.

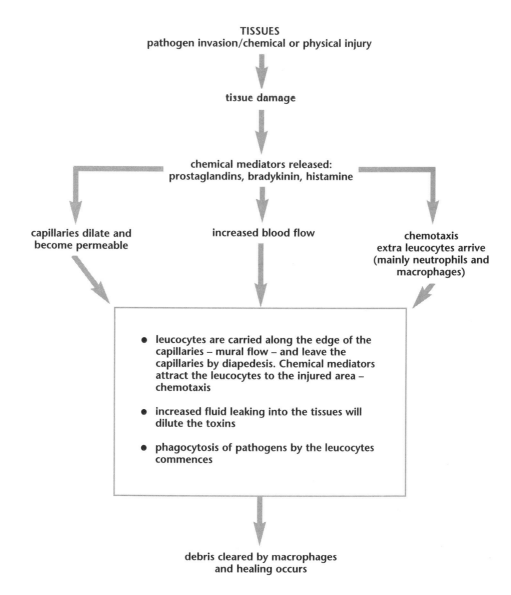

Figure 2.3   Events of inflammation – a summary

Eosinophils are weakly phagocytic, strongly cytotoxic cells not dependent on opsonins for their action. Enzymes released from their cytoplasmic inclusions are poured onto the surface of the pathogen, destroying it by perforating the cell

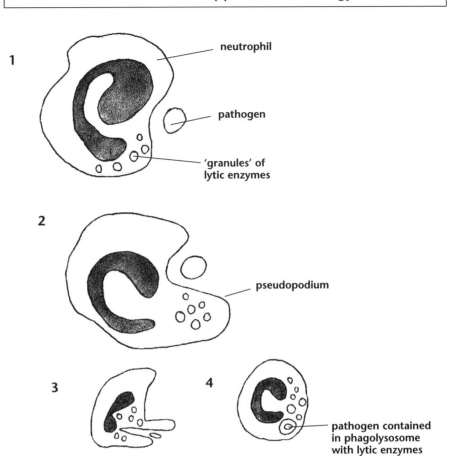

Figure 2.4   Phagocytosis

membrane. Their main activity appears to be the destruction of multicellular parasites too large for phagocytosis.

Natural killer (NK) cells do not appear in Figure 2.1 (above) as their origin is obscure. They make up less than 1 per cent of the total leucocyte count, but are powerfully cytotoxic against the host cells that have become infected with viruses. NK cells attach to these cells and release enzymes that destroy the membrane. Their activity is promoted by lymphokines and interferon, and they may play a role in controlling the differentiation of cells in the immune system.

Basophils and mast cells (basophils that migrate to the tissues) initiate inflammation by degranulation – the release of histamine from granules in response to the attachment of a particular antibody (IgE) to their membranes. Degranulation also requires a reaction between the antigen and the attached antibodies, and in some cases the action of complement proteins.

Interferons are proteins released by several types of leucocyte during the immune response. They inhibit viral replication by disrupting the transcription of DNA into RNA.

Clinical Application

Allergy (Hypersensitivity)

Approximately 10 per cent of the population show an abnormal, hypersensitive reaction to otherwise harmless materials (pollen, dust, fur and a range of foods including nuts and shell-fish, for example). This is the basis of allergy. Many allergic reactions involve the respiratory tract because potential allergens are so often inhaled and a large number of basophils and mast cells are present in the lungs. IgE present on the surface of the mast cells and basophils binds to the allergen (foreign material), leading to the release of histamine and bradykinin. Allergic reactions to the latex in rubber examination gloves is a growing problem among health professionals and patients (Mansell *et al.*, 1994). Protocols to reduce exposure have now been drawn up by some NHS Trusts (Trevelyan, 1996). Protocols should include the identification of other products that contain latex, for example catheters and some mattresses.

Complement comprises a group of 20 or so proteins present in an inactive form in body fluids. Activation of the first complement in the sequence occurs on exposure to polysaccharides present in bacterial cell wall, parasites, and by the 'labelling' actions of opsonins and antibodies, an example of interaction between the body's innate and adaptive defence mechanisms. A cascade is triggered in which each active complement component activates the next one in the chain (Figure 2.5), as in the blood clotting cascade. The final product is called a membrane attack complex. It perforates the cell walls of bacteria, destroying them. The attachment of complement to an antigen–antibody complex results in its destruction (complement fixation).

Table 2.1 shows that several complement proteins have additional functions important in the overall immune response, illustrating the highly complex and economic nature of immunity.

Table 2.1   Functions of the complement proteins

C3b	Potent opsoniser
C3a	Stimulates macrophages to release bactericidal agents and enhances mast cell degranulation
C5b	Chemotactic attractor for neutrophils and macrophages

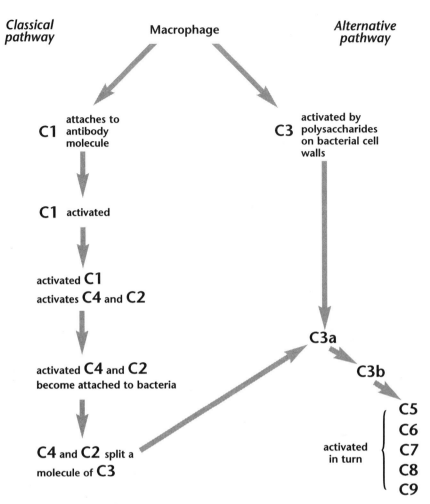

Figure 2.5   The complement cascade

Pyrexia – in response to infection

Pyrexia is an innate response to infection. It occurs in all vertebrates and is thought to play some beneficial role, perhaps by increasing the metabolic rate so that bacteria and their toxins are more rapidly eliminated from the body. In addition, the rate of tissue repair is increased and the immune response is heightened (Mackowiak, 1994). Pyrexia, however, has its disadvantages. Fever is exhausting, draining the body of energy at a time when the individual is anorexic.

Complications include:

■   A negative nitrogen balance – for every 1 ^{0}C rise in temperature above the norm, the adult pulse rises by approximately 10 beats per minute and the rate of breathing by seven respirations per minute. Glycogen stores become depleted, leading to nitrogen wastage as protein is catabolised to provide energy.

■ Rigors – uncontrollable attacks of violent shivering, often associated with the presence of bacterial toxins in the blood.

■ Febrile convulsions – these typically occur in young children (6 months to 5 years of age) and people with a history of epilepsy. Although transient, they are frightening and can be dangerous as they may lead to trauma, aspiration of secretions or asphyxia.

■ Delirium – this is most often seen in young children or older adults, or when pyrexia is marked. The patient becomes confused and restless. This may add to the difficulties of isolating infectious patients.

Temperature regulation and infection

Body temperature is controlled by the hypothalamus. An increase in body temperature is a systemic effect of the inflammatory response. Fever is induced by prostaglandins and proteins called pyrogens released by the leucocytes.

The temperature-regulating centre is often compared to a thermostat. Human core temperature is fixed at about 37 ^{0}C in most people, deviations detected by receptor cells in the skin being relayed to the hypothalamus along afferent nerves (Figure 2.6). If the temperature falls below the set point of 37 ^{0}C, heat-conserving mechanisms are initiated, while a rise above the set point triggers heat loss (Table 2.2).

Table 2.2   Mechanisms of heat loss and conservation

Heat loss	Heat conservation
Skin capillaries dilate	Skin capillaries constrict
Increases heat loss by:	Decreases heat loss by:
● convection	● convection
● conduction	● conduction
● evaporation (sweating)	Shivering (involuntary muscular activity)
Behavioural activities: removing clothes, stretching out, reducing activity	Behavioural activities: huddling up, putting on extra clothes

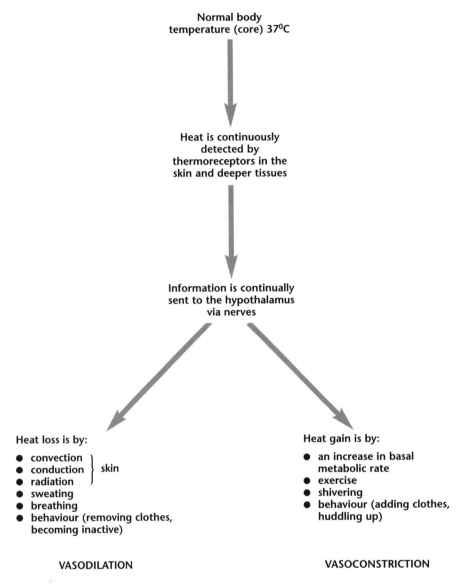

Figure 2.6

Thermoregulation

When infection supervenes, surface antigens on the bacteria or viruses 'reset' the thermostat to a higher set point by stimulating neutrophils to release pyrogens. Temperature is maintained at this level until the foreign antigens have been neutralised and eliminated. Vasoconstriction and shivering are accompanied by an increase in metabolic rate. The patient feels cold and huddles up irrespective of the number of blankets provided. The magnitude of the fever depends on the infective organism. Mild infections may have little or no effect, but some pathogens (for example, *Salmonella typhi*) stimulate pyrexia of as much as 39–40 ^{0}C. As the infection subsides, vasodilation and perspiration are stimulated. This promotes heat loss, and the patient feels hot and sticky. Some infections are associated with characteristic changes in body temperature that aid diagnosis. In patients with brucellosis, the temperature gradually rises and then resolves over 10 days or so before the cycle repeats.

Clinical Application

The Pyrexial Patient

As fever develops, the patient feels cold and will suffer if attempts are made to reduce the temperature. Antipyrexial drugs may mask symptoms indicating the need for a change in treatment (for example, an antibiotic) (Styrt and Sugarman, 1990). The kindest and safest option is to allow extra bedclothes, and the appropriate action is to assist in identifying the infection by careful observation and obtaining specimens to aid laboratory diagnosis. Appropriate antibiotics can then be prescribed. Once the temperature begins to fall, the patient will appreciate the removal of any heavy blankets, as well as cold drinks and the use of a fan. Key points on a care plan will include:

- Regularly monitoring the temperature, pulse and respiratory rate
- Preventing dehydration
- Ensuring adequate nutrition (with sufficient energy, protein, vitamins and minerals)
- Ensuring adequate rest (both physical and mental)
- Help with hygiene, including mouth care
- Careful observation for signs of disorientation (febrile convulsions in children under 5)
- The provision of bedclothes and equipment to ensure comfort at all times and heat loss when appropriate.

Adaptive immunity

Adaptive immunity occurs through the co-ordinated functioning of lymphocytes and macrophages in response to antigens – foreign cells or molecules that have a structure incorporating a ligand able to bind them to the membranes of lymphocytes or the products of lymphocytes (antibodies). Traditionally, two types of adaptive immune response are described: humoral immunity, mediated by B lymphocytes (B cells) and cell-mediated immunity, regarded as the property of T lymphocytes (T cells). However, as research progresses it is becoming increasingly obvious that the two interact closely, although for the sake of clarity they will be introduced separately here.

Humoral immunity

Humoral immunity refers to the activity of the B lymphocytes in body fluids (humors). They recognise and bind to antigens on the surface of pathogens, neutralising them. Figure 2.7 shows that binding takes place between antigen-binding sites on the surface of the B lymphocyte and a small region of the pathogen called the epitope, which has a complementary shape. The antigen receptor sites on the B lymphocytes are the antibodies (immunoglobulins) with a complementary shape. Antigens are covered with numerous epitopes, and if the cell is large more than one kind may be present.

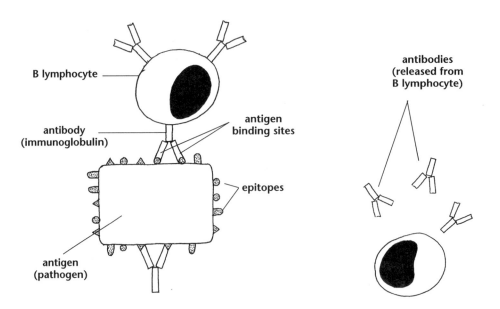

Figure 2.7 Simplified illustration of binding between B lymphocyte and antigen

Key features of adaptive humoral immunity include:

■ Antigen specificity
■ Clonal selection
■ Clonal expansion
■ Clonal suppression and the formation of memory cells
■ Antibodies (immunoglobulins).

Antigen specificity

B lymphocytes are able to recognise and respond to at least 10^8 different epitopes, so every different antigen encountered by the body is recognised independently of all the others. It is not possible for every single B lymphocyte to possess all the receptors necessary to recognise all the thousands of epitopes it could meet because there would be insufficient physical space on the surface of the cell to hold them and insufficient DNA to code for them all. Instead, each B lymphocyte carries receptor molecules of unique structure and specificity to allow the recognition of just a few epitopes of a similar configuration (shape).

Clonal selection

All B lymphocytes appear the same during microscopic examination, but there are thousands of different types, each type responding to the same limited range of epitopes. B lymphocytes responding to the same epitopes form a clone. The body contains thousands of different clones that are 'selected' when the epitopes they match invade. A large bacterial cell carrying numerous different epitopes could select several different B lymphocyte clones.

Clonal expansion

This process involves the rapid replication of B lymphocytes in response to the arrival and binding of antigens. It results in the production of thousands of B lymphocytes able to react to the particular pathogen that is invading.

Clonal suppression

Clonal suppression occurs once the antigen has been eliminated. The immune response is 'switched off' once it becomes redundant, conserving metabolic resources and preventing an excessive response. The number of B lymphocytes belonging to the clone diminishes, although a few remain circulating in the plasma as memory cells. These allow a further rapid clonal expansion in response to a second invasion by the same pathogen, explaining why the immune response following re-exposure to the same organism is swift and will usually prevent reinfection.

Antibodies (immunoglobulins)

Antibodies (immunoglobulins or Igs) are globular proteins carried on the surface of B lymphocytes, each B lymphocyte carrying about 10^5 immunoglobulins on its surface. Binding to the specific antigen takes place between the surface immunoglobulin molecule and a corresponding epitope (see Figure 2.7 above).

Immunoglobulin attachment is the signal for clonal expansion. Once a B-lymphocyte binds to its epitope, it secretes additional immunoglobulins into the blood and body fluids rapidly – at a rate of thousands per second. Secreted immunoglobulins have numerous functions:

Clinical Application

The Primary and Secondary Immune Responses

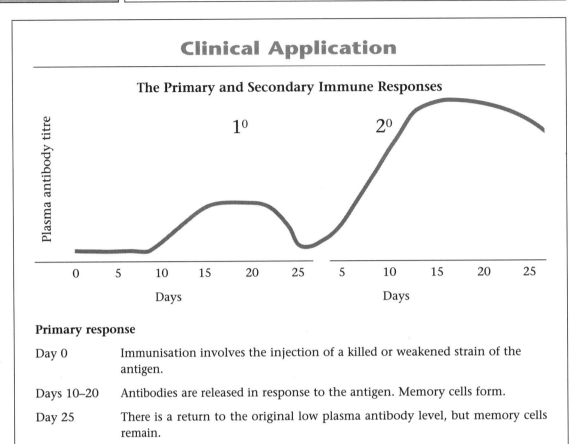

Primary response

Day 0   Immunisation involves the injection of a killed or weakened strain of the antigen.

Days 10–20   Antibodies are released in response to the antigen. Memory cells form.

Day 25   There is a return to the original low plasma antibody level, but memory cells remain.

Secondary response

Before Day 5   Exposure to the antigen has already resulted in a steep increase in the level of plasma antibodies, released from memory cells remaining from the primary response.

Days 10–20   The antibody titre is much higher than during the primary response. A sizeable and successful immune response is possible.

Day 25   The antibody level gradually wanes but is still relatively high for months or years.

■ They bind to their matching antigens. This does not destroy the antigen directly but results in clumping (agglutination) so that the resulting aggregates are more easily phagocytosed (see above).

■ Once bound, immunoglobulins function as opsonins, labelling the antigen as a target for phagocytosis.

■ Bound immunoglobulin enhances the cytotoxicity of NK cells and eosinophils (one example of the co-operation between innate and adaptive immunity).

■ Binding between immunoglobulin and antigen operates as one of the triggers for the complement cascade (see above). This generates C3a and C3b, contributing to the inflammatory response, another example of the overlapping functions of the innate and adaptive responses.

If these activities were evoked without the binding signal, the immune response would take place wastefully and dangerously.

There are several classes of immunoglobulins (IgG, IgA, IgM, IgD and IgE), they are found in different sites and perform a variety of functions (Table 2.3).

Table 2.3   The immunoglobulins

IgG	Structurally the simplest immunoglobulin
	The most abundant immunoglobulin
	Has a major role in the secondary immune response
	Neutralises toxins and binds to antigens
	Plasma levels provide an indication of recent exposure to antigens
	Crosses the placenta in the last 3 months (third trimester) of pregnancy
IgA	Protects mucous membranes
	Present in saliva, tears, breast milk and gut secretions
	Particularly active against bacteria and fungi
IgM	Exclusively found in serum
	Most abundant during the primary immune response
	Has a major role in agglutination and complement activity
IgD	Present on B lymphocytes, where it functions as the antigen receptor for the B lymphocyte
	May have other functions, but these are unclear
	Maximum levels occur during childhood
IgE	Present on basophils in the lungs, skin and mucous membranes
	Precipitates inflammation around parasites
	Plays a role in hypersensitivity (allergic) reactions

Cell-mediated immunity

Cell-mediated immunity is a function of the T cells. They are released from the red bone marrow and migrate to the thymus gland, where they reach maturation. The functions of cell-mediated immunity include:

- Protection against viral and fungal infections and parasites
- Intracellular protection against bacteria with resistant cell walls able to survive phagocytosis; once inside the living cells of the host, they are sheltered from humoral defence mechanisms
- Maintaining the inflammatory response in cases of chronic infection (for example, tuberculosis and leprosy)
- Surveillance against foreign cells, relevant in tumour detection and transplant rejection
- Regulation of the adaptive immune response.

Cell-mediated immunity is stimulated by the binding of an antigen to a receptor site on the surface of a T cell. The T cells respond by releasing chemical mediators called lymphokines. These activate macrophages, enhancing phagocytosis, and stimulate the activity of many other cells vital for the immune response.

Types of T cell

T cells proliferate rapidly following exposure to an antigen, and undergo differentiation. Numerous subsets exist:

- T cytotoxic cells destroy specific target cells carrying surface antigens that they recognise. These include virally infected cells and tumour cells (as cells that have undergone neoplastic changes develop surface antigens different from those present in health).

- T helper cells initiate the immune response by promoting the maturation of B and other T lymphocytes once these have been triggered by antigens. This function is executed only after they have been stimulated by chemicals called interleukins released from activated macrophages. It is thought that corticosteroids suppress fever by preventing the release of interleukins.

- T suppressor cells switch off the immune response by deactivating the T helper cells.

Individual variation in the immune response and predisposition to infection

The activity of the immune system is depressed in some people and varies between individuals, reflecting the influence of genetic control. Some infections are species

---

Clinical Application

T Cell Classification and Clinical Significance

In clinical settings, the T cells are generally classified according to the presence or otherwise of two surface molecules: CD4 and CD8. T helper cells are CD4 or T4 cells, T cytotoxic and T suppressor cells being CD8 or T8 cells.

The ratio of CD4 to CD8 cells is a useful guide to the progress of a person with established AIDS.

---

specific: distemper affects dogs, for example, but there are no recorded cases of transmission to a human host. Research on rhinoviruses, which cause the common cold, has never progressed well because so few laboratory species are susceptible to this illness. Some groups appear especially susceptible to certain infections, tuberculosis being particularly common among people of Asian extraction (Aditama, 1991). A genetic component appears to be operating in addition to environmental factors as it appears that if one twin of a monozygotic (identical) pair develops tuberculosis, the other is more likely to do so at some stage in his life than are other siblings who do not share all the same genes.

Some children are born with congenital or genetic deficiencies of the immune system and are highly susceptible to infection. Inherited lymphocytopenia (a low level of lymphocytes in the blood) and agammaglobulinaemia (the absence or deficiency of gammaglobulin in the blood) are X-linked disorders. Affected children (always males) rarely survive infancy. In chronic granulomatous disease, the affected subjects are highly susceptible to opportunistic infection because they have defective phagocytic enzymes and are unable to kill and digest bacteria.

Immunity throughout the lifespan

Immunity is also subject to variation throughout the lifespan and is influenced by a number of factors:

- **Age** – Infections occur less often between 20 and 40 years of age (Ayliffe *et al.*, 1977), the young and the very old being most at risk. Infants acquire antibodies via the placenta and in breast milk, but the effects are short lived (albeit valuable because they afford protection at a time when the adaptive system is still immature). At one time, antibody protection was thought to be impossible until the infant reached at least 3 months of age, but this is now disputed (Rudd, 1991). The ability to mount the inflammatory response and to form new antibodies declines with age (Weskler, 1980; Pahwa, 1981).

- **Drugs** – Corticosteroids depress the inflammatory response and inhibit anti-body formation. Antibiotics destroy the normal body flora, encouraging super-infection by extraneous strains of bacteria. The replacement of the normal flora in the bowel by pathogens may lead to diarrhoea and vomiting or more serious infections, superinfection with *Clostridium difficile*, for example, which is a serious complication of antibiotic treatment (Gammon, 1995).

- **Radiotherapy and chemotherapy** – These treatments depress the leucocyte count if the bone marrow or lymphatic tissues are involved. Patients with a depressed neutrophil count (neutropenia) are especially vulnerable to infection.

- **Metabolic disorders** – Such disorders reduce the immune response, but the mechanism by which they do this is unknown. Diabetes mellitus and malig-nant disease are both reported to have this effect. However, the mechanism increasing susceptibility to infection in patients with these two very different clinical conditions is unlikely to be the same (Young, 1981).

- **Malnutrition** – Obesity reduces the ability to heal (Roberts and Bates, 1992). Undernutrition interferes with all aspects of the immune response, as shown by the devastating effects of measles in parts of the world where food supplies are poor. In malnourished patients, the capacity of the gastrointestinal mucosa to act as a barrier against pathogens is impaired (Reynolds *et al.*, 1996).

- **Immobility** – Immobility contributes to susceptibility to infection because it inhibits the drainage of respiratory secretions, induces urinary stasis and increases the risk of pressure sores, which breach the normally intact cutaneous barrier and allow the entry of skin commensals that do not usually cause infection.

- **Psychological stress** – Stress appears to depress the immune response (Boore, 1978).

- **Specific and acquired immunity** – Immunity depends on the antigens to which an individual has been intentionally or accidentally exposed.

Immunity and community health

Herd immunity is the resistance to infectious disease exhibited by the population as a whole. High levels of herd immunity hinder transmission: epidemics are possible only when an infectious agent spreads throughout a susceptible popula-tion. The main source of herd immunity is exposure to naturally occurring infec-tions. Before vaccination was introduced, outbreaks of measles and pertussis (whooping cough) occurred cyclically every few years, sporadic cases arising in between. A large number of infections occurring simultaneously was possible only when an entire cohort of children lacking immunity had built up through a lack of previous exposure, the number of infections waning once they had all been infected. In community health terms, sporadic infection is significant as epidemics are possible as long as individuals lacking immunity remain and are promoted by the geographical or social clustering of susceptible people (Bedford, 1993). The aim of immunisation programmes is to induce acquired immunity in all susceptible people, preventing the development of outbreaks. It is generally believed that over 90 per cent of the population must be immune to a pathogen before a state of herd immunity can exist (Henderson, 1991).

The first vaccine was developed by Jenner in 1796 after his observation that milk-maids who had developed cowpox rarely contracted smallpox, a similar but much more serious infection. Jenner prepared a rudimentary vaccine from the cowpox virus that could induce immunity in people not previously exposed to cowpox or smallpox. This was a major scientific breakthrough as smallpox had claimed thousands of lives. For example, in 1629 over 3,000 people per million succumbed. The success of vaccination can be judged by the World Health Organization's declaration in 1980 that smallpox had been eradicated (Lochhead, 1991).

Childhood immunisation programmes against infectious disease were introduced in the UK from the 1940s onwards (Table 2.4). The terms 'vaccination' and 'immunisation' are sometimes used interchangeably, although vaccination is strictly defined as the act of administering the vaccine while immunisation is the result of vaccination. The types of vaccine available are shown in Table 2.5.

Table 2.4   Infectious diseases and the dates when vaccines were first introduced in the UK

Diphtheria	1940
Pertussis	1950s
Tuberculosis	1953
Tetanus	Mid-1950s
Poliomyelitis	1956
Influenza	Mid-1960s
Measles	1968
Rubella	1970
Hepatitis B	Early 1980s
Mumps	1988
MMR (measles/mumps/rubella)	1989
Hib (protects against *Haemophilus influenzae*)	1992
Group C Meningococcal Disease (long lasting vaccine)	1999/2000

Applied Microbiology for Nurses

Table 2.5   Types of vaccines

- **Killed vaccine** – The active organism is destroyed, usually by heat. A primary dose followed by two boosters is needed to induce immunity, for example against pertussis. These organisms are not infectious, and are therefore harmless, but the period of protection is relatively short.

- **Live vaccines** – Viable organisms are attenuated (weakened) so that they are unable to harm the recipient but can still induce immunity, as, for example, with yellow fever. One dose will usually confer immunity, except for polio, for which three doses are required. A second advantage is that after a single dose, they can spread naturally within a population, helping to produce herd immunity. Care must be taken if these are required for immunocompromised patients.

- **Toxoids** – Inactivated toxins derived from the pathogen are injected.

- **Subunit vaccines** – These use part of the virus or bacterium to induce immunity. Until recently, the hepatitis B vaccine was a subunit vaccine.

- **Conjugate vaccines** – These combine antigenic parts of different organisms, thus inducing immunity to two or more infections in a single vaccine. It may in future be possible to combine *Haemophilus influenzae* and *Meningococcus neisseriae* type B in this way.

Throughout the 1980s, there was concern about the uptake of the vaccines, especially for measles and pertussis (Peckham and Senturia, 1986). Attention was drawn to the social costs and benefits of immunisation and the dangers accruing to the population as a whole through a lack of compliance by a minority of parents refusing to present their children for vaccination through either ignorance or misplaced fears of side-effects associated with the vaccines (Orr, 1986). No vaccine can ever offer 100 per cent effectiveness, but the benefits of immunisation are demonstrable (Bedford, 1993). Immunisation against diphtheria and poliomyelitis has maintained a high degree of herd immunity within the population (Joce *et al.*, 1992), and the side-effects of measles vaccine are slight, especially compared with the lasting damage that may accrue from the infection itself (Peckham and Senturia, 1986).

Standard immunisation against infectious diseases

The current routine schedule for childhood immunisation is shown in Table 2.6.

Measles

Contrary to popular belief, measles is not always a harmless condition. Reports dating from the 1970s show that a significant number of children have been admitted to hospital with pneumonia or seizures. Death occasionally results from encephalitis arising as a late complication of measles infection (Miller, 1978). The vaccine was introduced in 1968, and since this time infection has typically arisen in those who have not received it. Immunity is established in over 95 per cent of immunised subjects.

Table 2.6   Routine schedule for immunisation – children and young people

Vaccine		Age	
Diphtheria/tetanus/pertussis (DTP)		1st dose:	2 months
Oral polio	Primary course	2nd dose:	3 months
Haemophilus influenzae type B (Hib)		3rd dose:	4 months
Measles/mumps/rubella (MMR)		12–15 months	
Diphtheria/tetanus	Booster	3–5 years	
Oral polio and MMR			
Bacille Calmette-Guérin (BCG) (after a tuberculin skin test – not required before 3 months of age)		10–14 years or infancy	
Tetanus, polio	Booster	13–18 years	
Low-dose diphtheria toxoid			

Notes

Hepatitis B vaccine is given to infants born to mothers who are hepatitis B positive. The World Health Organization and other authorities recommend that hepatitis B vaccine is routinely offered to all children.

A new vaccine effective against group C meningococcal disease became available in 1999. A phased immunisation programme has been put in place to target high-risk groups:

Initial phase

- Infants and children – three doses of the new vaccine with routine immunisations at 2, 3 and 4 months of age; or two doses between 4 months and 1 year; or a single dose with MMR at around 13 months.

- Young people – a single dose of the new vaccine for 15, 16 and 17-year-olds in school year 11, 6th form and colleges. 18 and 19-year-olds starting further/higher education programmes are offered the existing vaccine (effective for only 3 years).

Later phase

- Preschool children aged 14 months to 5 years – a single dose of the new vaccine.

- Schoolchildren aged 5–14 years – a single dose of the new vaccine.

- Young people – other 18–20-year-olds can request one dose of the existing vaccine.

Pertussis (whooping cough)

Pertussis may be accompanied by severe, occasionally fatal respiratory complications that are preventable by vaccination. Adverse publicity in 1975 led to a dramatic decrease in the uptake of vaccination with epidemics occurring throughout England and Wales. There were suggestions that children had suffered brain damage after receiving the vaccine, eventually later refuted by case control studies (Alderslade *et al.*, 1981). A similar association with sudden infant death syndrome has never been proved, and there are now suggestions that undiagnosed pertussis may in fact be the cause of some unexplained infant mortalities (Bedford, 1993).

Rubella

Rubella vaccination was introduced in the UK in 1970. The aim was initially to reduce the tragic consequences of infection during pregnancy rather than to eradicate the virus from the community, the vaccine being offered selectively to schoolgirls and susceptible women (Miller, 1990). Considerable success was achieved, so that by 1990 it was estimated that only 2–4 per cent of pregnant women were susceptible compared with 10–15 per cent before 1970. Congenital infections were, however, still reported to the Communicable Diseases Surveillance Centre, and as unvaccinated children were known to be operating as a reservoir of infection within the community, the immunisation programme was extended so that the vaccine could be offered during routine childhood immunisation. A major campaign to immunise schoolchildren in 1994 met with some opposition from religious groups objecting to the vaccine because the virus had been cultured on cells derived from fetal tissue.

Combined vaccines

The measles/mumps/rubella (MMR) vaccine for routine child immunisation introduced in 1989 was intended to eliminate measles, mumps, rubella and congenital rubella syndrome from the UK. The uptake of MMR has recently declined because of a perceived risk that it may be linked to the development of autism, although a large study (Public Health Laboratory Service, 1999) has not shown a causal association between MMR and autism.

Diphtheria, tetanus, poliomyelitis and pertussis vaccines have been offered at 2, 3 and 4 months of age, replacing an earlier, more widely spaced, schedule (Ramsay *et al.*, 1993). Preschool boosters are still recommended. This new approach has been welcomed as it is likely to increase the uptake of vaccination at baby clinics: many mothers have returned to full-time employment by the time that their children have reached 6 months of age, and attendance then becomes more difficult (Rudd, 1991). The poliomyelitis vaccine contains live organisms, so parents and other carers must be warned to pay particular attention to hygiene (for example, after changing nappies) as it is an enteric pathogen.

Hib vaccine

The Hib vaccine, which acts against *Haemophilus influenzae*, was first developed in the early 1970s but was then only effective in children over 2 years of age. Most cases, however, occur during infancy, when the levels of maternal antibodies have waned but the baby has yet to develop its own natural immunity.

Haemophilus influenzae is a Gram-negative organism often carried in the healthy throat. It has been associated with the development of respiratory infections and their associated side-effects of epiglottitis and otitis media. Infection is most damaging in young children and is the principal cause of bacterial meningitis in children under 5 years of age. It is a significant cause of mortality, and among survivors may cause neurological deficits including deafness, learning disability and poor motor co-ordination. Its onset is insidious. Infection often follows a cold and the symptoms are non-specific, so parents may not be aware that their child is becoming seriously ill (Lungmuss, 1989). A new Hib vaccine given in conjunction with the accelerated primary schedule is now available, being effective and well tolerated (Hodgson, 1992).

Group C meningococcal disease

A long acting vaccine became available in 1999 for vulnerable groups (Table 2.6).

Hepatitis B

See Chapter 12.

Tuberculosis

See Chapters 9 and 14.

Health promotion

Health promotion and immunisation form an important part of the work of health professionals employed in the community, especially health visitors, the efficiency with which immunisation programmes are implemented often being taken as a measure of the health visitor's efficiency (Orr, 1986). Compliance can be increased by programmes to promote public awareness, especially in relation to side-effects and safety. Uptake in the UK is now impressive, and fears expressed during the 1980s are waning (White *et al.*, 1992; Bedford, 1993). There is, however, evidence that when failure occurs it is more often caused by inadequate service provision or the misinterpretation of information than by a refusal to participate (Peckham *et al.*, 1989).

Professionals clearly need to know the contraindications to vaccination (Table 2.7) but tend to be poorly informed and to emphasise harmful effects in a manner likely to result in a failure of uptake among eligible children (Walker, 1990). There is little doubt that parents seeking information from more than one source and receiving contradictory advice are less likely to present their children for immunisation. One area in which there has been debate is the safety of vaccination in subjects for whom an allergy to egg has been reported, as the viruses are often cultured in eggs. Allergy is not, however, regarded as a contraindication (Ross, 1992; Aitken *et al.*, 1994).

Table 2.7   Contraindications to vaccination

- Febrile illness
- Active infection
- Pregnancy – live vaccines should be avoided
- Immunosuppression – live vaccines should be avoided

Clinical Application

The Nurse's Role in Administering Vaccinations

Nurses can immunise with or without the presence of a doctor providing that they are willing to be accountable for their actions. To be competent, they must be conversant with the indications for and contraindications to vaccination, and be able to recognise and treat anaphylaxis. Their employers must demonstrate that they have developed policies for those administering vaccination.

Environment, epidemics and vaccines

Environmental factors and epidemics

Environmental factors can play a major role in the promotion of epidemics in the human population:

- **Social factors** – overcrowding as people moved from rural areas to towns, for example, during the Industrial Revolution or are herded together in institutions.

- **The breakdown of previously successful control measures** – such as sanitation, resulting in epidemics of waterborne infection.

- **Altered behaviour** – human immunodeficiency virus (HIV) probably existed before the first reported cases in the late 1970s, but its incidence escalated in the early 1980s with an increase in high-risk activities such as unpro-

---

Clinical Application

Storage of Vaccines

Storage of vaccines involves placing each new batch under the conditions stipulated in the national guidelines (Longland and Rowbottom, 1989):

- The recommended temperature for polio vaccine is 0–4 ^{0}C, that for all other vaccines being 2–8 ^{0}C.
- A nominated, trained person should be responsible for storage, using the national guidelines, adapted as necessary to meet local needs.
- The temperature of the refrigerator should be monitored with a minimum and a maximum range thermometer, and should be recorded at regular intervals.
- Written procedures should be developed and followed if the refrigerator breaks down.
- The refrigerator should be defrosted regularly while the vaccines are placed in another refrigerator or cool box.
- Reconstituted vaccine should be used within the period recommended by the manufacturer, and partially used vials should be destroyed at the end of the clinic session.

---

tected intercourse with an infected person or the sharing of syringes and needles.

- **Geographical movement** – exposing people to pathogens that they have not encountered before. Travellers should seek expert advice about immunisation before embarking on their journey.

- **Exposure to mutant strains of pathogens** – mutant strains of pathogens can possess new antigenic properties to which the population may not have had the opportunity to develop herd immunity. New vaccines are periodically developed for influenza, which demonstrates this phenomenon of 'antigenic drift'.

Development of new vaccines

Factors influencing the development of new vaccines and their introduction are promoted by:

- **Changing patterns of disease within the community** – As new pathogens are identified, the search for disease prevention inevitably commences, although it usually takes many years. There is currently no effective vaccine for HIV (a 'new' disease) or for gonorrhoea (a significant community health problem that has been known since antiquity).

■ **Perceptions about existing infectious diseases** – One of the consequences of an effective immunisation programme is that a previously common disease becomes rare and the dangers of infection are forgotten (Bedford, 1993). Young health professionals and young parents, never having witnessed the effects of pertussis on a small baby, may be heavily influenced by media stories documenting complications associated with the vaccine.

■ **Changes in the sectors of the population at risk** – Since the eradication of smallpox, routine vaccination is no longer required.

The need for vaccination is greatest in developing countries (Bird, 1996).

Risks in hospital

Hospital patients are at particular risk of infection because they:

■ Experience high levels of physical and psychological stress, reducing their immune response
■ Have close contact with a large number of different hospital staff, increasing the risks of cross-infection
■ Are particularly likely to undergo invasive procedures and take drugs, both of which may depress the immune response
■ Share facilities for personal hygiene to a much greater extent than at home
■ Eat mass-produced food
■ Are exposed to micro-organisms not usually encountered.

Exposure to the above risk factors increases with the length of hospital stay and is greatest for those who are most sick. Immunisation is not yet possible because effective vaccines still have to be developed. It may always remain impractical owing to the large number of different organisms capable of causing nosocomial infection.

REVISION CHECKLIST: KEY AREAS

❏ Introduction to the immune response, immunity and immunology

❏ Types of immunity: Innate immunity – preventing invasion, Innate immunity – limiting spread, Adaptive immunity

❏ Individual variation in the immune response and predisposition to infection: Immunity throughout the lifespan

❏ Immunity and community health: Standard immunisation against infectious diseases, Health promotion, Environment, epidemics and vaccines, Risks in hospital

Activities – linking knowledge to clinical practice

1 **Draw** up a table, chart or other convenient device to compare and contrast the key features of innate and adaptive immunity. Using the same diagram, indicate where they interact.

2 **Select** one named human pathogen and explain to a colleague how the body evades its attack.

3 **Obtain** the latest information from journals and members of your local community health team to draw up the current schedule of childhood immunisation, including the ages at which vaccines and boosters are offered. How good is uptake in your locality?

SELF-ASSESSMENT

1. The bladder resists pathogenic invasion by the presence of a resident population of lactobacilli. True? ☐ False? ☐

2. The hallmarks of inflammation are:
   (a) . . . .
   (b) . . . .
   (c) . . . .
   (d) . . . .
   (e) . . . .

3. Briefly explain the following:
   (a) phagocytosis
   (b) chemotaxis
   (c) diapedesis

4. Basophils contain histamine. True? ☐ False? ☐

5. Complement is:
   (a) lipid ☐
   (b) mucopolysaccharide ☐
   (c) proteins ☐
   (d) leucocytes ☐

6. Clonal expansion is the rapid increase in the number of neutrophils arriving at the site of inflammation. True? ☐ False? ☐

7. Herd immunity is always a natural phenomenon. True? ☐ False? ☐

8. Corticosteriods increase the inflammatory response. True? ☐ False? ☐

9. Pyrexia is always beneficial. True? ☐ False? ☐

10. *Haemophilus influenzae* is the most common cause of childhood:
    (a) bacterial meningitis ☐
    (b) sore throat ☐
    (c) encephalitis ☐
    (d) influenza ☐
    (e) none of these ☐

References

Aditama TY (1991) 'Prevalence of tuberculosis in Indonesia, Singapore and the Philippines'. *Tubercle* **72**: 255–60.

Aitken R, Hill D and Kemp A (1994) 'Measles immunisation in children with allergy to egg'. *British Medical Journal* **309**: 223–5.

Alderslade R, Bellman MH, Rawson N *et al.* (1981) 'The National Childhood Encephalopathy Study' in *Whooping Cough. Reports from the Committee on Safety of Medicines and the Joint Committee on Vaccination and Immunisation.* HMSO, London.

Ayliffe GAJ, Brightwell KM, Babb BJ *et al.* (1977) 'Surveys of hospital infection in the Birmingham region'. *Journal of Hygiene* **79**: 299–313.

Bedford H (1993) 'Immunisation facts and fiction'. *Health Visitor* **66**: 314–16.

Bird C (1996) 'The battle continues'. *Nursing Times* **92**(27): 66–8.

Boore J (1978) *Prescription for Recovery.* RCN, London.

Gammon J (1995) 'The difficult bug to beat'. *Nursing Times* **91**(37): 57–8.

Henderson N (1991) 'Vaccination review'. *Practice Nurse* October: 271–4.

Hodgson S (1992) 'Primary prevention of *Haemophilous influenzae* type b'. *Health Visitor* **65**: 264–5.

Horan MA (1984) 'Outbreak of *Shigella sonnei* dysentery on a geriatric assessment ward'. *Journal of Hospital Infection* **5**: 210–12.

Joce R, Wood D, Brown D *et al.* (1992) 'Paralytic poliomyelitis in England and Wales'. *British Medical Journal* **305**: 79–82.

Lochhead YL (1991) 'Failure to immunise children under five years: a literature review'. *Journal of Advanced Nursing* **16**: 130–7.

Longland P and Rowbottom P (1989) 'Room temperature stability of medicines recommended pre cold storage'. *Pharmaceutical Journal* **4**: 584–94.

Lungmuss J (1989) 'Meningitis and epiglottitis: a new immunisation against *Haemophilous influenzae* type b infections'. *Health Visitor* **62**: 179–80.

Mackowiak P (1994) 'Fever: a blessing or a curse? A unifying hypothesis'. *Annals of Internal Medicine* **120**: 1037–40.

Mansell PI, Reckless JP and Lovell CR (1994) 'Severe anaphylactic reaction to latex rubber surgical gloves'. *British Medical Journal* **308**: 246–7.

Miller CM (1978) 'Severity of notified measles'. *British Medical Journal* **1**: 1253–5.

Miller E (1990) 'MMR and immunisation policies in the future'. *Midwife, Health Visitor and Community Nurse* **26**(7): 250–1.

Orr J (1986) 'Strong arm of the law'. *Nursing Times* **82**(34): 29–30.

Pawha SG (1981) 'Decreased *in vitro* humoral response in aged persons'. *Journal of Clinical Investigation* **47**: 1094–101.

Peckham CS and Senturia Y (1986) 'Why we're missing the point'. *Nursing Times* **82**(34): 29–30.

Peckham CS, Bedford H, Senturia Y *et al.* (1989) *The National Immunisation Study: Factors Affecting Immunisation Uptake in Childhood.* Action Research, Horsham.

Public Health Laboratory Service (1999) MMR vaccine and autism: no epidemiological evidence for a causal relationship. PHLS http://www.phls.co.uk/news/pressreleases

Ramsay MEB, Rao M, Begg NT *et al.* (1993) 'Antibody response to accelerated immunisation with diphtheria, tetanus, pertussis vaccine'. *Lancet* **342**: 203–5.

Reynolds JV, O'Farrelly C, Feighery C *et al.* (1996) 'Impaired gut barrier function in malnourished patients'. *British Journal of Surgery* **83**: 1288–91.

Roberts JV and Bates T (1992) 'The use of the body mass index in studies of abdominal wound infection'. *Journal of Hospital Infection* **20**: 217–20.

Ross EM (1992) 'MMR vaccine'. *Maternal and Child Health* **3**: 76–80.

Rudd P (1991) 'Childhood immunisation in the new decade'. *British Medical Journal* **302**: 481–2.

Sawyer SM, Bowes G and Phelan PD (1994) 'Vulvovaginal candidiasis in young women with cystic fibrosis'. *British Medical Journal* **308**: 1609–10.

Styrt B and Sugarman B (1990) 'Antipyresis in fever'. *Archives of Internal Medicine* **150**: 1597–8.

Trevelyan J (1996) 'Glove allergies'. *Nursing Times* **92**(42): 42–5.

Walker D (1990) 'Pertussis immunisation: professional attitudes and knowledge'. *Health Visitor* **63**: 386–7.

Weskler ME (1980) 'The immune system and the aging system'. *Proceedings of the Society of Experimental Biology and Medicine* **165**: 200–5.

White JM, Gillam SJ, Begg NT *et al.* (1992) 'Vaccine coverage: recent trends and future prospects'. *British Medical Journal* **304**: 682–4.

Young LS (1981) 'Nosocomial infections in the immunocompromised adult'. *American Journal of Medicine* **70**: 398–404.

Further reading and information sources

Cohen IR (1988) 'The self, the world and autoimmunity'. *Scientific American* **258**(4): 34–42.

Knowles HE (1993) 'The experience of the infectious patient in isolation'. *Nursing Times* **89**(30): 53–6.

Maclenan WJ, Watt B and Elder AT (1994) *Infections in Elderly People*. Edward Arnold, London.

Weir DM and Stewart J (1997) *Immunology* (8th edn). Churchill Livingstone, Edinburgh.

Westwood OMR (1999) *The Scientific Basis for Health Care*. Mosby, London.

White IR (1997) 'Setting standards for product selection: allergy prevention'. *European Journal of Surgery* **579**: 27–8.

Young DE and Chon ZA (1988) 'How killer cells kill'. *Scientific American* **258**(1): 28–34.

3 The microbiology laboratory

CHAPTER OUTCOMES

After reading this chapter you should be able to:

- State the functions of the hospital microbiology department
- Explain what happens when a specimen is processed in the hospital microbiology department
- Discuss the role of the nurse in obtaining specimens for microbiological examination
- Identify good practice during specimen handling and storage

---

Introduction to the microbiology laboratory

Staff in the microbiology department diagnose infection and give advice on the most effective treatment. Their work involves isolating and identifying bacteria and other organisms from specimens of blood, urine, faeces, sputum, pus and cerebrospinal fluid (CSF), and swabs taken from infected sites. Nurses need to understand the work of the medical microbiology laboratory in order to:

- Provide information to patients about diagnostic tests
- Collect specimens – success depends on good practice when the patient is prepared for the test, on when the specimen is obtained and on the way in which it is stored and handled before it reaches the laboratory (Higgins, 1994)
- Understand the findings expressed on laboratory reports.

Clinical Application

Near-patient Testing

Developments in technology have paved the way for newer, more rapid ways of performing laboratory tests known as near-patient testing. These are particularly used in premises away from laboratories when organisms present in the specimen could perish during transport, especially in situations where patients may be reluctant to return for follow-up. The nurse collects specimens and analyses the results, which are available immediately. For example, a 2-minute test can be performed for C reactive protein (CRP); this is used to identify whether a patient with a sore throat should receive antibiotics. The results, cross-checked with later laboratory findings, give an accurate and reliable indication of the presence of bacterial infection.

Diagnostic laboratory services

When a specimen arrives in the laboratory, it is first examined macroscopically and then with a microscope. Detailed identification requires the culture (growth) of the bacteria in a suitable medium. If the specimen has been obtained from a site where other organisms will be present (for example, skin or faeces), special techniques are used to isolate those causing infection. Additional biochemical and serological tests may be necessary to confirm the identification. Sensitivity tests are performed to determine the most effective antibiotic.

Following the various examinations and special tests, the laboratory produces a report (Figure 3.1) for the clinician. Interim results and those of special significance may be relayed by the telephone or facsimile.

Initial examination

Some information on the nature of the infection can be obtained by an initial inspection: odour and appearance can offer some clues. Foul-smelling, purulent material suggests the presence of anaerobes (for example, *Bacteroides*). CSF or urine that appears cloudy probably contains neutrophils, which indicate active infection. Mucus or blood in a stool suggests dysentery, and many roundworms and the segments of tapeworms are visible to the naked eye.

Microscopic examination

Wet films

A drop of fluid taken from the specimen is placed on a microscope slide beneath a cover slip and examined at low power (x400). This technique is used to look at:

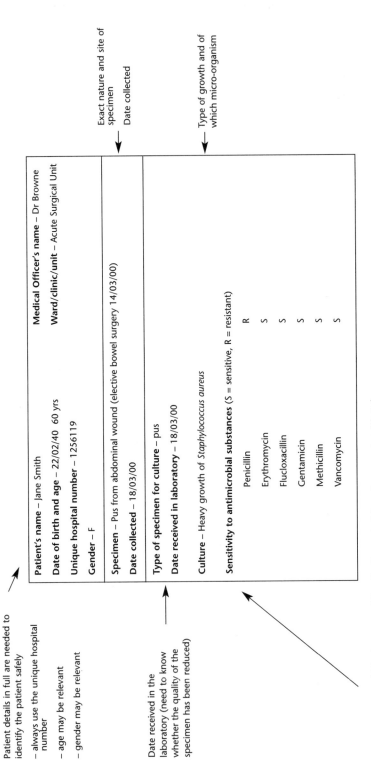

Patient details in full are needed to identify the patient safely

– always use the unique hospital number

– age may be relevant

– gender may be relevant

Date received in the laboratory (need to know whether the quality of the specimen has been reduced)

Exact nature and site of specimen

Date collected

Type of growth and of which micro-organism

Patient's name – Jane Smith   **Medical Officer's name** – Dr Browne

Date of birth and age – 22/02/40   60 yrs   **Ward/clinic/unit** – Acute Surgical Unit

Unique hospital number – 1256119

Gender – F

Specimen – Pus from abdominal wound (elective bowel surgery 14/03/00)

Date collected – 18/03/00

Type of specimen for culture – pus

Date received in laboratory – 18/03/00

Culture – Heavy growth of *Staphylococcus aureus*

Sensitivity to antimicrobial substances (S = sensitive, R = resistant)

Penicillin	R
Erythromycin	S
Flucloxacillin	S
Gentamicin	S
Methicillin	S
Vancomycin	S

Which antimicrobial substances will be effective against the micro-organism (S) and those which will not be effective (R)

NB. Methicillin is not used clinically.
NB. Most hospital-acquired *Staphylococcus aureus* infections are resistant to penicillin.

Figure 3.1   A laboratory report

- Body fluids – where pus cells or whole organisms may be present – for example, urine, CSF and vaginal secretions
- Faeces, to detect ova or cysts
- Scrapings from hair, skin or nails to detect fungal infection

Dry films

Dry films provide more detailed information about bacterial infection. A higher magnification is usually necessary (x1000), and stains are added to help to identify the bacteria. A thin film taken from the specimen is added to a microscope slide and the material is 'fixed' by passing it through the flame of a Bunsen burner. Gram staining is most often used (see Chapter 1): Gram-positive organisms appear deep purple, and Gram-negative bacteria stain pink.

Special microscopy techniques

Special techniques are necessary to identify specific bacteria:

1. **Acid-fast (Ziehl–Neelsen) technique** – this technique is used to identify *Mycobacterium* spp. These organisms do not respond well to Gram staining because their thick cell walls are impermeable to the dyes. Instead, they are identified by the acid-fast or acid/alcohol-fast staining technique (Table 3.1).

2. **Dark ground microscopy** – this technique is used to identify spirochaetes. These tiny bacteria, which react poorly to traditional staining methods, are best visualised at high magnification against a dark background. Wet films made from a recently collected specimen are used because spirochaetes die rapidly outside the tissues.

Table 3.1   Acid-fast (Ziehl–Neelsen) staining technique

- The smear on the slide is covered with hot carbol fuchsin stain for 5 minutes
- The slide is decolourised with an acid/alcohol solution (hydrochloric acid and ethanol)
- The slide is counterstained with methylene blue or malachite green
- Acid-fast bacilli (or AFBs) resist decolourisation and appear red or yellow on a dark background

NB. Acid/alcohol decolourisation is used because *Mycobacterium tuberculosis* is distinctive in that it resists decolourisation by both acid and alcohol. *Mycobacterium tuberculosis* is therefore referred to as being acid/alcohol fast

Identifying bacteria

Many related bacteria appear identical under the microscope. Identification involves growing them in special culture media and performing various tests.

Cultures

Solid media are produced by mixing nutrients with agar. A variety of culture media are used, blood agar being the one most commonly encountered in hospital laboratories. The concentration of different chemicals added to the medium alters its properties so the growth of a particular organism is encouraged while others are suppressed. This makes it easier to identify the pathogen. For example, MacConkey's medium contains a small amount of lactose and a pH indicator. Bacteria able to grow on MacConkey agar and to ferment lactose produce acid, turning the pH indicator red while species that do not ferment lactose remain colourless.

A special technique is used to inoculate culture media with bacteria taken from the specimen (Figure 3.2).

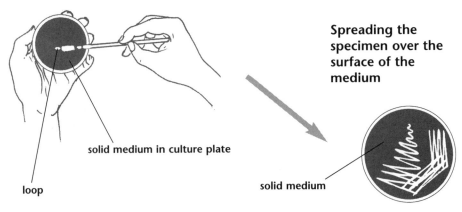

Introducing the specimen to the solid medium

Spreading the specimen over the surface of the medium

solid medium in culture plate

loop

solid medium

Figure 3.2   Technique for inoculating a culture medium

Following the inoculation of the culture medium, the specimen is incubated at an appropriate temperature for a certain period of time. Most bacteria able to cause human infection grow steadily at 37 ^{0}C, producing visible colonies on the surface of the agar within 24–48 hours (Figure 3.3). However, some bacteria (for example, *Mycobacterium*) grow much more slowly. Such cultures are kept and re-examined for several weeks. If the specimen is likely to contain anaerobes (for example, if it arises from a wound), a portion is cultured in a special container free of oxygen (an anaerobic jar).

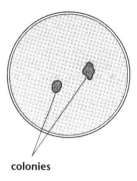

colonies

Figure 3.3   Bacterial colonies

Colonies result when bacteria are cultured on solid media. Each cell multiplies over and over again until a clump visible to the naked eye appears. All the bacteria in the colony are of the same type. The size, colour and shape of colonies vary according to the type of bacteria and can be used to help to identify the different species. For example, *Pseudomonas aeruginosa* produces characteristic green colonies and *Serratia marcescens* red ones. Haemolytic bacteria such as *Streptococcus pyogenes* release enzymes that destroy erythrocytes in blood agar; as a result, each colony becomes surrounded by a clear halo.

Biochemical tests

Biochemical tests are used to confirm the identity of many bacteria. Most tests are designed to detect the presence of specific enzymes and have been developed so that a visible, easily detected change, usually the production of gas or a change in pH, occurs. This is demonstrated by an indicator incorporated into the medium. *Shigella* species are differentiated by their ability to ferment carbohydrates, releasing bubbles of gas. Commercially prepared kits are available so that biochemical tests can be conveniently performed.

Antibiotic sensitivity

It is vital to establish which antibiotics destroy the pathogen so that the appropriate drug can be prescribed. Antibiotic sensitivity tests are performed by the disc diffusion method. The bacteria are inoculated onto solid media, a paper disc impregnated with different antibiotics is placed over them, and the culture is incubated. Where the bacteria are sensitive to a particular antibiotic, the agar remains clear of growth.

Serological tests

Serological tests are used to identify bacteria based on their immunological reactions. Portions of the specimen containing the organism to be identified are exposed to several different known antibodies, these antibodies being specific to antigens on the surfaces of particular species of bacteria. If the antigens and antibodies belong to the same species, the antibody binds to the bacterial cells, which causes visible clumping (agglutination).

Typing bacteria

During outbreaks, additional, more specialised 'typing' procedures are used to establish whether the same strain is responsible for cross-infection. These tests are usually performed at specialist Public Health Laboratories. Tests distinguish between related strains belonging to the same species by determining their susceptibility to bacteriophages (viruses) or whether they have identical surface antigens. Phage typing is used to identify different strains of methicillin-resistant *Staphylococcus aureus* (also known as MRSA). If all cases are being caused by the same strain, infection must be coming from a common source, which can be identified as a step towards control.

Virology – identifying viral infections

Specimens for virology are transported to the laboratory in a solution containing antibiotics to inhibit bacterial growth. Viral infection is diagnosed either by directly detecting the virus particles using the electron microscope, by culture or by serological tests to detect viral antibodies in the patient's blood.

Electron microscopy

Electron microscopy at high magnification is required to visualise virus particles. These are identified according to their characteristic shape once they have been stained. It is possible to identify rotavirus and herpes viruses using the electron microscope. The absence of virus particles in a specimen cannot, however, be taken as conclusive evidence that no infection is present because the particles are minute and, unless present in large numbers, can easily be overlooked.

Viral culture

Viruses cannot be cultured outside living cells. In the laboratory, sheets of cells grown in nutrient medium can be used to culture some viruses. The presence of a particular virus is indicated by the characteristic way in which it changes the shape of the cells.

Serological tests for viruses

Viral infection stimulates the appearance of specific antibodies in the blood, their presence forming the basis of diagnostic testing. The most widely used method is the enzyme-linked immunosorbent assay (or ELISA). Specific antigen is mixed with the patient's serum. If the antigen and antibody are from the same virus, they combine. A second antibody attached to the enzyme is added. The conjugate becomes attached to the antibody bound to the original antigen, causing a visible change in the test solution as a result of the enzyme's action.

Identifying fungal infections

Fungi may be detected in stained films during the routine examination of sputum, swabs and vaginal secretions. Most species will grow in the same types of media as those used to culture bacteria, but apart from a few species that grow quickly (for example, *Candida albicans*), colonies do not appear until after the usual incubation period of 24–48 hours. Where fungal infection is suspected, special cultures are set up and examined at intervals of 2–3 weeks. A medium containing antibiotics to inhibit bacterial growth, usually Sabouraud's glucose agar, is used. Identification is generally based on the characteristic appearance of the fungus on the surface of the agar and its microscopic appearance.

Taking and processing specimens

The success of diagnostic testing depends on good practice when the patient is prepared, on when the specimen is obtained and on the way in which it is stored and handled on its way to the laboratory. Nurses obviously have a vital role to play in ensuring that specimens are obtained correctly and reach the laboratory in good condition.

Urine specimens

Urine specimens must be collected as free of contamination as possible. In health, urine is sterile, but it is easily contaminated during collection by contact with the perineum or the hands. Extraneous Gram-negative bacteria multiply rapidly, especially if the specimen is stored, leading to a result that is falsely positive or difficult to interpret.

The risk of error can be reduced by collecting a 5–10 ml midstream specimen. Male patients are instructed or helped to withdraw the foreskin; the urethral meatus is then cleansed and the middle portion of the flow collected directly into the sterile receptacle. Collecting an uncontaminated urine specimen from a female patient is never easy, and there are particular problems when the patient is bed bound or too disorientated to co-operate. The patient is required to micturate with the labia separated, catching the middle part of the stream in the sterile container. The procedure has traditionally involved cleansing the perineum before obtaining the specimen in a sterile receptacle, but there is little evidence that this procedure yields specimens of any higher quality than when patients have simply passed

Clinical Application

Taking Specimens: General Points To Ensure Good Practice

- **Good sampling technique** – the specimen should contain organisms only from the site being investigated; saliva, for example, should not be substituted for sputum.
- **Sufficient material should be provided for examination** – for example, rectal swabs should not replace a specimen of faeces because there will be insufficient material for culture.
- **Time of collection** – except in an emergency, the specimen should be obtained before antibiotics are given.
- **Use the appropriate specimen container** – for example, viruses do not survive well in transport media intended for bacteria.
- **Correctly label the specimen and request card** – particular care is needed when patients on the same ward have similar names or initials. Use unique identification, for example, the hospital number.
- **Provide adequate data on the request form** – clinical signs and details of antibiotic therapy.
- **Transport to the laboratory without delay, at the correct temperature** – wherever possible, specimens should be obtained just before a pick-up is due.
- **Maintain safety** – specimens must be transported in robust, leak-proof containers, with the request card separate from the specimen container. The container should not be contaminated with blood or any other body fluid and must not be overfilled: fermentation may occur, especially with faeces, leading to the accumulation of gas and a build-up of pressure sufficient to force off even a tightly fitting lid. Staff handling specimens should be aware of the hazards attached to spillage, should wear overalls and should know that they must wash their hands frequently. Leak-proof trays should be available for transport (see the Clinical Application box on transporting specimens safely, below).

urine into a clean container. Even without cleansing and collection in a sterile receptacle, most specimens are satisfactory (White, 1992).

For catheterised patients, a freshly passed specimen is obtained by aspiration with a needle and syringe from the special self-occluding sleeve on the catheter tubing. The drainage apparatus and catheter should never be disconnected to collect a specimen because of the risk of introducing infection. Urine from the drainage bag will not yield satisfactory results because it may be heavily contaminated from environmental sources.

Specimens from infants are more likely to be free of contamination if they are obtained by aspiration with a syringe from the compressed fibres of wet, disposable nappies than if they are obtained from special collection bags, providing the baby has been changed within the last 4 hours and there is no faecal soiling (Ahmad *et al.*, 1991).

All specimens should be examined within 3 hours of collection, before any contaminating bacteria not responsible for the infection have had time to multiply, distorting the results. If examination is likely to be delayed, the specimen must be stored at 4 ^{0}C until it reaches the laboratory bench.

In the laboratory, the specimen is inoculated onto nutrient agar and incubated overnight. The colonies are counted and the number of bacteria present in 1 ml of the urine is calculated the next day. Counts of 10^5 or more organisms per ml suggest that infection is present, especially in the presence of neutrophils (pus cells). A lower count suggests contamination rather than genuine infection.

Specimens from wounds

Specimen collection from wounds sometimes yields poor results because the swab of pus or exudate dries out and the bacteria are dead before they reach the laboratory. This especially occurs if the specimen is stored before it is examined. Whenever possible, pus should be aspirated from a wound, or a small portion of excised tissue should be obtained. If swabbing is the only practical method, two or three specimens are better than one: the first can be stained for microscopy, the others used to inoculate the culture medium. Two agar plates are inoculated – one to grow aerobes, the other to grow anaerobes.

Stool specimens

Stool specimens are obtained to identify bacteria (for example *Salmonella* or *Campylobacter*) or viruses (for example, Rotaviruses) that may be causing infection as well as to identify parasites. Protozoa and the eggs of parasitic worms are always microscopic, but the adult forms of many worms are clearly visible to the naked eye. If their presence is suspected, the specimen should be examined as soon as possible: the ova of parasites survive desiccation and cold, but the worms themselves and protozoa become sluggish on cooling and are more difficult to detect.

Rectal swabs are not acceptable in place of stool specimens because they provide insufficient material for culture. Stools usually contain millions of bacteria, and interpreting the results requires skill. It is not easy to identify those responsible for enteric infection, and several specimens may be necessary before the pathogen is isolated and identified.

Sputum specimens

Sputum is the secretion produced by the mucous membranes lining the lower airways. Its function is to trap inhaled foreign material, including bacteria. About 100 ml are secreted daily, but this is not usually apparent in health, when the sputum is normally swallowed. Excess production occurs when the airways become inflamed. This frequently occurs with infection but, even in the case of severe infection, sputum is often difficult to obtain in sufficient quantity to be examined and cultured. Sputum from an intubated patient is obtained by tracheal aspiration. Other patients must be encouraged to cough to produce a specimen. Saliva from the oropharynx is frequently sent to the laboratory instead of sputum. The help of a physiotherapist can be enlisted to overcome this difficulty. Many of the organisms responsible for infection of the lower respiratory tract do not survive well outside the host, so specimens should be dispatched to the laboratory immediately.

Throat swabs

Exudate from the throat is obtained by passing the tip of the swab over the tonsils and the posterior pharyngeal wall while the tongue is depressed with a spatula (Figure 3.4). A good source of illumination is necessary to avoid contaminating the swab by contact with the oral mucosa. Patients usually find this procedure unpleasant and should be warned in advance about the gag reflex. Children may be more co-operative if the help of a parent is enlisted. Wrapping the child in a blanket helps to restrict movement.

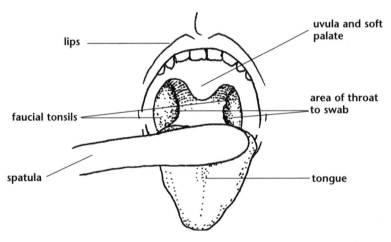

Figure 3.4   Taking a throat swab

Nasal swabs

Nasal swabs are taken with the patient's head tilted, rotating the previously moistened swab to ensure that as much secretion as possible is collected. Both nostrils are swabbed. For infants and very young children, a fine wire swab-holder may be used instead of a wooden swab-stick. Great care is necessary to avoid damaging the delicate epithelium. When healthy people are screened to exclude staphylococcal carriage, the tip of the swab is moistened with sterile water because, in health, the nasal mucosa is usually dry.

Pernasal swabs are used to confirm a presumptive diagnosis of pertussis. *Bordetella pertussis* is most readily recovered from the posterior nasopharynx, especially if the specimen is obtained immediately after coughing. The tip of the swab is connected to a fine, flexible wire so that it can be introduced into the space without contamination (Figure 3.5).

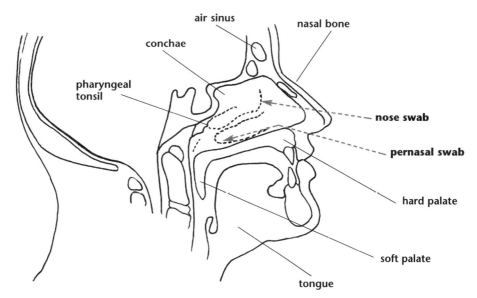

Figure 3.5   Taking a pernasal swab

Eye swabs

Eye swabs often yield poor results because lysozyme (an antibacterial enzyme), naturally present in tears, destroys bacteria. Instead, conjunctival scrapings can be obtained with a plastic loop and inoculated directly onto culture media. This procedure is usually undertaken by staff who have received special training.

Blood cultures

Blood cultures require strict aseptic technique during their collection. Two bottles containing liquid culture media are inoculated, one for aerobic culture and the other for anaerobic culture. The procedure is strictly aseptic to avoid contamination with skin flora. Any patient likely to be septicaemic is very ill, so there should be no delay in sending the specimens to the laboratory: most provide an incubator to receive blood cultures outside normal working hours.

Specimens of CSF

CSF is obtained by lumbar puncture. This is a highly invasive procedure usually performed on a very sick patient who is likely to be anxious, possibly disorientated and unco-operative. It is undertaken by a doctor, assisted by a nurse. The specimen is collected by strict aseptic technique to avoid introducing infection and to prevent the CSF becoming contaminated with skin organisms. Three consecutive tubes are filled with CSF, which must be sent to the laboratory at once. The specimens must be maintained at 37 ^{0}C until they are examined, which must occur no later than 2–4 hours after collection.

Vaginal and cervical swabs

Most pathogens recovered from the female genital tract survive poorly in the environment, so contamination is less problematic than with other specimens. Special transport media (Stuart's or Amies' medium) are used. Storage at room temperature may be helpful to the laboratory staff since *Trichomonas vaginalis* will multiply and is more easily detected. When refrigerated, the protozoa become immobile and difficult to detect. *N. gonorrhoeae*, however, survives so poorly outside the tissues that it is advisable for all specimens to be examined immediately when this infection is suspected. Most genitourinary medicine clinics have satellite laboratories so that specimens can be examined at once. It is usual to obtain more than one swab so that culture plates can be inoculated, permitting antibiotic sensitivity testing. This is essential owing to the increasing number of gonococci that have been found to be resistant to penicillin, the drug of choice for this condition.

General points important for obtaining specimens have been outlined in the Clinical Applications box above. Safe transport is equally important, as shown below.

Clinical Application

Transporting Specimens Safely

All specimens contain potentially infectious material and therefore present a hazard during transport. To reduce the risks to handlers during transport, the Health Services Advisory Committee (1991) recommends the use of leak-proof boxes and agreed protocols for dealing with spillages. The use of biohazard labels is recommended to indicate to handlers and laboratory staff that a specimen may contain particularly hazardous pathogens. The indications for their use vary between hospitals. However, they should be applied to specimens that may contain *Mycobacterium tuberculosis* or parenterally transmitted viruses (DoH, 1990).

The interpretation of laboratory results

Interpreting laboratory reports combines the results of microbiological findings (see Figure 3.1 above) with clinical evaluation. Some of the bacteria isolated may be contaminants or part of the normal flora that do not cause infection at that site. Thus, the diagnosis of infection must also take into consideration the patient's signs and symptoms. For example, *Staphylococcus epidermidis* from the skin may contaminate a blood specimen but there will be no evidence of pyrexia.

Environmental sampling

Bacteria are present throughout the environment. Most are not pathogens, those on the floor, walls and so on being unlikely to harm patients. The number of bacteria isolated from a swab will depend on the site sampled. Routine sampling is expensive, time consuming and (as little is known about the level of contamination that should be taken as unacceptable) uninformative. It is occasionally initiated by the control of infection team during an outbreak, when it may help to identify environmental reservoirs or test the efficacy of the ventilation system in a newly commissioned theatre suite, for example. This process involves the use of an air sampler to measure the number of organisms per cubic centimetre of air. Agar 'settle plates' are not a useful substitute because the results are difficult to interpret and may not accurately reflect the level of contamination (Holton and Ridgeway, 1993).

REVISION CHECKLIST: KEY AREAS

❑ Introduction to the microbiology laboratory

❑ Diagnostic laboratory services: Initial examination, Microscopic examination, Identifying bacteria, Virology – identifying viral infections, Identifying fungal infections

❑ Taking and processing specimens: Urine specimens, Specimens from wounds, Stool specimens, Sputum specimens, Throat swabs, Nasal swabs, Eye swabs, Blood cultures, Specimens of CSF, Vaginal and cervical swabs, The interpretation of laboratory results, Environmental sampling

Activities – linking knowledge to clinical practice

1 **Visit** your local microbiology laboratory. Observe the procedure for receiving and storing specimens before they are processed, their initial examination, microscopy, culture, antibiotic testing and the return of the results to the clinical areas.

2 **Find** out how urine specimens are obtained from female patients in your clinical area. (a) Is this practice evidence based? Identify any steps that you consider fail this criterion. (b) Think about ways in which you would improve the quality of specimens obtained from patients who are immobile or confused.

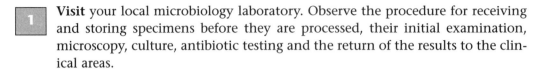

SELF-ASSESSMENT

1. A high magnification is always needed to observe microbiological specimens.
   True? ☐ False? ☐

2. State three techniques used to examine microscope slides.

3. Explain why all the bacteria in a colony are of the same type.

4. Explain how laboratory methods used to identify fungi and viruses differ from those used to identify bacteria.

5. List five points to ensure safe specimen handling.

References

Ahmad T, Vickers D, Campbell S, Coulthard MG and Pedler S (1991) 'Urine collection from disposable nappies'. *Lancet* **338**: 674–6.

Department of Health, Advisory Committee on Dangerous Pathogens (1990) *Categorisation of Pathogens According to Hazard and Categories of Containment*. HMSO, London.

Health Services Advisory Committee (1991) *Safe Working and Prevention of Infection in Clinical Laboratories*. HMSO, London.

Higgins C (1994) 'An introduction to the examination of specimens'. *Nursing Times* **90**(47): 29–32.

Holton J and Ridgeway GL (1993) 'Commissioning operating theatres'. *Journal of Hospital Infection* **23**: 153–60.

White S (1992) 'Choosing the right container'. *Nursing Times* **88**(6): 64–5.

Further reading and information sources

Visit the Health and Safety Executive web site at http://www.open.gov.uk/hse/hsehome. htm for up-to-date guidelines on dangerous pathogens and the handling and transport of specimens.

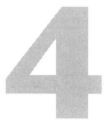

Treating infectious disease

CHAPTER OUTCOMES

After reading this chapter you should be able to:

- Define the terms: 'antibiotic', 'bactericidal' and 'bacteriostatic'

- State the aims of antibiotic therapy in the treatment of established infection and in chemoprophylaxis

- Name the main groups of antibacterial agent and explain how they exert their effects

- Discuss the consequences of indiscriminate antibiotic use

- Explain the mechanisms that give rise to antibiotic-resistant strains of bacteria

- Explain the difficulties associated with the treatment of viral and fungal infections and name the drugs in current use

---

Introduction to antibiotics

Antibiotics are, strictly speaking, defined as naturally produced chemicals released by living organisms that are able to inhibit the growth of other organisms. However, the term is now used to refer to any antimicrobial chemotherapeutic agent: those produced naturally, synthetic compounds and the semi-synthetic antibiotics created by modifying natural drugs (for example, cloxacillin and ampicillin produced from 6-aminopenicillanic acid). Antibiotics are widely prescribed to treat established infection and as chemoprophylaxis (the prevention of infection by giving antibiotics before signs and symptoms appear; Table 4.1) when the risk of developing an infection is significant. Their use is increasing, the number of prescriptions in England doubling between 1980 and 1991 (Davey *et al.*, 1996). Nurses are the main group of health professionals responsible for administering medication, including antibiotics. To educate patients about the possible side-effects, nurses need to understand:

- The aims of antibiotic treatment
- How antibiotics act
- Their side-effects
- The dangers of indiscriminate antibiotic use.

Table 4.1 Situations in which chemoprophylaxis is appropriate

- Surgery involving the large bowel to prevent infection by the normal gut flora, especially anaerobes. **Suitable chemoprophylaxis:** metronidazole with gentamicin or a cephalosporin

- Major orthopaedic surgery to prevent the infection of a prosthesis. **Suitable chemoprophylaxis:** flucloxacillin with gentamicin or a cephalosporin

- Major cardiac surgery, especially to prevent infection of implanted valves. **Suitable chemoprophylaxis:** flucloxacillin with gentamicin or a cephalosporin

- Amputation of an ischaemic limb to avoid the serious risk of infection with *Clostridium perfringens* (gas gangrene). **Suitable chemoprophylaxis:** penicillin, or erythromycin for those sensitive to penicillin

- Dental treatment for patients with a history of infective endocarditis to reduce the risk of streptococcal infection. Streptococci are invariably released into the blood during any dental procedure. **Suitable chemoprophylaxis:** a single large dose of amoxycillin immediately before the procedure

- Contacts of patients with meningococcal meningitis. **Suitable chemoprophylaxis:** (see Chapter 14)

- Travellers to malaria-endemic regions. **Suitable chemoprophylaxis:** (see Chapter 14)

The purpose of antibiotic therapy

The purpose of antibiotic treatment is to cure the patient or to effect chemoprophylaxis while causing minimum side-effects and discomfort. This is necessary in the case of severe infectious illness but is not considered good practice in the case of trivial infections or if the condition could be caused by a virus against which antibiotics have no effect (for example, a viral sore throat). In 1998, the Department of Health issued recommendations to prescribers regarding the use of antibiotics, including the recommendation that antibiotics should not be prescribed for viral sore throats, colds and simple coughs (DoH, 1998). Unnecessary prescription is dangerous because it promotes the emergence of antibiotic-resistant strains and may cause side-effects (Davies, 1994).

Clinical Application

Helping To Reduce the Inappropriate Use of Antibiotics and Bacterial Resistance

A recent report (DoH, 1998) makes recommendations for the prescribing of antibiotics in an effort to reduce the development of resistant strains of bacteria. The main recommendations include:

- No prescribing of antibiotics for colds, simple coughs and sore throats caused by viruses
- Prescribing antibiotics over the telephone in only exceptional situations
- Prescribing antibiotics for only 3 days for uncomplicated cystitis in otherwise healthy women
- Increasing understanding in professionals and the public about the prescribing of antibiotics.

Nurses, midwives and health visitors have an important role in educating the general public and junior medical staff with regard to the proper use of antibiotics. The pressure on prescribers to provide antibiotics for patients suffering from minor viral conditions can be very intense. Antibiotic use could be reduced if the general public and prescribers had information about conditions in which such antibiotic use is justified. Community nursing staff, practice nurses and those working in emergency departments are particularly well placed to provide this information for the public.

Historical development of antibiotic therapy

Despite the hazards of side-effects and bacterial resistance, antibiotics still feature among the greatest triumphs of modern medicine. Down the ages, there have been strenuous efforts to control infectious disease, but until the beginning of the 20th century, none were successful. The search to find a cure encompassed every kind of substance imaginable, from toxic chemicals to home-made remedies. Mercury, for example, was used to treat syphilis even though its long-term effects were as severe as the disease itself. A breakthrough at the beginning of the 20th century was made possible because the germ theory of disease had been accepted and advances in the chemical industry permitted the development of previously unknown organic compounds.

The first major advance was made in 1910 by the German scientist Paul Ehrlich, who synthesised 605 derivatives of arsenic before isolating neoarsphenamine '606'. This could kill *Treponema pallidum,* although a long course of treatment was necessary to cure syphilis. Nevertheless, it was for many years the main treatment.

Further progress was made by Gerhard Domagk in Germany in 1935. His research with dyestuffs yielded a compound called sulphamidochrysoidin able to resolve infection in experimental animals. The active component was sulphanilamide, the forerunner of a group of synthetic drugs called sulphonamides. The potential effectiveness of dyes as antibacterial agents stemmed from an awareness that dyestuffs used in the clothing industry exerted their effects by uniting with the protein in wool, suggesting that they might similarly bond to and destroy bacterial protein. Over the next 20 years, other sulphonamides became available. Although these were eventually superseded by penicillins, their success was considerable. However, the sulphonamides were associated with potentially severe side-effects: nausea, rashes and fever. The drugs precipitate out of solution in the urinary tract, leading to obstruction in severe cases. Only a few of the sulphonamides are still used (Table 4.2), having largely been replaced, first by penicillins and then by newer antibiotics.

Table 4.2   Sulphonamides in common use

Name of drug	Important properties	Indications
Sulphadimidine	Good oral absorption	Urinary infections
Sulphasalazine	Releases sulphapyridine (antibacterial) and 5-aminosalicylic acid (anti-inflammatory drug) in the gut	Chronic Crohn's disease, ulcerative colitis, rheumatoid arthritis
Sulphacetamide	Non-irritant in solution	Used as eye drops
Silver sulphadiazine		Applied topically as a cream after severe burns to prevent infection

The discovery of penicillin in 1928 predated Domagk's work. It had been known since the 19th century that fungi could inhibit bacterial growth. The discovery of penicillin, the first naturally occurring antibiotic to be identified, is attributed to Sir Alexander Fleming, working at St Mary's Hospital in Paddington. His laboratory on the corner of the hospital building overlooking a busy street was draughty, and dust was apt to swirl into the room. Spores of the fungus *Penicillium notatum* carried by the air currents settled onto a culture that had been inoculated with *Staphylococcus aureus.* The mould took over, producing a chemical that inhibited the growth of the staphylococci. Fleming was unable to isolate the antibiotic produced by *P. notatum*, this being left to Ernst Chain and Sir Howard Florey working in Oxford. The first penicillin was isolated in 1939. The Second World War had provided the impetus for research leading to the development of commercially available antibacterial agents to treat the large number of infections associated with trauma and communicable diseases among the troops, but penicillin did not become universally available in the UK until the war was over. Throughout the war, the further development of penicillin took place in the USA.

Antibiotics revolutionised the treatment of infection. UK childhood mortality statistics show that in 1940, when the earliest antibacterial agents were just becoming available, 3000 children per million died of infectious conditions every year. By 1970, the mortality from childhood infectious disease had declined to 450 per million because of the ready availability of treatment. The triumph of antibiotic therapy must, however, be judged in the light of other social and medical advances made towards the end of the 19th and throughout the early 20th centuries: better social conditions, improved hygiene and immunisation programmes. Social historians argue that the development of medicine, despite spectacular advances in the fields of therapeutics and immunology, is insufficient to explain the increase in the rate of infant survival and the decline in mortality that occurred as the 19th century drew to a close (McKeown, 1979). For example, smallpox was conquered and antibacterial drugs became widely available at a time when the health of the nation was already improving, better health occurring secondary to industrial and economic developments such as improved nutrition, education and hygiene. Nevertheless, the contribution of antibiotics should not be underestimated.

The discovery of other antibiotics

Following the widespread, successful use of penicillin, the search commenced for other naturally occurring antibacterial agents. Soil, the normal environment of fungi, was subjected to intensive investigation, leading to the discovery of chloramphenicol, streptomycin and the tetracyclines (1940s), erythromycin and rifampicin (1950s), and gentamicin and sodium fusidate (1960s). The forerunner of the cephalosporin group of antibiotics was isolated from a fungus growing in sewage effluent in 1948. Most of the naturally occurring antibiotics are produced by fungi or *Streptomyces,* a few being made by *Bacillus* spp. and actinomycetes. Each new drug was initially welcomed as a broader-spectrum alternative to any of the antibacterials already available, but in reality none has fulfilled these claims, owing to the emergence of antibiotic-resistant strains.

Range of antibiotic action

Antibiotics can be classified according to the type of bacteria against which they act. There are three groups:

1. Drugs active mainly against Gram-positive organisms, for example penicillins, erythromycin and lincomycin

2. Drugs mainly active against Gram-negative organisms, for example polymyxin and nalidixic acid

3. Broad-spectrum antibiotics active against Gram-positive and Gram-negative organisms, for example tetracyclines, chloramphenicol, ampicillin, cephalosporins and sulphonamides.

There are, however, exceptions. *Neisseria* spp. are Gram negative yet they are usually sensitive to penicillin and erythromycin. The natural susceptibility of many bacteria may be altered by resistance developing through exposure to antibiotics. This occurs much more rapidly with some types of bacteria than others. *Mycobacterium tuberculosis* is able to develop resistance to antibiotics within 6 weeks, this being the rationale behind the use of combined chemotherapy to treat tuberculosis. Tetracyclines are effective against chlamydias, rickettsiae and mycoplasmas.

Mode of antibiotic action

Antibiotics either kill bacteria or prevent them multiplying:

- **Bactericidal agents** – for example, aminoglycosides, cephalosporins and polymyxin – kill bacteria rapidly
- **Bacteriostatic agents** – for example, sulphonamides, tetracyclines and chloramphenicol – prevent bacteria replicating but do not kill them.

Many antibiotics that operate principally as bacteriostatic agents can become bactericidal in favourable circumstances. Influential factors include the concentration of the drug and the number and type of bacteria present. Where only a few highly sensitive organisms are present and the drug is given in a high dose, an agent such as penicillin that is usually bacteriostatic becomes bactericidal. The mechanisms of antibiotic action are shown in Table 4.3.

Antibiotics exert their effects directly on the bacterial cell wall or penetrate it to disrupt metabolism at the intracellular level. In all bacteria, the cell wall is composed of layers of protein molecules bound together by cross-linkages, but the fine structure depends on whether they are Gram positive or Gram negative, this influencing susceptibility to the different groups of antibiotic. For example, erythromycin penetrates the cell walls of Gram-positive bacteria and is effective in the treatment of some staphylococcal and streptococcal infections, but it has no effect on Gram-negative bacteria.

Table 4.3   Mechanisms of antibiotic action

Action on micro-organism	Example
Prevents cell wall formation	Penicillins Cephalosporins Vancomycin
Alters permeability of cell membrane	Antifungal agents, for example amphotericin
Disrupts protein synthesis	Aminoglycosides Tetracyclines Chloramphenicol Erythromycin
Disrupts nucleic acid synthesis	Quinolones
Disrupts cell metabolism	Trimethoprim Sulphonamides

Specific antibiotics – mode of action

Some of the diverse ways in which the different groups of antibiotics exert their effects are illustrated below:

- **Sulphonamides** have a molecular structure similar to that of a metabolite called para-aminobenzoic acid (PABA) essential for the growth of many bacteria. If a sulphonamide is present, it is absorbed instead of PABA but cannot be metabolised, so the bacteria cease to multiply. This phenomenon is known as competitive inhibition.

- **Trimethoprim** inhibits the action of a bacterial enzyme called dihydrofolate reductase but has no effect on the corresponding human enzyme. It interferes with the metabolism of folic acid and ultimately prevents the bacteria synthesising DNA. Trimethoprim and the sulphonamides operate at different points in the same metabolic pathway.

- The **penicillins**, the **cephalosporins** and **vancomycin** inhibit the formation of cross-links between protein molecules in the bacterial cell wall, which gradually weakens, eventually bursting as the cell grows.

- The **tetracyclines, chloramphenicol, streptomycin** and the **aminoglycosides** interfere with protein synthesis within the cell by attaching themselves to the ribosomes (cell organelles concerned with protein synthesis) thus inhibiting protein synthesis and bacterial replication.

- **Quinolones** disrupt the structure of bacterial DNA by inhibiting an enzyme that allows transcription (part of protein synthesis) or DNA replication.

Adverse reactions to antibacterial drugs

Toxicity to antibacterial drugs falls into two broad categories:

1. Direct chemical toxicity
2. Superinfection arising through prolonged or inappropriate antibiotic treatment.

Direct chemical toxicity

Direct chemical toxicity can be mediated through side-effects specifically related to the drug. Examples include the nephrotoxic (that is, toxic to renal tubule cells) and ototoxic (toxic to cells in the cochlea and vestibular structure) action of gentamicin, and the much-publicised but rare depressant effect of chloramphenicol on the bone marrow. These effects are well established, and it is usually possible to find an alternative treatment. If no alternative is readily available, antibiotic assays are required to ensure that the plasma level does not exceed safe limits. Additionally, some individuals develop type 1 hypersensitivity (allergic) reactions to particular drugs, often penicillins or cephalosporins. Type 1 hypersensitivity reactions are mediated by IgE (see Chapter 2). The allergen binds to IgE on the surface of the mast cells and basophils, and chemical mediators (for example, histamine and bradykinin) are released. Symptoms include nausea, vomiting and diarrhoea if the drug is taken orally, or contact erythema if it is applied topically or injected, and may persist after it is stopped. Anaphylactic shock is a more severe complication, which can be life-threatening.

Clinical Application

Hypersensitivity Reactions

It is difficult to predict who will develop a hypersensitivity reaction. Clinical observations suggest that patients with a history of allergy are more susceptible, but all patients should be asked about allergies and sensitivity to drugs before the first dose is administered. A note of any history of allergy or side-effects to drugs should be recorded in the nursing and medical records.

Superinfection

Superinfection occurs when the body's normal commensal flora is suppressed by antibiotics and replaced by drug-resistant organisms. It may follow treatment with any antibiotic but is most commonly seen with broad-spectrum antibiotics such as the tetracyclines, especially if they are administered for a long time. In the upper respiratory tract, the normal flora is replaced with drug-resistant coliforms. Suppression of the normal vaginal flora causes superinfection with yeasts. The normal gut flora is replaced with *Klebsiella*, *Pseudomonas*, yeasts and staphylococci.

Clinical Application

Antibiotic Assays

An antibiotic assay (a measurement of the concentration of a particular antibiotic in human body fluids) is necessary in the following circumstances:

- To confirm that adequate levels of the antibiotic are being attained in the tissues. This might be necessary in the case of a patient severely ill with meningitis or when an individual taking an oral drug is known to have some defect of the intestinal tract that could impair its absorption.
- To ensure that the plasma level does not exceed the limits of safety when the patient is receiving a drug with known toxic effects (for example, gentamicin)
- During the investigation of a new drug. Assay of the body fluids will provide information about absorption, the way in which the drug becomes distributed through the tissues and its rate of excretion.

Patients complain of a sore mouth, vomiting and diarrhoea, which can lead to non-adherence to a drug regimen.

These problems have been documented since the 1970s, but more recently super-infection with *Clostridium difficile* has become a major problem. This organism is usually present in small numbers, but suppression of the rest of the gut flora allows it to multiply and release cytoxins (Gammon, 1995). Large areas of the intestinal epithelium necrose, and the patient develops profuse, watery diarrhoea. This condition, known as pseudomembranous colitis, is potentially life-threatening. During investigations of hospital outbreaks, asymptomatic carriers have been identified (Degl'Innocenti *et al.*, 1989), and the person-to-person spread of clostridia and infection from spores in environmental reservoirs have been documented (Wilcox, 1996). The development of pseudomembranous colitis appears to be exacerbated if patients receive injectable antibiotics that are not completely absorbed, reaching a high level in the gut. Cefamandole and ceftriaxone attain high concentrations in the bile, which then delivers them to the gut where they are not fully absorbed. Superinfection with these antibiotics is more marked than that seen with the oral cephalosporins. *Clostridium difficile* superinfection can be treated with vancomycin or metronidazole.

Bacterial resistance to antibiotics

Antibiotic-resistant micro-organisms are defined as those not inhibited or killed by antibiotics at the drug concentration achieved in the body after a therapeutic dose (Kelly and Chivers, 1996). This is not a recent phenomenon: Ehrlich, working in the early 1900s, noticed that neoarsphenamine had to be administered in an increasing dose because the treponemes gradually became less susceptible. The first major concern was expressed by Miles (1944), who predicted that the incidence of drug-resistant organisms, particularly Gram-negative bacteria, might increase as more patients received sulphonamides and penicillin to treat Gram-positive infections. These fears were confirmed 3 years later when Florey *et al.* (1947) reported that 50 per cent of traumatic wounds treated in hospital became colonised with coliforms, the major predisposing factor being antibiotic treatment. The ability of *Pseudomonas* to cause cross-infection in critical care units soon became apparent, a situation further exacerbated by the introduction of broad-spectrum antibiotics (Colebrook *et al.*, 1948).

Staphylococci first became significant as nosocomial pathogens during the 1940s, replacing streptococci, which had previously been responsible for most cases of cross-infection. Penicillin-resistant strains were first reported during the 1950s. The new synthetic penicillins initially helped to control the problem, but strains resistant to methicillin were reported before the end of the decade (Shanson, 1985). Methicillin itself is of limited therapeutic value because its oral absorption is poor, but methicillin resistance is of enormous clinical significance because methicillin-resistant strains of bacteria are inevitably also resistant to cloxacillin, flucloxacillin and the cephalosporins. New synthetic antibiotics at first brought about a dramatic improvement in the treatment of infection. The disappearance of methicillin-resistant *Staphylococcus aureus* (MRSA) during the 1970s was greeted with complacency, which evaporated in the 1980s when persistent outbreaks of MRSA were reported world wide (Cafferkey *et al.*, 1985). The control of MRSA is now regarded as one of the major challenges facing infection control experts (Cox *et al.*, 1995).

Enterococci are an increasingly common cause of infection in hospitalised patients (Beaumont, 1998). Over the past decade, there has been a worrying escalation in the development of multiresistant strains of enterococci. Many enterococci, especially *Enterococcus faecium*, are now resistant to vancomycin – so-called vancomycin-resistant enterococci (VRE). Treatment options are extremely limited, and bacteraemia caused by VRE carries a high mortality rate. VRE are discussed further in Chapter 6.

A further hazard for vulnerable patients in intensive care settings is infection with *Acinetobacter*. This aerobic bacterium can develop resistance to many antibiotics and is responsible for a wide range of infections, for example pneumonia and wound infection. *Acinetobacter* is spread via the hands of staff, on which it is capable of surviving for some time. The organism also thrives in damp conditions such as humidification devices. It is vital, therefore, that equipment is stored dry.

Bacterial resistance may be described as:

- **High level** – when the drug is completely ineffective

Clinical Application

Preventing the Spread of *Clostridium difficile*

The spread of *Clostridium difficile* can be prevented by meticulous attention to hand hygiene and by ensuring that the environment does not become contaminated with spores spread from infected individuals (symptomatic or asymtomatic).

Preventive measures include:

- The isolation of patients with diarrhoea (which can be stopped after 2 days of normal stools) to stop cross-infection and environmental contamination
- Wearing plastic aprons and gloves for any contact with faeces and during environmental cleaning procedures
- Thorough handwashing by staff and visitors following any patient contact
- Handwashing by patients both before and after meals
- The proper disposal of used linen in red aliginate bags
- Frequent changes of bed linen – at least every 24 hours
- The proper disposal of waste in yellow bags for incineration
- High standards of general cleaning, with frequent monitoring
- Avoiding the transfer of patients between wards and to or from other hospitals
- Thorough environmental cleaning to remove spores once the patient is free from infection
- Liaison with the infection control nurse
- Informing and educating all concerned.

- **Partial** – when a high tissue concentration can still be effective. This may not, however, be feasible, for example if the drug is toxic if given in a high dose. Gentamicin is nephrotoxic in high doses and is therefore not suitable for patients with renal impairment.

Bacterial resistance to antibacterial drugs falls into two broad categories: intrinsic resistance and acquired resistance.

Intrinsic resistance

Intrinsic resistance is the innate property of the organism determined by the structure of the cell wall. Gram-positive bacteria are more susceptible to antibiotics than Gram-negative bacteria because their cell walls are less complex and lack the natural sieve effect against large antibiotic molecules that is shown by Gram-negative organisms. This explains why *Pseudomonas aeruginosa* has always been resistant to flucloxacillin.

Clinical Application

Antibiotic-resistant Bacteria in Hospital and the Community

Antibiotic resistance is recognised as a major problem in hospital because broad-spectrum antibiotics are commonly prescribed for the critically ill, contributing to the well-documented problems of superinfection and cross-infection. Antibiotic resistance is, however, not a problem restricted to hospitals. Patients who become colonised in hospital may continue to carry antibiotic-resistant strains of bacteria and cause problems when they are readmitted. Infection control procedures have now become necessary in nursing homes to help to contain spread (Cox *et al.*, 1995). Antibiotics are also prescribed very widely for patients with minor infections, both systemically and as topical creams, ointments and powders. Patients who use these unsupervised at home may not recognise the dangers presented to the environment if antibiotics are spilled and may unknowingly contribute to the emergence of resistance by failing to complete a course of medication, exposing the bacteria to subclinical doses.

Nurses employed in general practice have a role educating the public about the safe use of antibiotics, and antibiotic policies should be implemented in health centres as well as in hospitals (See the Clinical Application box on: Helping to reduce the inappropriate use of antibiotics and bacterial resistance, above).

Acquired resistance

Bacteria become resistant either by spontaneous chromosomal mutation and selection, or by the transfer of a plasmid carrying genes that code for antibiotic resistance.

Mutation is the chance genetic change in one cell resulting in the synthesis of an altered protein. Mutation is often lethal but occasionally results in a bacterium able to withstand the action of a particular antibiotic better than its parent cell. For example, the production of an altered protein in the ribosomes accounts for the ability of some bacteria to withstand streptomycin (Friedland and McCraken, 1994). When exposed to the antibiotic to which it has become resistant, the mutant will have obvious advantages over the rest of the bacterial population and will be free to multiply without competition for nutrients and space. The indiscriminate use of antibiotics promotes the multiplication of antibiotic-resistant mutants that then spread to other people by cross-infection.

Plasmid transfer occurs by conjugation, transformation or transduction (Chapter 1). Transformation does not appear to be clinically important in the dissemination of resistance. However, streptococci, staphylococci and clostridia readily undergo conjugation, and transduction plays an important role in the transmission of resistant genes between staphylococci and *Streptococcus pyogenes*.

Factors contributing to bacterial resistance include:

- The misuse of antibiotics in chemoprophylaxis. Antibiotics should be restricted to those cases in which the advantages outweigh the risks (see Table 4.1 above).

- Employing antibiotics used to treat systemic infection in topical preparations. This practice promotes plasmid-mediated resistance in the normal skin flora.

- Adding antibiotics to animal feeds. This practice is still common in some countries because it improves the yield of meat as well as protecting the livestock against infection.

Clinical Application

Principles of Antibiotic Therapy

To ensure adequate treatment for the individual patient and to reduce the exposure of organisms to antibiotics, promoting resistance:

1. The use of antibiotics should be restricted to occasions when they are genuinely necessary. They should not be used for trivial infections or viral infections.
2. Antibiotic chemoprophylaxis should be reserved for patients identified as being at risk of developing bacterial infection known to present a specific threat (see Table 4.1 above), and not used as part of a blanket policy. Chemoprophylaxis is no substitute for good infection control practice.
3. Treatment should be based on a sound bacteriological diagnosis, specimens being obtained for laboratory examination if possible before the first dose of antibiotic is administered.
4. Broad-spectrum antibiotics are not indicated for infections against which an antibacterial drug with a more specific range could be used.
5. Antibiotics should be administered for a full therapeutic period (usually a minimum of 3 days). If the patient's condition has not responded to treatment towards the end of this time, the following possibilities should be considered:
   - The bacteria are resistant to the antibiotic and further specimens must be sent to the laboratory
   - The drug is not reaching the organisms because they are sheltered in an abscess or a blood clot; further investigation is required
   - The patient has not been taking the drug, and the possibility of non-adherence and the reasons for it must be explored.
6. Antibiotics used in preparations for topical application should not be the same as those used to treat systemic infections. Antibiotics commonly used in topical preparations include mupirocin, polymyxin and bacitracin.
7. The spillage of antibiotic solutions and powders should be avoided because exposure may induce hypersensitivity reactions in some people.
8. Antibiotic policies should be adopted in hospital and general practice.

Antibiotic policies

Policies have been developed to encourage the efficient, safe and economical use of antibiotics, their purpose being to reduce the emergence of antibiotic-resistant strains. In most hospitals, a local formulary is drawn up to reserve the use of particular drugs. Most local policies adopt the following general format:

■ A section that includes a single member of each of the main groups of antibiotic. Each of these can be prescribed without a formal procedure and is held as ward stock.

■ A reserve section containing alternatives, including the most newly developed antibiotics. These are not usually prescribed without liaison with the infection control team and are not held as ward stock.

Policies need regular updating and reviewing to take account of new drugs and changing patterns of microbial behaviour.

Clinical Application

Antibiotic Policies

The purpose of an antibiotic policy is to limit prescription to just a few antibiotics so that bacteria lack the opportunity to develop resistance. The decision to prescribe any other antibiotic is usually taken between the doctor and medical microbiologist.

Main groups of antimicrobial drugs

Penicillins

Penicillins (Table 4.4) belong to the beta-lactam group of antibiotics, their molecular structure including the beta-lactam ring – the part exhibiting antibacterial properties (Figure 4.1). Penicillins are still effective against most of the common pathogens and, apart from their ability to induce hypersensitivity reactions in susceptible individuals, are generally less toxic than many of the other antibiotics currently in clinical use. Their value has, however, been seriously undermined by the ability of many bacteria to synthesise beta-lactamase (penicillinase) enzymes. These degrade the beta-lactam ring so that it becomes ineffective. Ninety per cent of staphylococci and approximately a third of *Escherichia coli* are now resistant to penicillin.

Table 4.4   The penicillins

Drug	Indications	Comments
Benzylpenicillin	Diphtheria, tetanus, syphilis, endocarditis, meningitis	Parenteral
Phenoxymethylpenicillin (Penicillin V)	Soft tissue infections	Oral
Ampicillin	Pneumonia, bronchitis, urinary infection	Broad spectrum Oral
Amoxycillin	Pneumonia, bronchitis, urinary infection	Broad spectrum Oral Parenteral Well absorbed
Beta-lactamase resistant		
Flucloxacillin	Staphylococcal infection (tissue, bone, joint)	Oral Parenteral
Mezlocillin	Systemic Gram-negative sepsis	Parenteral Broad spectrum
Piperacillin	Systemic Gram-negative sepsis and anaerobic infection	Parenteral Broad spectrum
Azlocillin	*Pseudomonas*	Parenteral Broad spectrum

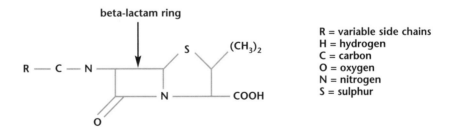

beta-lactam ring

R = variable side chains
H = hydrogen
C = carbon
O = oxygen
N = nitrogen
S = sulphur

Figure 4.1   The beta-lactam antibiotics

Clavulanic acid is a naturally occurring beta-lactamase compound. It has little antibacterial activity when used alone but is a powerful inhibitor of many of the beta-lactamase enzymes and can be combined with other antibiotics to destroy strains that would otherwise show resistance. Amoxycillin combined with clavulanate is prescribed as Augmentin; ticarcillin combined with clavulanate is prescribed as Timentin.

Cephalosporins

The cephalosporins (Table 4.5) are chemically related to the penicillins as they also contain the beta-lactam ring. Thus, they share many of the properties of the penicillins: they may cause hypersensitivity reactions, and resistance may develop if the bacteria can produce beta-lactamase enzymes. It has, however, been possible to produce different 'generations' of cephalosporins to achieve a wider antibacterial spectrum than is possible with the penicillins, and resistance is less marked. The newer cephalosporins are valuable in the treatment of septicaemia and other severe infections. Cefotaxime and ceftazidime can be used to treat meningitis because they cross the blood–brain barrier effectively. The chief drawbacks associated with the cephalosporins are their comparatively high cost compared with other antibiotics, and superinfection, which develops because no individual member of the group has a complete antibacterial spectrum.

Table 4.5   The cephalosporins

Drug		Indications	Comments
Oral	Cefalexin and cefradine	Moderately severe infections. Active against Gram-positive but less effective for Gram-negative infection	First generation. Wide spectrum, good oral absorption
	Cefaclor	Urinary and respiratory infections	Second generation. Wider spectrum, active orally
	Cefpodoxime proxetil	Respiratory infections	Third generation. More resistant to beta-lactamase
Parenteral	Cefazolin	Moderate to severe infection including respiratory, urinary and septicaemia. Surgical prophylaxis	First generation. Active against a broad range of infections
	Cefuroxime	As above plus meningitis and gonorrhoea	Second generation. Wide range of activity. Also given orally
	Cefotaxime*, ceftazidime and ceftizoxime	Greater effect against Gram-negative infections	Third generation. May cause superinfection
	Cefsulodin	Used for Pseudomonas infections only	Third generation. Narrow spectrum

*Cefotaxime is used for some types of meningitis, and as a single dose treatment for gonorrhoea.

Aminoglycosides

The aminoglycosides (Table 4.6) are a group of bactericidal antibiotics effective against a wide range of Gram-negative aerobic bacteria. They are also effective against many Gram-positive bacteria, although not to the same extent as many other antibiotics. Their range of action can be extended by combining treatment with other antibacterials (for example, cephalosporins). The aminoglycosides are associated with a number of potentially severe and highly undesirable side-effects, inducing renal and auditory impairment. Patients should have their blood level of the drug monitored to ensure that a toxic concentration is not reached, and diuretics should if possible be avoided.

Table 4.6   The aminoglycosides

Drug	Indications	Comments
Gentamicin	Serious Gram-negative infection	Parenteral Assays needed
Tobramycin and netilmicin	Gentamicin-resistant organisms	
Amikacin	Similar to gentamicin	See gentamicin
Neomycin	Usually topical use only	Toxic if absorbed
Streptomycin	Tuberculosis	Given as combined therapy to avoid resistance

Tetracyclines

The tetracyclines are broad-spectrum antibiotics whose use has declined in recent years as bacterial resistance has increasingly become a problem. They are, however, still used to treat genitourinary, respiratory and dermatological infections (Table 4.7). One of their chief advantages is that they are effective against chlamydial, rickettsial and *Mycoplasma* infections against which other antibiotics would have no action. Caution must be exercised when the tetracyclines are prescribed because they may be deposited in developing bones and teeth, and can have a teratogenic effect. Patients taking tetracyclines may complain of gastrointestinal upsets resulting from superinfection, and existing renal failure may be exacerbated.

Table 4.7   The tetracyclines

Drug	Indications	Comments
Tetracycline oxytetracycline and doxycycline	Respiratory and genital infections	Superinfection Renal failure exacerbated

> ## Clinical Application
>
> ### Safer Use of Tetracyclines
>
> Tetracyclines are deposited in developing bones and teeth. This can occur both before birth and during childhood, and can result in staining of the teeth and bone deformities. These potential problems can be avoided by ensuring that tetracyclines are not prescribed during pregnancy, during lactation or for children under the age of 12 years.

Antituberculosis drugs

Treatment with antituberculosis drugs is complicated by the lack of compliance and the emergence of multidrug resistant tuberculosis (MDR-TB – see Chapter 14). The effectiveness of medication depends on prescribing drugs that are still able to destroy the mycobacteria, and on ensuring patient adherence. Traditionally, three drugs are given in combination (Table 4.8). This strategy is adopted to achieve rapid destruction in the shortest time possible (8–10 weeks), thus limiting exposure to the drugs as resistance to a single antibiotic can develop within 6 weeks. This regimen is followed by a continuing phase of treatment involving the use of two effective antibiotics for at least 6 weeks. Antituberculosis drugs have a number of toxic side-effects that may be serious, including disturbed gastrointestinal and hepatic function. This and the length of treatment reduce adherence to the regimen. Intermittent drug administration under supervision for longer periods may be more effective than daily administration and may need to involve outreach community projects to encourage adherence (Taylor, 1996).

Other antibiotics

Chloramphenicol

Chloramphenicol is a broad-spectrum antibiotic that exerts its antibacterial effects in a similar way to the tetracyclines. It is potentially a very valuable drug as it is absorbed readily from the gastrointestinal tract and crosses the blood–brain barrier into the cerebrospinal fluid, but its usefulness is limited by its highly toxic, albeit rare, effects on the bone marrow, reducing the leucocyte count to a dangerously low level. Prescription is limited to those patients for whom a useful alternative is not available. Chloramphenicol is sometimes used to treat typhoid and para-typhoid fevers and *Haemophilus influenzae* meningitis because of its ability to cross the blood–brain barrier.

Table 4.8   Chemotherapy for tuberculosis

Pulmonary tuberculosis – initially, the following once daily:
  Rifampicin*
  Ethambutol* (if the organism is thought to be a resistant form)
  Isoniazid*
  Pyrazinamide*

* first-line drugs

Then:
  Rifampicin and isoniazid for 4 months

NB. Second-line drugs – cycloserine, capreomycin and streptomycin – are used when the organism is resistant to the first-line drugs or these drugs have caused side-effects

Genitourinary tuberculosis
  Isoniazid for 4 months
  Rifampicin for 4 months
  Pyrazinamide for 2 months

Tuberculous meningitis – initially, the following once daily for 8 weeks:
  Isoniazid
  Rifampicin
  Pyrazinamide

Then daily for 10 months:
  Isoniazid
  Rifampicin

Macrolides

The macrolides include erythromycin, the most commonly prescribed member of the group, and a number of newer drugs, including clarithromycin and azithromycin. Erythromycin is a bacteriostatic drug, first introduced in 1952, effective in the treatment of Gram-positive infections including *Legionella* and *Mycoplasma* infections. Erythromycin is useful for patients who are allergic to penicillin because its range of action is similar. Unfortunately, bacteria readily become resistant.

Other antimicrobial agents

Nitrofurans

Nitrofurantoin is the only member of this group still in routine use. It has a fairly wide antibacterial spectrum, becomes concentrated in the urine and is effective in the treatment of urinary tract infections. It has few side-effects, but nausea is sometimes reported. Nitrofurantoin is not suitable for patients with impaired renal function because accumulation to toxic levels will occur. It may also cause gastrointestinal upsets.

Nalidixic acid

Nalidixic acid is a bactericide effective against most Gram-negative urinary pathogens apart from *Pseudomonas*. It concentrates in the urine and is valuable in the treatment of urinary tract infection because its action is not affected by pH. Resistance develops rapidly. Occasional toxic reactions include urticarial rashes and gastrointestinal disturbances.

Quinolones

The quinolones operate by interfering with an enzyme essential for the division of bacterial cells (see modes of action, above). They are a new, rapidly expanding group of antibacterial agents. Ciprofloxacin is effective against a wide range of bacteria, although it is generally less successful for Gram-positive infections. It can be used to treat infections resistant to the older antibacterial drugs and as chemoprophylaxis for people who have been in contact with meningococcal meningitis. Adverse reactions include gastrointestinal upsets and rashes.

Co-trimoxazole: trimethoprim and sulphamethoxazole

Like the sulphonamides, trimethoprim interferes with bacterial metabolism by disrupting the production of folic acid. The combination of a sulphonamide and trimethoprim is very effective because it prevents bacterial division and is also bactericidal. Co-trimoxazole is effective against the same range of organisms as the sulphonamides: *Haemophilus influenzae* and *Salmonella*. It has been used widely and successfully to treat chronic bronchitis, urinary infections, *Pneumocystis* infections in the immunocompromised and occasionally salmonellosis, but its usefulness is restricted by the number of side-effects that can occur: nausea, vomiting and – more rarely but also more seriously – blood disorders and Stevens–Johnson syndrome, characterised by a bullous rash, fever and ulceration of the mouth. This latter condition can be fatal.

Trimethoprim can be used on its own and has superseded co-trimoxazole in the treatment of urinary tract infections because it causes fewer side-effects.

Clindamycin

Clindamycin is used to treat staphylococcal infections involving the bones and joints, and in cases of severe intra-abdominal sepsis. Its value is reduced by its tendency to cause superinfection, leading to *Clostridium difficile* infection (see Superinfection above).

Colistin

Colistin is active against Gram-negative bacteria, including *Pseudomonas*. It is not absorbed orally but is used to destroy the skin and gastrointestinal flora of severely immunocompromised patients. If administered by injection, it causes severe toxic effects involving the neurological system, vertigo and muscle weakness.

Polymyxin

Polymyxin is similar to colistin. It is occasionally used in cases of systemic and urinary infection.

Fucidin

Fucidin is a narrow-spectrum antibiotic able to penetrate all tissues, especially bone. It is used mainly to treat penicillin-resistant staphylococcal infection, for example in cases of osteomyelitis. Bacterial resistance may develop rapidly, a problem overcome by the simultaneous administration of another antibiotic. Side-effects involve the gastrointestinal system and the liver.

Vancomycin

Vancomycin is effective against most Gram-positive bacteria and is of particular value in the treatment of resistant strains such as MRSA. It may be given orally to treat pseudomembranous colitis, and by slow intravenous infusion: if it is given too quickly, the patient may develop a sensitivity reaction characterised by hypotension and the appearance of a rash over the face and trunk. The side-effects of vancomycin – ototoxicity and nephrotoxicity – are severe. Plasma assays are essential during treatment.

Teicoplanin

Teicoplanin is similar to vancomycin but is associated with fewer side-effects. It has been used to control MRSA.

Metronidazole

Metronidazole was originally introduced as an antiparasitic drug but is also highly effective in the treatment of anaerobic infections arising after gynaecological and gut surgery, and in the treatment of pseudomembranous colitis. Side-effects are uncommon, but patients taking metronidazole at home are advised to avoid alcohol because of possible interactions. Metronidazole is also used in combination with other drugs to eradicate *Helicobacter pylori*, the organism implicated in the aetiology of gastritis and peptic ulceration.

Antiviral drugs

Problems associated with treating viruses

Treating viral infections is difficult because:

- Viruses are minute, intracellular particles so it is difficult for chemotherapeutic agents to reach and attack them
- Infection is usually well established before the patient develops symptoms
- Many of the agents currently used have severe toxic side-effects.

Acyclovir

Acyclovir is used to treat local and systemic herpes simplex and varicella zoster infections. It can be given topically, orally or by slow intravenous infusion. Renal function must be carefully monitored.

Idoxuridine

Idoxuridine is used to treat herpes infection and, until the availability of acyclovir, was the only effective drug for this condition. It is applied topically. Other forms of administration have been associated with severe haematological toxicity.

Vidarabine

Vidarabine is similar to idoxuridine, but its side-effects tend to be less severe so that it can be used parenterally to treat infections in immunocompromised patients.

Amantidine

Amantidine is used in prophylaxis against the influenza type A virus. It is given orally and has been associated with relatively few side-effects.

Ganciclovir

Ganciclovir is effective for serious infections caused by cytomegalovirus (CMV) in immunocompromised patients. Leucocyte and platelet counts are depressed, but recovery usually occurs spontaneously when the drug is stopped.

Zidovudine

Zidovudine (Azidothymidine, AZT) inhibits the replication of human immuno-deficiency virus (HIV) in laboratory tests. It cannot, however, arrest the onset of AIDS, although it slows the development of symptoms arising through opportunistic infection, and increases life expectancy (see Chapter 13). Suppression of the bone marrow is a severe side-effect.

Didanosine

Didanosine became available in 1994. It is licensed for patients with HIV disease whose condition has begun to deteriorate. The most severe side-effect is pancreatitis.

Ritonavir

Ritonavir is an example of a protease inhibitor, a newer type of drug used in the management of HIV disease. Protease inhibitors cause the production of faulty virus particles that are unable to infect host cells.

Interferons

The interferons are a group of naturally occurring protein substances that help the body to defend itself against virus infections (Chapter 2). Interferons can be produced synthetically and have been used to treat neoplastic disease, particularly leukaemia, as well as infectious disease. Here, their success has been limited.

Antifungal drugs

Most serious fungal infections warranting treatment occur in patients who are immunocompromised, especially if they have received powerful broad-spectrum antibiotics resulting in superinfection. The main antifungal drugs currently available are indicated in Table 4.9.

Table 4.9   Antifungal drugs

Drug	Indications	Comments
Nystatin	Oral and vaginal candidiasis	Topical application Too toxic for parenteral use
Amphotericin	Systemic and topical fungal infection	Oral, topical and parenteral Severe toxic effects: fever, hypokalaemia and nephrotoxicity
Clotrimazole	Topical fungal infection	
Miconazole	Topical fungal infection	Poor response if used for systemic infection Topical, oral and parenteral
Ketoconazole	Systemic fungal infection	Not as effective as amphotericin. Hepatic toxicity
Griseofulvin	Dermatophyte fungal infection	Oral Concentrates in keratin so is the drug of choice for intractable fungal infection of the skin
Flucytosine	Systemic yeast infection	Oral and parenteral Not effective against *Aspergillus* or dermatophytes

---

REVISION CHECKLIST: KEY AREAS

- ❏ Introduction to antibiotics: The purpose of antibiotic therapy, Historical development of antibiotic therapy, Range of antibiotic action, Mode of antibiotic action, Adverse reactions to antibacterial drugs, Bacterial resistance to antibiotics, Antibiotic policies

- ❏ Main groups of antimicrobial drugs: Penicillins, Cephalosporins, Aminoglycosides, Tetracyclines, Antituberculosis drugs, Other antibiotics, Other antimicrobial agents

- ❏ Antiviral drugs

- ❏ Antifungal drugs

Activities – linking knowledge to clinical practice

1   **Obtain** the antibiotic policy currently used in your clinical area and identify those drugs which are in unrestricted and restricted use:

(a) Is there any rationale for the categorisation of the drugs included?
(b) How often is the document updated?
(c) Who is responsible for updating it?
(d) Is any system of audit in progress?

2   **Debate** the relative advantages and disadvantages associated with chemo-prophylaxis.

3   **Plan** a teaching session for a patient being discharged from hospital with a 7-day course of antibiotics.

4   **Identify** a critical incident concerning the inappropriate use of antibiotics. Reflect upon the factors involved and plan ways in which this type of incident could be avoided in the future.

SELF-ASSESSMENT

1. A bactericidal agent kills bacteria.
   True? ☐   False? ☐

2. In ideal circumstances, chemoprophylaxis is restricted to ....

3. Streptococci are usually resistant to penicillin.
   True? ☐   False? ☐

4. Which of the following bacteria exhibit a high level of natural resistance to many antibiotics?
   (a) staphylococci ☐
   (b) *Pseudomonas* ☐
   (c) *Streptococcus pyogenes* ☐
   (d) *Klebsiella aerogenes* ☐

5. Which of the following drugs contain a beta-lactam ring within their molecular structure?
   (a) macrolides ☐
   (b) cephalosporins ☐
   (c) penicillins ☐
   (d) beta-blockers ☐

6. Which of the following drugs are effective against *Chlamydia*?
   (a) macrolides ☐
   (b) cephalosporins ☐
   (c) tetracyclines ☐
   (d) beta-blockers ☐

7. Superinfection arises when ....

8. Explain why virus infections are difficult to treat.

References

Beaumont G (1998) 'Resistance movement'. *Nursing Times* **94**(37): 69–75.

Cafferkey MT, Coleman D, McGrath B *et al.* (1985) '*Staphylococcus aureus* in Dublin'. *Lancet* **2**: 705–8.

Colebrook L, Duncan JM and Ross WPD (1948) 'The control of infection in burns'. *Lancet* 1093–9.

Cox RA, Mallaghan E, Conquest E *et al.* (1995) 'Epidemic methicillin resistant *Staphylococcus aureus*: controlling the spread outside hospital'. *Journal of Hospital Infection* **29**: 107–19.

Davey PG, Bax RP and Reeves D (1996) 'The growth of the use of antibiotics in the community in England and Scotland in 1980–1993'. *British Medical Journal* **312**: 613–4.

Davies J (1994) 'Antibiotic resistance and the dissemination of resistance genes'. *Science* **264**(5157): 375–82.

Degl'Innocenti R, De Santis M, Berdondini I *et al.* (1989) 'Outbreak of *Clostridium difficile* diarrhoea in an orthopaedic unit: evidence by phage typing for cross infection'. *Journal of Hospital Infection* **13**: 309–14.

Department of Health (1998) *The Path of Least Resistance. Report on the Impact of Clinical Prescribing on Antibiotic Resistance* (98/361). Standing Medical Advisory Committee, DoH, London. http://www.open.gov.uk/doh/dhhome.htm

Florey ME, Ross RWNL and Turton EC (1947) 'Infection of wounds with Gram-negative organisms: clinical manifestation and treatment'. *Lancet* **2**: 855–61.

Friedland IR and McCracken GH (1994) 'Management of infections caused by antibiotic- resistant *Streptococcus pneumoniae*'. *New England Journal of Medicine* **331**: 377–82.

Gammon J (1995) 'Difficult bug to beat'. *Nursing Times* Infection Control Supplement **91**(37): 57–60.

Kelly J and Chivers G (1996) 'Built in resistance'. *Nursing Times* **92**(2): 50–4.

McKeown T (1979) *The Role of Medicine.* Blackwell Science, Oxford.

Miles AA (1944) 'Epidemiology of wound infection'. *Lancet* 809–14.

Shanson DC (1985) 'Control of a hospital outbreak of methicillin-resistant *Staphylococcus aureus*: the value of an isolation ward. *Journal of Hospital Infection* **6**: 285–92.

Taylor D (1996) 'Promoting compliance with tuberculosis drug therapy'. *Nursing Standard* **10**(20): 33–5.

Wilcox M (1996) 'Cleaning up *Clostridium difficile* infection'. *Lancet* **348**: 767–8.

Further reading and information sources

Molyneux R and Chadwick C (1997) 'Vancomycin-resistant enterococci: implications for infection control'. *Professional Nurse* **12**(9): 641–4.

Visit the Department of Health website at http://www.open.gov.uk/doh/dhhome.htm for up-to-date guidelines on treating infections.

5 Infection control policies

CHAPTER OUTCOMES

After reading this chapter you should be able to:

- Define the terms 'cleaning', 'disinfection' and 'sterilisation', giving examples of when each procedure would be appropriate and the most suitable method for the task

- Discuss the role of the hands in cross-infection and the steps that may be taken to reduce the transmission of micro-organisms via this route

- Outline strategies used to collect, contain and dispose of waste materials in hospital and community premises

- State the measures taken to decontaminate laundry

- Debate the role of protective clothing in the prevention of infection (note that gloves are discussed in Chapter 12)

- List the special precautions taken to control infection in theatres and other high-risk units

- Discuss effective policies for patient isolation

- Identify specific circumstances in which cross-infection may occur and suggest appropriate methods of control

Introduction to strategies that prevent infection

The strategies that prevent infection fall into three categories:

■ **Individual patient care** – identifying factors increasing susceptibility to infection or constituting an infection risk and delivering the appropriate care tailored to meet individual need

■ **Policies and procedures** – to reduce the risk of infection to all the patients and staff in the hospital, health centre or clinics where they are implemented (for example, antibiotic policies and cleaning policies)

■ **Community/public health measures** – policies to promote the health of the entire community: the notification of infectious diseases to the Public Health Laboratory Services, immunisation programmes and the inspection of premises where food is produced or sold.

Risk factors associated with hospital admission

Risk factors (see Chapter 2) when patients are admitted to hospital include:

■ Shared facilities
■ Contact with different members of staff carrying bacteria, especially antibiotic-resistant strains
■ Mass-produced food
■ Physical and psychological stress, reducing resistance to infection, very sick and long-stay patients being at particular risk.

Very sick patients are handled more often, and by a larger number of people, undergo more invasive procedures (mechanical ventilation and catheterisation, for example) and are more likely to receive antibiotics.

Long-stay patients have a greater exposure to the hospital flora. They are more likely to succumb to infection and to operate as reservoirs of antibiotic-resistant hospital strains, presenting an infection risk to others.

Preventing the spread of infection – hospital and community

Knowing how to prevent the spread of infection is relevant to all nurses irrespective of the clinical setting in which they work. Although most of the existing literature pertains to the hospital environment, the potential for cross-infection also exists in clinics and in the home, especially with the present move toward community care (Johnson and Harker, 1996). Here, there is much room for improvement.

There is disturbing evidence that in GP surgeries, relevant equipment and staff training are not currently available (Foy *et al.*, 1990).The early discharge of acutely ill patients may increase the number of infections caused by hospital strains of micro-organisms in the community. Infection control policies will have to be adapted or new ones developed to meet this challenge. Many community-acquired infections are already caused by antibiotic-resistant bacteria.

In hospital and general practice, infection control policies should address the following:

- Fundamental hygiene, including hand decontamination
- Policies for the use of cleaning agents, disinfection and sterilisation, including guidance on the use of equipment such as autoclaves
- The disposal of clinical waste
- The disposal of soiled laundry
- The use of protective clothing
- Universal precautions, and the proper handling and disposal of sharps
- Procedures to be followed in the case of accidents, especially needlestick injury and exposure to blood and body fluids
- The isolation of potentially infectious patients.

Policies and procedures to prevent infection

Standard and high-risk situations

The hospital environment consists of everything on the premises: all fixtures, fittings, equipment, patients and staff. It is possible to differentiate between two settings – those where the risk of infection is exceptionally high and extraordinary precautions are necessary (theatres and critical care units), and all others, where hazards certainly exist but are not of the same magnitude. However, the same principles of infection prevention are vital everywhere (Table 5.1). Table 5.2 indicates situations where the risk of contamination and subsequent infection is high.

Risk management

Risk management (Figure 5.1) may be effectively incorporated into programmes designed to control infection. Risk management is a systematic process of identifying and analysing the accepted risks that may occur in a given situation, deciding the action required and evaluating the potential and actual risks (DoH, 1993a), thus providing a mechanism for reducing risk of infection and avoiding economic loss. It is necessary because of the increasing need to provide safe and effective health services within the developing relationships between Primary Care Groups/Trusts and their secondary care providers, the increasing number of claims made against healthcare providers and the cost of court settlements. Its objectives are to minimise the number of risks occurring, to enhance quality of care and to reduce costs to the organisation.

Table 5.1 Controlling infection in the hospital environment

General principles include:

- Providing an environment hostile to the growth and multiplication of micro-organisms: clean, dry, well ventilated and with good lighting, as the ultraviolet rays in sunlight destroy bacteria

- Protecting susceptible patients/sites from contamination, for example by dressing wounds and employing isolation precautions to protect immunosuppressed patients

- Containing sources of infection: avoiding spillage and using colour-coded systems for waste disposal, for example

- Decontamination

Table 5.2 Situations in which risk of contamination is high

- Situations in which there is potential for contact with organic waste (for example blood, body fluids, waste food, raw food and cleaning fluid)

- Handling materials that have been in contact with an infected site (for example soiled dressings, sharps, linen, body fluids and laboratory specimens)

- The immediate environment of patients who are infectious

- The immediate environment of highly susceptible patients (for example critical care units, neonatal units, burns units and theatres)

Decontamination

Decontamination is achieved at three levels:

- Cleaning
- Disinfection
- Sterilisation.

Each level becomes progressively more effective but also more expensive, more difficult to perform and more likely to damage the item concerned. Considerable time and money can be spent performing unnecessary rituals (Axnick and Yarborough, 1984), which is not acceptable in the present cost-conscious climate of health care. Thus, the method of decontamination chosen should be not more complex or expensive than necessary. In addition to expense, other important

IDENTIFYING THE RISK

depends on a knowledge of:

■ The nature of the service provided in a particular setting

■ The equipment and supplies required

■ The legislation and regulations affecting provision

■ The potential liability that may be incurred (based on previous reports or audit)

ANALYSING ACTUAL AND POTENTIAL RISKS

■ Likelihood of risk

■ Severity (from previous claims)

■ Previous trends of occurrence

■ The cost of eliminating or reducing risk

■ Deciding whether any immediate action is required

IDENTIFYING POSSIBLE RISK SOLUTIONS

■ Dispense with the procedure

■ Implement new protocols/new equipment (staff training being necessary)

■ No immediate action necessary

MONITORING/EVALUATING

■ The number and nature of accidents

■ The number and nature of injuries

■ The number of claims

Figure 5.1 The risk management process

factors to consider include the nature of the item to be decontaminated and the circumstances in which decontamination will be performed. Key questions to ask are, 'How soon will recontamination occur?', 'Will the equipment withstand the procedure chosen?' and 'Will contact with the cleaning or disinfecting agent be possible for long enough to achieve the desired outcome?'

How soon will recontamination occur?

Some items become recontaminated so rapidly that disinfection is pointless, cleaning thus being sufficient. Floors, drains, sluice hoppers and toilets become recontaminated so swiftly that it is wise to regard them as permanent, albeit unlikely, sources of potential pathogens (Ayliffe *et al.*, 1967). Infection rates are not reduced by routinely disinfecting in hospital (Danforth *et al.*, 1987). Sinks in hospital become heavily contaminated and are recontaminated quickly after disinfection. Despite this, the inanimate environment contributes little to infection risk (McGowan, 1981).

Will the equipment withstand the procedure chosen?

Metal surfaces are corroded by hypochlorite disinfectants and delicate equipment will not withstand autoclaving. Even when sterility is essential, some other method must be chosen.

Will contact with the cleaning or disinfecting agent be possible for long enough?

Disinfectants require time to take effect, the length of time varying between different agents.

Cleaning

Cleaning maintains the appearance, structure and efficient functioning of the clinical environment and its contents. It contributes to infection control by reducing the number of micro-organisms present and preventing their transfer (Table 5.3). The safe removal of cloths, mop heads and cleaning fluids is essential as they may become heavily contaminated, inefficient practices leading to the redistribution of micro-organisms (Table 5.4). These may also be spread if the cleaning materials are used again without decontamination. In the clinical environment, cleaning is a skilled activity undertaken by domestic staff who should receive special training. Good practice includes:

- The use of disposable cloths
- Autoclaving equipment when possible
- Storing equipment (for example, mops and buckets) clean and dry between uses
- Damp-dusting to avoid the dispersal of micro-organisms into the air
- Avoiding splashes to reduce risks of contamination and accidents (for example, falls on slippery floors)

■ Drying surfaces after damp-cleaning as moisture supports the growth of bacteria
■ Regularly changing the cleaning solution.

In hospital, nurses or technicians are responsible for looking after equipment that is too delicate or expensive for domestic staff to handle and for items directly involved in patient care that need regular cleaning to avoid heavy contamination. In many community settings (health centres and family planning clinics, for example), nurses take responsibility for the routine cleaning and decontamination of all clinical equipment.

Table 5.3   Outline policy for good cleaning practice

1. Use a new cleaning solution for each task, checking that it is of the required dilution

2. Apply it evenly to all surfaces, ensuring that all equipment (for example, mops and wipes) is clean and dry before use. Avoid applying excess solution as it can seep into joins and cracks, thus damaging equipment, and it makes drying more difficult

3. Change the solution at regular intervals during cleaning to prevent the accumulation of bacteria, leading to recontamination

4. Allow sufficient time for the solution to penetrate surface soiling

5. Dispose without splashing to prevent environmental contamination. Use a sluice hopper rather than washbasins adjacent to clinical areas

6. Dry the surface thoroughly as bacteria thrive in moisture and slippery surfaces are dangerous

7. Wash the hands

Table 5.4   Items in the clinical environment that may become heavily contaminated

Baths	Boycott (1956)
Bedclothes	Overton (1988)
Bedpans	Block *et al.* (1990)
Catheter drainage bags	Glenister (1987)
Flannels	Sanderson and Rawal (1987)
Hoists	Murdoch (1990)
Mattresses	O'Donoghue and Allen (1992)
Urinals	Curie *et al.* (1978)
Washbowls	Greaves (1985)

Clinical Application

Long-stay Care Environment

Units and wards providing long-term care for older adults or disabled people pose a special challenge in terms of infection control. The aim of nursing care is to promote the independence and dignity of all individuals, enabling them to lead lives as normal as possible in a homely environment, but this may conflict with the implementation of essential infection control policies and procedures. For example, it is desirable for every patient to have his or her own clothing, but few garments withstand the laundering processes employed to decontaminate hospital bedclothes. Personalised laundry systems can be implemented on individual wards and units, but they must be able to cope with the volume of laundry and decontaminate it adequately (incontinence may be a problem), and facilities for drying must exist. Cross-infection is likely where articles for personal hygiene (soap, flannels and skin creams) are shared. Providing sufficient articles for personal hygiene on a regular basis for a ward full of long-stay residents, many without families, may severely tax the budget.

The precleaning of instruments is essential before disinfection or sterilisation as the first step in decontamination. All items should be washed in warm water and detergent using a brush, and then thoroughly rinsed. Care is necessary as brushing can produce contamination through aerosols or splashing. Brushes must be sterilised every day and stored dry. Staff should wear protective clothing such as plastic aprons and gloves appropriate to the cleaning tasks.

Clinical equipment should be stored clean and dry wherever possible. Soaking in disinfectant solutions is poor practice as the fluid is rapidly inactivated by organic matter and becomes heavily contaminated, setting up a reservoir of infection (Burdon and Whitby, 1967).

Disinfection

Disinfection is the destruction of vegetative micro-organisms but not their spores. Infection is likely to supervene when a large number of micro-organisms is present. The aim of disinfection is to reduce this number to a level below the infective dose. It is difficult and expensive to destroy all the micro-organisms present, so a compromise is usually reached by attempting to destroy most of them, bearing in mind the limitations of the chosen method. There are two methods: heat and chemical disinfection.

Heat disinfection (pasteurisation)

Heat disinfection is the method of choice. It is rapid, cheaper than chemical disinfection and more easily controlled. Micro-organisms vary considerably in their

Clinical Application

Disinfection

'Safe' levels of micro-organisms are likely to vary according to circumstance. This will depend on:

■ **The patient** – Someone who is very sick will be more susceptible. A level of bacteria that would not be harmful to a healthy individual might, for example, cause fatal infection in a leukaemic child.

■ **The virulence** – Some species of micro-organism are more readily destroyed than others. The spores of Gram-positive bacteria (such as *Bacillus* and *Clostridium*) are particularly resistant.

ability to withstand high temperatures, but nearly all species of clinical significance are destroyed by exposure to moist heat between 50 and 70 ^{0}C for 20–30 minutes. The current recommendation is 65 ^{0}C for 10 minutes, 71 ^{0}C for 3 minutes or 80 °C for 1 minute (DoH, 1993b); spores are more resistant to heat and some will not be destroyed. The disinfection temperature and time commonly used ranges from 60 ^{0}C for 10 minutes to 80 ^{0}C or above for one minute. Extra time is needed for cold instruments to reach the disinfection temperature and to become cool enough for handling afterwards.

In hospital, nurses are unlikely to be responsible for heat disinfection, but in community settings they may be required to operate hot-water disinfectors. The correct procedure involves:

■ Precleaning all items
■ Placing them on the tray within the disinfector, completely covering them with water and ensuring that no air bubbles are trapped
■ Checking that the hot-water disinfector is not overloaded
■ Ensuring that the water returns to the boil for at least 5 minutes after the items have been added, using a timer for accuracy
■ Raising the tray holding the items with clean forceps
■ Placing the items on a clean surface and leaving them covered while they cool
■ Storing clean items in a dry, clean container
■ Changing the water in the boiler daily.

Cleaning and disinfection are often combined in dishwashers, washing machines and bedpan washers. Most of the contaminants are removed by the mechanical action of cleaning, those remaining being destroyed by heat.

Chemical disinfectants

The ideal disinfectant is effective, does not damage equipment or harm people and is inexpensive. No chemical incorporating all these properties exists, and the entire

Clinical Application

Maintaining Equipment

Maintaining equipment in good working order is of paramount importance in the successful control of infection. Bedpan washers and macerators pose special problems. Surveys have shown that a high proportion do not function adequately (Block *et al.*, 1990), typical problems including poor water pressure, blockage by solid material, attachment to pipes of the wrong size and lack of drainage. Breakdown is common and has been implicated as one of the factors contributing to outbreaks of nosocomial infection (Curie *et al.*, 1978). This problem is most acute when patients are immunocompromised (Chadwick and Oppenheim, 1994). Macerators may create aerosols when the lid is slammed and may leak if overfilled. Environmental contamination results (Bentham, 1979). Routine maintenance checks are necessary for all equipment.

process of chemical disinfection is at best an uncertain process. Many chemical disinfectants are toxic, corrosive, unstable in solution and readily deactivated by organic matter, plastics, rubber detergents and hard water. When there is no alternative to chemical disinfection, compromise is required, taking into consideration the factors in Table 5.5. Soaking equipment in disinfectant is poor practice as solutions may support the growth of Gram-negative bacteria, leading to heavy contamination (Burdon and Whitby, 1967).

Table 5.5   Factors that determine the effectiveness of chemical disinfectants

- **Satisfactory contact** – Disinfection is not possible unless the solution has direct and complete contact with all surfaces. Precleaning and complete immersion, expelling trapped air bubbles, are important precautions

- **Avoiding neutralisation** – Hard water, plastic, rubber, organic waste and many detergents reduce the effectiveness of many chemical disinfectants

- **Concentration** – A solution reconstituted below the recommended strength will not be fully effective while higher concentrations are not necessarily more efficacious but are a waste of resources. For example, 100 per cent alcohol evaporates too rapidly to disinfect

- **Stability** – Dilutions may deteriorate with age. The expiry date on the container must be checked before use

- **Speed of action** – Some chemical disinfectants destroy micro-organisms more readily than others. Hypochlorites and alcohol act rapidly; glutaraldehyde disinfects slowly

- **Range of action** – Chemical disinfectants do not all destroy the same range of micro-organisms. Consideration must be given to the pathogens likely to be present

- **Cost** – Using a chemical disinfectant inappropriately is expensive and inefficient: chlorhexidine is too expensive and has too narrow a spectrum for satisfactory use as an environmental disinfectant

Clear soluble phenolics

Clear soluble phenolics (Clearasol, Stericol and Hycolin) are suitable as environmental disinfectants at concentrations of 1–2 per cent. They are toxic and corrosive but stable in solution, are not easily neutralised, are cheap and destroy a wide range of micro-organisms, although not spores or viruses.

Hypochlorites

Hypochlorites (Domestos, Milton, bleach, Presept and Vinusorb) are marketed at different solutions, expressed as parts per million (ppm) of available chlorine (Table 5.6). Hypochlorites destroy a wide range of micro-organisms and are effective against the hepatitis B and human immunodeficiency (HIV) viruses. Their activity is reduced in the presence of organic matter. They are corrosive at concentrations necessary for environmental disinfection.

Table 5.6   Hypochlorites and their uses at different dilutions

	Dilution (%)	Available chlorine (ppm)
Blood/body fluids	1.0	10 000
General environmental use	0.1	1000
Infant feeding equipment	0.0125	125

Milton (125–140 ppm) can be safely used in food preparation and to clean infant feeding bottles, but articles should not be left soaking because the solution is readily neutralised by organic matter. The contamination of feeds may occur in hospital milk kitchens (Ayliffe, 1970); this may be avoided by heat sterilisation or purchasing commercially prepared feeds.

Glutaraldehyde

Glutaraldehyde (Cidex) is used as a 2 per cent solution to decontaminate expensive, precision items, principally fibreoptic equipment that would be damaged by heat or more corrosive chemicals (Wicks, 1994). Disinfection is achieved after a contact time of 20 minutes. Prolonged contact of 3 hours or more will destroy spores, acid-fast bacilli (AFBs) and viruses, achieving sterilisation. Glutaraldehyde is toxic and corrosive, and causes dermatitis if it is allowed to contact skin. Its use is, however, justified as numerous outbreaks of infection have resulted through failure adequately to decontaminate endoscopes and other fibreoptic equipment (Martin and Reicheldfer, 1994). Glutaraldehyde must be used in conjunction with Department of Health Guidelines for the Control of Substances Hazardous to Health (COSHH, 1988). This involves:

- Wearing goggles, plastic aprons and nitrile rubber gloves: ordinary rubber and latex are permeable to glutaraldehyde
- Working in well-ventilated conditions to avoid the accumulation of toxic fumes. An extraction system or fume cupboard is recommended
- Keeping the container covered.

The Health and Safety Commission recommends that, whenever possible, a substitute disinfectant should be used in place of glutaraldehyde. Where this is not possible, glutaraldehyde should be used in enclosed equipment or with local exhaust ventilation (HSC, 1998).

Disinfection/sterilisation with glutaraldehyde involves:

- Complete immersion so that contact with every surface is achieved
- Covering the container to prevent the escape of fumes
- Using a timing device, 3 hours being required for sterilisation
- Removing the items using the aseptic technique and rinsing them thoroughly with sterile water
- Replacing the solution regularly after preparation. The length of time it can be used depends on the commercial preparation; if it is in continuous use, changes must be more frequent.

Alcohol

Alcohol (isopropanol or ethanol) in 70 per cent solution is suitable to rapidly disinfect physically clean surfaces and clinical equipment (dressing trolleys and thermometers, for example). It evaporates quickly, leaving the surfaces dry, and penetrates organic matter poorly. Alcohol destroys most viruses but not spores. A contact time of at least 2 minutes is necessary to destroy HIV (Hanson *et al.*, 1989). Alcohol is convenient because it can be incorporated into sprays, impregnated into swabs or combined with emollients into handrubs.

Chlorhexidine

Chlorhexidine (for example Hibitane) is formulated to disinfect human tissue. It is a non-toxic, non-corrosive but relatively expensive fluid, more effective against Gram-positive than Gram-negative bacteria. It continues to destroy organisms for some time after application (Russell and Day, 1993). Chlorhexidine has slight activity against AFBs but does not destroy spores. It is readily inactivated by organic matter and chemicals. Its expense and narrow range of bactericidal activity make it unsuitable for environmental use. It is incorporated into alcoholic handrub and is sometimes used preoperatively as a skin antiseptic.

Iodophors

Iodophors (povidine iodine) are marketed as Betadine and Disadine. They have a broader spectrum than chlorhexidine and destroy spores.

Hexachlorophane

Hexachlorophane (Ster-Zac) is used as a skin antiseptic, especially on neonatal units. It destroys bacteria and some viruses but not spores. Once extremely popular, it is now used with caution following reports of central nervous system damage to infants.

Quaternary ammonium compounds

Quaternary ammonium compounds destroy most Gram-positive and negative bacteria, but not AFBs or spores. These compounds are rapidly inactivated by organic matter and many other chemicals. The most widely used member of the group is cetrimide, which has natural detergent properties. It is sometimes used as a wound disinfectant. Cetrimide and chlorhexidine are marketed in combination as Savlon, a wound and skin disinfectant.

Disinfectant policies

A typical hospital disinfectant policy will include:

- A detergent for general domestic purposes
- A phenolic for 'heavy' environmental use
- A hypochlorite for situations where contamination with blood or body fluids is possible
- Isopropanol 70 per cent for cleaning physically clean clinical equipment
- Glutaraldehyde for endoscopes and other precision equipment.

The number of agents used is generally limited both for simplicity and because large quantities can be purchased more cheaply on contract. Staff training is important to the success of the policy, and auditing is recommended (Coates and Hutchinson, 1994).

Hand hygiene

The hands are the main vectors of infection in hospital wards (Reybrouck, 1983), strains colonising patients' skin and nurses' hands invariably being the same. Rates of infection and colonisation have fallen following the introduction of stringent hand decontamination protocols (Casewell and Phillips, 1978). The aim of ward hand hygiene is to remove transient micro-organisms before their transfer to susceptible patients. Cross-infection is possible as the nurse moves from one patient to another or handles different sites on the same patient (for example, giving an injection after bed-bathing). Hands should be decontaminated frequently both between patients and between sites. Gloves (see Chapter 12) give added protection in situations where heavy contamination occurs (such as bathing incontinent patients or changing stoma bags) and washing is unlikely to remove the bacteria effectively (Kjolen and Andersen, 1992). Decontamination is still necessary because gloves may puncture or leak (Kotilainen *et al.*, 1990). Even if they remain intact, hands can become contaminated during removal of the gloves (Linden, 1991).

Hand decontamination

Hand decontamination is recommended:

- Between different patients unless contact has been superficial
- Before aseptic procedures
- After handling patients
- After handling any items that are or could be soiled
- Before handling food
- As soon as the hands become visibly soiled.

Soap, antiseptics and alcoholic handrubs containing 60–70 per cent ethanol or isopropanol are available. It is difficult to demonstrate that one particular product destroys more organisms than another. Laboratory studies to test bactericidal effectiveness are performed under tightly controlled conditions that allow comparisons but do not necessarily reflect the clinical situation. When soap is used, the mechanical action of washing and drying removes micro-organisms. Antiseptics destroy organisms providing that the contact time is sufficient, which it is often not (Sprunt et al., 1973).

The choice of hand decontamination depends on the type of activity undertaken and the susceptibility of the patient:

- **Soap** is adequate for most routine tasks (for example, helping patients with hygiene, and bed-making).

- **Antiseptics** are recommended before invasive procedures (such as catheterisation and tracheobronchial suction).

- **Handrubs** are recommended by manufacturers for application to physically clean hands but are not otherwise suitable because they have no detergent properties and will not remove grime. They are often routinely used in critical care units when invasive procedures are frequently performed because they give added protection to conventionally washed hands.

When using a handrub for decontamination, the correct technique involves the following steps:

1. **Dispense** – 3 ml of solution into the cupped hands
2. **Massage thoroughly** – until no trace of moisture remains
3. **Take particular care** – to contact all hand surfaces with handrub. Alcohol lacks viscosity and this may result in insufficient contact (Ojajarvi et al., 1977).

Clinical Application

Handwashing Technique

Effective handwashing technique (Figure 5.2) incorporates the following:

- Using elbow- or foot-operated taps to avoid transferring organisms either to the clean hands when the tap is switched off or to the next person
- Using the product from a dispenser as bar soap may be heavily contaminated with Gram-negative rods. Dispensers should not be 'topped up' as this introduces the risk of contamination (Graf *et al.*, 1988; Gould and Chamberlain, 1997)
- Moistening the hands before the agent is added. This helps to reduce contact with harsh chemicals that can damage the skin
- Vigorously rubbing all the surfaces (dorsum, palm and interdigital spaces) with lather for at least 10 seconds. This is often poorly executed (Taylor, 1978; Gould and Ream, 1993)
- Thorough drying as damp hands transfer bacteria more readily than dry ones (Marples and Towens, 1979; Gould, 1984), and residual dampness contributes to soreness
- Disposal of the paper towel into a bin without touching the lid, in order to avoid recontamination.

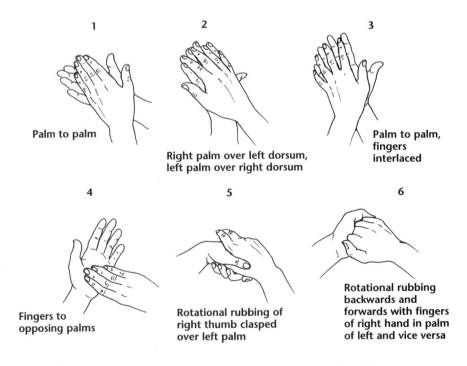

1 Palm to palm

2 Right palm over left dorsum, left palm over right dorsum

3 Palm to palm, fingers interlaced

4 Fingers to opposing palms

5 Rotational rubbing of right thumb clasped over left palm

6 Rotational rubbing backwards and forwards with fingers of right hand in palm of left and vice versa

7 Hands and wrists rubbed until end of 30-second period

Figure 5.2 Hand decontamination technique

The advantages of using a handrub include:

- **Reduced damage to the skin** – This increases compliance (Ojajarvi, 1991). Emollients may be incorporated to further reduce dryness and soreness, both well-documented hazards of frequent decontamination (Larson and Killien, 1982).

- **Increased bactericidal effectiveness** – Dry, cracked skin increases the number of bacteria present because they are more difficult to dislodge by the friction of conventional washing. This defeats the aim of decontamination.

- **Convenience** – The hands are decontaminated more often when handrub is available at the bedside, especially when the workload is high and valuable time would be expended making trips to the nearest sink (Gould and Ream, 1993).

Care of the hands is important in reducing infection. Soreness and dryness induced by frequent decontamination can be reduced by using a good-quality hand cream from a tube reserved for individual use, as communal dispensers can become contaminated (Morse and Schonbeck, 1968). Cuts and abrasions should be covered with waterproof dressings in order to avoid the risk of parenterally transmitted infection. Septic lesions must be occluded to prevent cross-infection. Advice from the occupational health department should be sought, and antibiotics may have to be prescribed. Wearing rings is not advisable as this encourages the growth of Gram-negative bacteria on the underlying skin (Hoffman *et al.*, 1985); an optimal handwashing technique is required to remove these organisms (Jacobson *et al.*, 1985). The nails should be kept short as bacteria beneath them are leached out by sweating after gloves have been worn so more are present on the surface of the hands, contributing to the risk of cross-infection (Peireira *et al.*, 1990). The frequency, appropriateness and technique of hand decontamination can be monitored by periodic auditing.

Sterilisation

Sterilisation is the destruction of all micro-organisms and spores. It is necessary when the small number surviving disinfection would be able to establish infection, either because the organisms themselves are highly virulent or because the patient is very susceptible (Table 5.7). Sterilisation is rarely absolute, and quality control is essential to ensure that an adequate number of micro-organisms and spores is destroyed.

Dry heat sterilisation (Table 5.8) is possible at 160 ^{0}C for 60 minutes or for shorter periods at higher temperatures. It is suitable only for items that are very heat resistant; this excludes plastics, rubber and many fabrics. The items are placed in a hot-air oven after precleaning. Ovens should be fan assisted to ensure an even distribution of heat to all items. Items enter cold so heating time must be added to the period of sterilisation.

Table 5.7   Situations in which sterilisation is necessary

- Equipment that will be used to breach the body's natural barriers to infection (for example, surgical instruments, urinary catheters, injection needles and intravenous fluid sets)

- Dressing materials and topical applications in contact with areas of the body that would normally be free of micro-organisms

- Situations in which contamination is possible with a large number of bacterial spores (for example, exposure to *Clostridium spp.* or *Bacillus anthracis*)

- Equipment that has been in contact with extremely virulent pathogens (for example, in the viral haemorrhagic fevers)

Table 5.8   Methods of sterilisation

- **Heat**
  Dry heat – incineration, hot-air ovens, infrared convectors
  Moist heat under pressure – autoclaves

- **Radiation**
  Ultraviolet irradiation
  X-rays
  Gamma rays

- **Chemicals**
  Ethylene oxide gas
  Formaldehyde gas
  Glutaraldehyde solution

- **Filtration**
  Filters to remove all vegetative bacteria, spores and viruses from commercially prepared solutions

Autoclaving employs moist heat (steam under pressure) to sterilise. It is more efficient than dry heat because steam penetrates fabrics and porous objects rapidly, a property enhanced by increased pressure. In the autoclave, air is removed by suction to create a vacuum before the steam enters, thus ensuring contact with every surface; failure of contact results in failure of sterilisation. Sterilisation is achieved at:

- $121\,^{0}C$ for 15 minutes
- $126\,^{0}C$ for 10 minutes
- $134\,^{0}C$ for 5 minutes.

In hospital, equipment is autoclaved in large batches by technicians. In outpatient departments, where the same small items of equipment are required in rapid succession, and in clinics in the community, nurses may have to operate the autoclaves. The procedure involves:

Clinical Application

Single-use Items

Single-use items cannot be heat sterilised and should be discarded after use. The range of products marketed for single use is increasing; they are convenient, especially in busy clinics and domiciliary settings. The Consumer Protection Act (1987) would be contravened if an item marked for single use only was recycled.

- Precleaning all items.

- Arranging them within the autoclave. They should not touch one another because this could impede steam penetration. Hinged instruments should be opened to allow the maximum exposure of all surfaces, and items should not be wrapped or placed inside one another.

- Items should be removed from the autoclave by sterile forceps and placed in a sterile container.

- They should be used as soon as possible. Resterilisation is necessary if they are not used within 3 hours.

- Autoclaves should be serviced on a regular basis in line with the timing recommended by the manufacturer.

- Routine testing to ensure efficient function should be performed at least weekly, recording the results in a log book.

- Small autoclaves of the type used in GP surgeries are not suitable for sterilising porous loads (such as dressings or fabrics).

Other methods of sterilisation – radiation, chemicals and filtration – are outlined in Table 5.8 above. Chemicals such as ethylene oxide are used to sterilise items that will be damaged by high temperature. Ethylene oxide is rarely used and then usually only within specialist units. Radiation is used commercially to sterilise single-use items such as syringes or needles.

Disposing of waste, dealing with laundry and other contaminated items

Waste disposal policies

Waste forms part of the hospital and care environment and contains potentially pathogenic material. Inappropriate handling or disposal may lead to environmental contamination or a reduction in socially acceptable or aesthetic standards. To avoid this problem, waste must be contained in colour-coded bags (Health Services Advisory Committee Recommendations for Disposal of Waste, 1987; Table 5.9):

- **Black bags** – for normal household waste
- **Yellow bags** – for clinical waste to be incinerated
- **Light blue/transparent bags (with light blue inscriptions)** – waste to be autoclaved before disposal.

High-risk clinical waste is autoclaved before incineration. There is no advantage in double-bagging (Maki *et al.,* 1986).

Table 5.9   Legislation covering the disposal of waste

Date	Legislation	Contents
1990	Environmental Protection Act	Places a 'duty of care' on those dealing with controlled waste
1991	Waste Management: A Duty of Care	Approved code of practice
1992	Controlled Waste Regulations	
1996	Special Waste Regulations	Defines 'special waste'

Waste awaiting collection must be stored in a secure, washable, covered area to discourage the attention of drug misusers and pests (rodents or feral cats). This is much easier on hospital premises than when patients are nursed at home. The amount of waste generated in hospital is enormous, but, as more acutely sick people are cared for at home and in other community settings, the disposal of clinical material from community premises will increase, giving rise to new problems of storage, collection and transport. Under the Environmental Protection Act 1990 (see Table 5.9 above), a duty of care has been placed on those dealing with waste, who must prevent:

- Waste causing environmental pollution or harm to human health, secure packaging being essential at all times
- Handling by those unauthorised to receive waste. Controlled waste should only be dealt with by a registered waste carrier or someone holding a disposal licence. When waste is transferred, a transfer note describing the content should be given to the recipient, labelled to identify the source.

Laundry policies

Laundry falls into three categories (DHSS, 1987):

1.   Used (soiled and fouled)
2.   Infected
3.   Heat-labile fabrics such as wool and synthetic materials.

Linen is considered to be infected only if it has been used by patients who have or are suspected of having an enteric infection, hepatitis, open pulmonary tuberculosis, HIV or any of the notifiable diseases. In this case, it should be placed directly into a water-soluble bag without sorting. This bag is sealed and placed within a red laundry bag. A national colour code is recommended for linen bags and their containers:

■   Used (soiled and fouled) – a **white** bag. To be laundered at 65 ^{0}C for 10 minutes or 71 ^{0}C for 3 minutes
■   Infected, heavily bloodstained – a water-soluble bag enclosed in a **red** bag
■   Heat-labile fabrics damaged by thermal disinfection – white bags with a prominent **orange** stripe. To be laundered at 40 ^{0}C.

The holding area where linen is stored before collection must be dry and covered. In the laundry, dirty and infected linen should be received separately and dealt with in a machine designated for its use.

Crockery and cutlery

Crockery and cutlery should be heat disinfected. In ideal circumstances, this will involve removal from the clinical area to a central kitchen and processing in a dishwasher operating at a minimum temperature of 60 ^{0}C, with a final rinse at a minimum temperature of 82 ^{0}C.

Specific details of policies concerning antibiotics, the handling and disposal of sharps and universal precautions are not provided in this chapter. Readers are directed to the following:

■   Antibiotic policies – Chapter 4
■   Sharps handling and disposal policies – Chapter 12
■   Universal precautions – Chapter 12.

Protective clothing

Protective garments should:

■   Protect clothing from contamination by pathogens that could subsequently be transferred to other people, from patient to nurse or vice versa

- Prevent the direct transfer of pathogenic organisms from patient to nurse or vice versa
- Prevent clothing becoming soiled, wet or stained.

In the past, the use of protective clothing appeared to have been given undue emphasis in infection control programmes. Today, research findings suggest that clothes are of secondary importance to hands in the dissemination of infection and that considerable time and money could be saved by applying evidence-based practice to the use of protective garments. There are, however, situations in which adequate protection is necessary, and the regulations of the Health and Safety Executive (1993) require employers to provide it, to ensure that staff are instructed in the correct use of protective clothing and to ensure that it is worn appropriately.

The use of gloves is discussed in Chapter 12.

Aprons, gowns and tabards

Research concerning protective clothing for use in theatres and burns units has now become specialised, resulting in the manufacture of sophisticated garments (Mackintosh, 1982). Their use in these settings is justified because patients are particularly vulnerable. However, in the wards the hazards of airborne spread from skin scales on clothes have been exaggerated, and less expensive precautions are usually sufficient for most patients (Rahman, 1985). Even when the clothes are heavily contaminated, there is minimal threat to other patients (Babb *et al.*, 1983).

Plastic aprons are more suitable than cotton gowns as cotton weave is permeable and plastic aprons carry fewer bacteria than cotton ones because they cannot adhere readily to cold, slippery surfaces and they dry out quickly. Plastic aprons are cheap and should be used as intended by the manufacturers – being discarded between patients or after activities that may result in heavy soiling (Curran, 1991).

Tabards worn to cover the uniform in paediatric areas are usually made of cotton. They should be changed daily, being laundered at 65 ^{0}C for at least 10 minutes or at 71 ^{0}C for at least 3 minutes to achieve adequate disinfection (DHSS, 1987).

Surgical masks

Most studies to evaluate the effectiveness of surgical masks have been performed either by analysing postoperative infection rates or by laboratory studies. Early simulation tests to examine the risk of contamination after sneezing, coughing and speech indicated that paper masks were superior to fabric ones (Madsen and Madsen, 1967). Even if they incorporate filters, their efficiency is imperfect because bacteria-laden particles can escape around the sides (Davis, 1991). The routine use of masks outside theatre is unnecessary and, except in high risk situations such as orthopaedic surgery or burns units, masks may eventually be abandoned (Tunevall,

1991). The same number of bacteria is shed into the environment whether masks are worn properly to cover both nose or mouth, or leave the nose exposed (Berger *et al.,* 1993).

Hair covering

Hair is a source of staphylococci (Summers *et al.,* 1965), but disposable hair coverings have no effect on bacterial air counts under ventilated conditions (Humphreys *et al.,* 1991). There is now some suggestion that the use of headgear by non-scrubbed staff could be abandoned. However, it seems advisable for the surgeon and his or her assistants to cover their hair because of their close proximity to the operative field. Hair coverings are of no value on wards. Cross-infection is possible when staff suffer from scalp infections, but in these circumstances they should not anyhow be at work (Dineen and Drusin, 1973).

Overshoes

Overshoes contribute to the risk of infection rather than help to prevent it. Bacteria from the floor are seldom responsible for infection, but handling footwear without washing the hands provides a route for cross-infection (Carter, 1990). 'Sticky mats' outside theatres or isolation cubicles are of no value (Meddick, 1977).

Theatre precautions

The operating theatre is a special high-risk environment because the body's tissues are exposed, vastly increasing the opportunity for infection. In wards, bacteria are not disseminated to any great extent via the airborne route, but in theatre airborne staphylococci can cause wound infections, especially during lengthy procedures and orthopaedic surgery (Ayliffe and Lowbury, 1982). The insertion of an orthopaedic prosthesis poses a special risk because the operation is usually lengthy and complex, and because a small number of bacteria is able to cause deep-seated infection within the implanted device (Whyte *et al.,* 1990).

Staff and patients are the main source of airborne bacteria in theatre. During walking, 10^4 skin scales are shed per minute, about 10 per cent of which carry clusters of bacteria of sufficient number to generate infection (Hambraeus, 1988). The bacteria usually settle onto drapes and are transferred into the open wound on instruments and via the hands. Ventilation is important to reduce postoperative infection (see Chapter 8), to maintain a comfortable working environment for staff and to disperse anaesthetic gases. This is reflected in the prominence afforded to ventilation systems in theatre design and to the conduct recommended for staff during operations.

Infection risks in theatre are controlled by:

- Maintaining the environment through regular cleaning and safety checks
- Precautions taken by staff, especially when operations are in progress (Table 5.10)
- The design of the operating suite (Table 5.11), especially the demarcation between clean and dirty areas.

Table 5.10   Reducing the risks of infection in theatre

The environment

- The theatre should be thoroughly cleaned daily
- Floors and surfaces should be damp-dusted between cases and any visible soiling and spillage of blood or body fluids should be removed
- The ventilation system should be switched on daily before the list commences. It must be checked at regular intervals by hospital engineers

Staff precautions

- Gowns and overshoes (note the comments made in the text regarding their effectiveness) are required by all visitors to the theatre suite
- Theatre staff should wear:
  - filter masks
  - shoes reserved for use in theatre
  - dresses or trouser suits changed at least daily
  - gloves, worn by all scrubbed staff and changed whenever there is evidence of puncture
- Illness, (for example boils and stomach upsets) among staff should be reported to the occupational health department

Conduct during operations

- Aseptic technique must be strictly observed
- Movement within theatre needs to be kept to a minimum to keep the number of airborne particles to a minimum
- The number of people in the operating room should be as low as possible: a viewing gallery should be available for educational purposes
- Incidents and breaches in asepsis should be monitored
- The infection rate of clean wounds should be monitored (see Chapter 8)

It is conventional for the theatre suite to be divided into four zones (MRC, 1962). These are:

1. **The aseptic zone** – the operating room and the layout room
2. **The clean zone** – the anaesthetic rooms and scrub area
3. **The protective zone** – the reception area and changing facilities
4. **The disposal zone** – where the sluice is situated.

The zonal layout focuses attention on the importance of good practice and helps to prevent the entry of an excessive number of people (Humphreys *et al.*, 1991).

Table 5.11 Requirements for the design of operating theatres

- Division into clean and dirty zones is considered desirable according to Medical Research Council recommendations (MRC, 1962)
- Doors should be self-closing; windows should be hermetically sealed and accessible for cleaning
- Floors should be durable, easily cleaned and free of horizontal ledges
- Ventilation systems should comply with official recommendations (DHSS, 1983) This involves:
  - Ensuring that the air source is as far as possible from sources of bacterial contamination and protected from the weather
  - Ensuring that there is a pressure gradient from the sterile to all other areas so that air moves from the cleanest to the least clean areas and corridors
  - Ensuring that the air filters are correctly sited and sealed to prevent air escaping around the sides

Many current recommendations are based on clinical judgement as much as on research findings because sound scientific evidence is not available (Humphreys *et al.*, 1991). This situation is inevitable because of the quantity of data that would be required to reveal a significant reduction in the postoperative infection rate associated with clean wounds.

Isolation policies

Isolation was introduced as a method of preventing the spread of infection in hospitals early in the 20th century. Special fever hospitals were built to accommodate those with infectious disease. In general hospitals, the lack of cubicles on long 'Nightingale' wards was compensated for by the erection of physical barriers such as sheets soaked in disinfectant and by staff wearing the full range of protective clothing. Physical barriers served mainly to remind staff to take 'barrier nursing' precautions, but these were distressing to patients and the complicated rituals performed were often superfluous to requirements. They were practised in view of the widely held belief that infectious particles could easily become airborne and be readily transferred to patients in other parts of the ward. It has gradually become apparent that most infections are transmitted primarily in body secretions and that the hands, and to a lesser extent other fomites, rather than airborne spread, are the route of transmission. In most cases, airborne transmission, if it occurs at all, takes place over a relatively short distance.

Today, isolation policies designed to contain infection have become much simplified, falling into two main categories – disease-specific isolation precautions and isolation based on categories of infection.

Disease-specific isolation precautions

Disease-specific isolation precautions involve breaking the chain of infection by taking precautions specific to the particular infection. For example, in the case of enteric organisms such as *Salmonella*, spread by the faecal-oral route, precautions would include wearing protective clothing when handling excreta and washing the hands after patient contact. Operating this system when an infectious patient is admitted would involve routine assessment to establish:

- The probable cause of infection.

- The mechanism of dissemination.

- Articles likely to become heavily contaminated that could readily transmit infection and that would require careful disposal or decontamination.

- The need for a single room. A single room might be desirable but not practical; an older patient with an infected pressure sore might become upset or confused if nursed in isolation, even if visited frequently by the nurse: the experience of isolation can itself be distressing (Knowles, 1993).

- Any other circumstances peculiar to that individual. A patient with HIV does not need to be isolated but may prefer privacy, especially during terminal care, with close friends and family in constant attendance.

- The susceptibility of other patients and staff. Precautions required on a ward where immunosuppressed patients are nursed will not be appropriate on a general ward.

Disease-specific isolation is cost-effective as it eliminates unnecessary rituals and the wasteful use of equipment such as masks, which are usually unnecessary. The disadvantage is that all nurses need a very good knowledge of the way in which each type of infection is spread. Non-specialist nurses frequently do not have this information, so for the system to operate successfully, there must be good communication with the infection control team, with opportunities for regular updating (Gould, 1985). Additional problems occur when the infection is difficult to diagnose or it becomes apparent that the patient has been carrying an infectious organism for some time.

Categories of isolation

With this system, patients are assigned to a particular category of isolation according to the mode of transmission of the organism they are carrying. A system of colour-coded cards provides guidelines for specific source isolation (Control of Infection Group, Northwick Park Hospital, 1974). This approach is effective if staff and visitors follow the instructions but can be criticised for a number of reasons:

- It results in mechanistic, task-oriented care, not in keeping with the spirit of patient-oriented, individualised care
- It is necessary to display the instruction card on the door of the patient's room. The precise nature of the infection is not disclosed, but it will be immediately apparent to any casual observer that he or she has an infection.

For people carrying parenterally transmitted infections, the card system is redundant. Isolation in a single room is not usually necessary for those carrying such infections because their carrier status should be irrelevant if universal precautions are taken, and confidentiality is breached by labelling them (see Chapter 12).

Protective isolation

Protective isolation is required for patients with a high risk of developing infection because their immune system is compromised. This includes patients with prolonged neutropenia as a result of chemotherapy for leukaemia, lymphoma and bone marrow transplantation. For these patients, infection can be life-threatening. Early attempts to nurse them focused on the provision of a 'germ-free' environment in a specialist unit, with sterile food and contact only with fully gowned staff. This approach was distressing for patients and their families, expensive, time-consuming and not always effective as it focused on the prevention of infection by extrinsic organisms spread by cross-infection from other people. However, considerable risk comes from the patient's own flora, especially the gastrointestinal tract, and a 'germ-free' state is not attainable. Today, stringent precautions are reserved for patients undergoing bone marrow transplantation. For other patients, a less stringent approach, possibly outside specialist transplant units, is recommended (Fenelon, 1995).

Simple protective isolation

- **Accommodation** in a single room is not likely to have a protective effect but may help by reminding staff and visitors that special precautions are required, and may be appreciated owing to the considerable stress experienced by patients (Knowles, 1993). There is no reason to exclude visitors unless they have an infection, and providing they will not have contact with the patient, there seems no logical reason for them to wear protective clothing.

- **Handwashing** should be thorough (see above) before patient contact to reduce the risk of cross-infection.

- **Protective clothing** is of secondary importance to handwashing in the prevention of cross-infection but is of value in preventing the patient's own flora gaining access to a vulnerable site. Gloves and aprons used during contact with blood and body fluids should be changed before contact with a wound or any invasive device, and the hands should be washed.

■ **Food** contains organisms that are not harmful if their numbers are small. Salads are a well-known source of Gram-negative bacteria that may be a threat to immunocompromised patients, and raw food may harbour *Listeria*. It thus seems logical to exclude those items (Fenelon, 1995). Eggs, as a possible source of *Salmonella*, should be thoroughly cooked.

■ **Invasive procedures** are a major threat to immunosuppressed patients as they have a very high rate of bacteraemia (bacteria in the blood). Today, good protocols for care exist, which are particularly important for these patients (see Chapters 7, 8, 9 and 10).

Staff who are pregnant should not have contact with immunosuppressed patients who may be carrying a large number of organisms that could damage the fetus.

Critical care units

Patients in critical care units (intensive and neonatal units) are immunocompromised and at high risk of infection. Particular care must thus be taken with hand hygiene. In some units, theatre dress is worn by staff with direct patient contact, and it has in the past been common policy to insist that all visitors wear a gown or a plastic apron. This does not, however, contribute to the prevention of infection (Nyström, 1981; Haque and Chagla, 1989).

Improving care and increasing knowledge

Infection control is the responsibility of everyone involved in patient care. Specialists in public health and members of the infection control team provide expertise, but their advice is of limited value unless it is reflected in the care provided by staff with direct patient contact. Considerable research has been undertaken in the field of infection control and has contributed to the development of protocols to prevent infection. A brief glance at the reference list at the end of this chapter will reveal that, although the best of recent research findings have been represented, much of our knowledge in this field is not new, even though it is still of clear relevance in contemporary patient care. There is, however, also disturbing evidence that compliance with infection control protocols often remains poor. Much work remains to be done; important tasks requiring immediate attention include finding effective ways of increasing compliance and auditing infection control procedures.

REVISION CHECKLIST: KEY AREAS

- ❏ Introduction to strategies that prevent infection: Risk factors associated with hospital admission, Preventing the spread of infection – hospital and community

- ❏ Policies and procedures to prevent infection: Standard and high-risk situations

- ❏ Decontamination: Cleaning, Disinfection, Hand hygiene, Sterilisation

- ❏ Disposing of waste and dealing with laundry and other contaminated items: Waste disposal policies, Laundry policies, Crockery and cutlery

- ❏ Protective clothing: Aprons, Gowns and tabards, Surgical masks, Hair covering, Overshoes

- ❏ Theatre precautions

- ❏ Isolation policies: Disease-specific isolation precautions, Categories of isolation, Protective isolation, Improving care and increasing knowledge

---

Activities – linking knowledge to clinical practice

1   **Obtain** the infection control policy currently in use in your clinical area. How adequate is the provision for each of the following (where relevant)?

(a) Handwashing
(b) Use of autoclaves
(c) Cleaning mattresses
(d) Cleaning thermometers
(e) Isolating a patient with diarrhoea and vomiting.

2   **Select** a procedure/piece of equipment widely used in your practice area. How adequate is the guidance for this procedure or the care of this piece of equipment?

3   **Your** department is about to be rehoused in a new building, and you have been asked to provide infection control advice when it is commissioned. Identify the key areas and make suggestions. Try to identify which are essential and which constitute desirable but not essential additonal features.

SELF-ASSESSMENT

1. Bactericides:
   (a) destroy micro-organisms ☐
   (b) destroy only spores ☐
   (c) destroy only viruses ☐

2. Sterilisation is the destruction of all micro-organisms and their spores. True? ☐ False? ☐

3. Chemical disinfection is superior to disinfection by heat. True? ☐ False? ☐

4. Chlorhexidine is effective against:
   (a) Gram-positive bacteria ☐
   (b) spores ☐
   (c) viruses ☐
   (d) *Mycobacterium tuberculosis* ☐

5. Which of the following should be taken into consideration when choosing an appropriate disinfectant?
   (a) potential harmfulness to users ☐
   (b) potential harmfulness to patients ☐
   (c) bacterial effectiveness ☐
   (d) potential harmfulness to the environment ☐

6. Sterilisation is achieved at 121 ^{0}C moist heat for 15 minutes. True? ☐ False? ☐

7. Handwashing is necessary:
   (a) before aseptic procedures ☐
   (b) after handling patients ☐
   (c) after handling any items that are or could be soiled ☐
   (d) before handling food ☐

8. Which of the following are the most likely to disseminate infection?
   (a) nurses' uniforms ☐
   (b) hands ☐
   (c) hair ☐
   (d) not wearing a mask during the general surgical list in theatre ☐

9. It is good practice for all visitors entering a critical care unit to wear an apron. True? ☐ False? ☐

10. Surgical instruments may be effectively sterilised by immersion in boiling water. True? ☐ False? ☐

References

Axnick KJ and Yarborough M (1984) *Infection Control: An Integrated Approach.* Mosby, Toronto.

Ayliffe GAJ (1970) 'Contamination of infant feeds in a Milton milk kitchen'. *Lancet* **1**: 559–60.

Ayliffe GAJ and Lowbury EJ (1982) 'Airborne infection in hospital'. *Journal of Hospital Infection* **3**: 217–40.

Ayliffe GAJ, Collins BJ and Lowbury EJ (1967) 'Ward floors and other surfaces and reservoirs of hospital infection'. *Journal of Hygiene* **65**: 515–37.

Babb JR, Davies JG and Ayliffe GAJ (1983) 'Contamination of protective clothing and nurses' uniforms in an isolation ward'. *Journal of Hospital Infection* **4**: 149–57.

Bentham AJ (1979) 'An investigation into a cross-infection problem in a cardiovascular unit'. Proceedings of the Tenth Annual Symposium of the Infection Control Nurses Association.

Berger SA, Kramer M, Nagar H *et al.* (1993) 'Effect of surgical mask position on bacterial contamination of the operative field'. *Journal of Hospital Infection* **23**: 51–4.

Block C, Baron O, Bogkowski B *et al.* (1990) 'An in-use evaluation of polypropylene versus steel bedpans'. *Journal of Hospital Infection* **16**: 331–8.

Boycott JA (1956) 'A note on the disinfection of baths and basins'. *Lancet* **2**: 678–9.

Burdon DW and Whitby JL (1967) 'Contamination of hospital disinfectants with *Pseudomonas* species'. *British Medical Journal* **2**: 153–4.

Carter R (1990) 'Ritual and risk'. *Nursing Times* **86**: 63–4.

Casewell MW and Phillips I (1978) 'Epidemiological patterns of *Klebsiella* colonisation and infection in an intensive care unit'. *Journal of Hygiene* **80**: 295–300.

Chadwick PR and Oppenheim BA (1994) 'Vancomycin-resistant enterococci and bedpan washer machines'. *Lancet* **344**: 685

Coates D and Hutchinson DN (1994) 'How to produce a hospital disinfection policy'. *Journal of Hospital Infection* **26**: 57–68.

Control of Infection Group, Northwick Park Hospital (1974) 'Isolation system for general hospitals'. *British Medical Journal* **2**: 41–6.

Curie K, Speller DCE, Simpson RA *et al.* (1978) 'A hospital epidemic caused by gentamicin-resistant *Klebsiella aerogenes*'. *Journal of Hygiene* **80**: 115–23.

Curran E (1991) 'Protecting with plastic aprons'. *Nursing Times* **87**(38): 64–68.

Danforth D, Nicolle K and Hume N (1987) 'Nosocomial infections on nursing units with disinfectant compared with detergent'. *Journal of Hospital Infection* **10**: 229–35.

Davis WT (1991) 'Filtration efficiency of surgical face masks: the need for meaningful standards'. *American Journal of Infection Control* **19**: 16–18.

Department of Health (1988) Control of Substances Hazardous to Health (COSHH) *Statutory Instrument No 1657*. DoH, London.

Department of Health (1993a) *Risk Management in the NHS*. HMSO, London.

Department of Health (1993b) *Guidance on Decontamination: Sterilisation, Disinfection and Cleaning of Medical Equipment*. HMSO, London.

Department of Health and Social Security (1983) *Ventilation of Operating Departments: A Design Guide*. HMSO, London.

Department of Health and Social Security (1987) *Hospital Laundry Arrangements for Used and Infected Linen*. HMSO, London.

Dineen P and Drusin L (1973) 'Epidemics of post-operative wound infections associated with wound carriers'. *Lancet* **2**: 1157–9.

Fenelon LE (1995) 'Protective isolation: who needs it?' *Journal of Hospital Infection* (Supplement) **30**: 218–22.

Foy C, Gallagher M, Rhodes T *et al.* (1990) 'HIV and measures to control infection in general practice'. *British Medical Journal* **300**: 1048–9.

Glenister H (1987) 'The passage of infection'. *Nursing Times* **83**(22): 68–73.

Gould DJ (1984) 'The significance of hand drying in the prevention of infection'. *Nursing Times* **80**(47): 33–5.

Gould DJ (1985) 'Isolation procedures in one health district'. *Nursing Times* **81**(7): 47–51.

Gould DJ and Chamberlain A (1997) 'The use of a ward-based educational teaching package to enhance nurses' compliance with infection control procedures'. *Journal of Clinical Nursing* **6**(1): 55–67.

Gould DJ and Ream E (1993) 'Assessing nurses' hand decontamination performance'. *Nursing Times* **89**(25): 47–50.

Graf W, Kersh D and Scherzer P (1988) 'Medical contamination of liquid soap wall dispensers with one-way bottles'. *Zentral Bacteriologie, Microbiologie und Hygiene* **186**: 166–79.

Greaves A (1985) 'We'll just freshen you up, dear'. *Nursing Times* **81**(36): 1–4.

Hambraeus A (1988) 'Aerobiology of the operating suite'. *Journal of Hospital Infection* (Supplement A) **11**: 68–76.

Hanson PJ, Gor D and Jeffries DJ (1989) 'Chemical inactivation of HIV on surfaces'. *British Medical Journal* **298**: 862–4.

Haque KN and Chagla AH (1989) 'Do gowns prevent infection in neonatal intensive care units?' *Journal of Health Hospital Infection* **14**: 159–62.

Health and Safety Commission (1998) 'Glutaraldehyde and you: guidance for the healthcare sector'. *HSC* **3**: 98.

Health and Safety Executive (1993) *Personal Protective Equipment at Work Regulations. Guidance on Regulations.* HSE, Leeds.

Health Services Advisory Committee (1987) *Recommendations for the Disposal of Waste.* HSC, London.

Hoffman PN, Cooke EM, McCarville MR *et al.* (1985) 'Micro-organisms isolated from skin under wedding rings worn by hospital staff'. *British Medical Journal* **290**: 206–7.

Humphreys H, Russell HJ, Marshall HJ *et al.* (1991) 'The effect of surgical theatre headgear on bacterial counts'. *Journal of Hospital Infection* **19**: 175–80.

Jacobson G, Thiele JE, McCune JHJ *et al.* (1985) 'Handwashing, ringwearing and number of micro-organisms'. *Nursing Research* **34**: 186–8.

Johnson H and Harker M (1996) 'An overhaul of home loans'. *Nursing Times* **92**(10): 33–4.

Kjolen H and Andersen BM (1992) 'Handwashing and disinfection of heavily contaminated hands; effective or ineffective?' *Journal of Hospital Infection* **21**: 61–71.

Knowles HE (1993) 'The experience of infectious patients in isolation'. *Nursing Times* **89**(30): 53–6.

Kotilainen HR, Avato JL and Gantz NM (1990) 'Latex and vinyl non-sterile examination gloves: status report on laboratory evaluation of defects by physical and biological methods'. *Applied Environmental Microbiology* **56**: 1627–30.

Larson E and Killien M (1982) 'Factors influencing handwashing behaviour of patient care personnel'. *American Journal of Infection Control* **10**: 93–9.

Linden B (1991) 'Protection in practice'. *Nursing Times* **87**(11): 59–63.

McGowan JE (1981) 'Environmental factors in nosocomial infection – a selective focus'. *Review of Infective Diseases* **3**: 760–9.

Mackintosh CA (1982) 'A testing time for gowns'. *Journal of Hospital Infection* **3**: 5–8.

Madsen P and Madsen R (1967) 'A study of disposable surgical masks'. *American Journal of Surgery* **114**: 431–5.

Maki DG, Alvarado C and Hassemer C (1986) 'Double-bagging items from isolation rooms is unnecessary as an infection control measure: a comparative study of surface contamination with single and double bagging'. *Infection Control* **7**: 535–7.

Marples RR and Towers A (1979) 'A laboratory model for the contact transfer of micro-organisms'. *Journal of Hygiene* **82**: 237–48.

Martin AM and Reicheldfer M (1994) 'Association of Professionals in Infection Control and Epidemiology Guidelines 1994'. *American Journal of Infection Control* **22**: 19–38.

Meddick MM (1977) 'Bacterial contamination control mats: a comparative study'. *Journal of Hygiene* **79**: 133–40.

Medical Research Council (1962) 'Design and ventilation of operating room suites for control of infection and for comfort'. *Lancet* **2**: 945–51.

Morse P and Schonbeck LE (1968) 'Hand lotions – a potential nosocomial hazard'. *New England Journal of Medicine* **278**: 376–7.

Murdoch S (1990) 'Hazards in hoists'. *Nursing Times* **86**(49): 68–70.

Nyström B (1981) 'The contamination of gowns in an intensive care unit'. *Journal of Hospital Infection* **2**: 167–70.

O'Donoghue MAT and Allen KD (1992) 'Costs of an outbreak of wound infections in an orthopaedic ward'. *Journal of Hospital Infection* **22**: 73–9.

Ojajarvi J (1991) 'Handwashing in Finland'. (Supplement B) *Journal of Hospital Infection* **18**: 35–40.

Ojajarvi J, Makela P and Rantasolo I (1977) 'Failure of hand disinfection with frequent hand-washing: a need for prolonged field studies'. *Journal of Hygiene* **72**: 109–19.

Overton E (1988) 'Bedmaking and bacteria'. *Nursing Times* **84**(9): 69–71.

Peireira LJ, Lee GM and Wade FJ (1990) 'The effect of surgical handwashing routines on the microbial counts of operating room nurses'. *American Journal of Infection Control* **18**: 354–64.

Rahman M (1985) 'Commissioning a new hospital isolation unit and assessment of its use over five years'. *Journal of Hospital Infection* **6**: 65–70.

Reybrouck G (1983) 'The role of hands in the spread of nosocomial infections'. *Journal of Hospital Infection* **4**: 103–11.

Russell AD and Day MJ (1993) 'Antibacterial activity of chlorhexidine'. *Journal of Hospital Infection* **25**: 229–38.

Sanderson PJ and Rawal P (1987) 'Contamination of the environment of spinal cord injured patients by orqanisms causing urinary tract infection'. *Journal of Hospital Infection* **10**: 173–8.

Sprunt K, Redman W and Leidy G (1973) 'Antibacterial effectiveness of routine handwashing'. *Paediatrics* **52**: 264–71.

Summers MM, Lynch PF and Black T (1965) 'Hair as a reservoir of staphylococci'. *Journal of Clinical Pathology* **18**: 13–15.

Taylor LJ (1978) 'An evaluation of handwashing techniques'. *Nursing Times* Part 1: **74**(2): 54–5; Part 2: **74**(3): 108–9.

Tunevall TG (1991) 'Post-operative wound infections and surgical masks: a controlled study'. *World Journal of Surgery* **15**: 383–8.

Whyte W, Hamblen DI and Kelly IG (1990) 'An investigation into occlusive polyester surgical clothing'. *Journal of Hospital Infection* **15**: 363–74.

Wicks J (1994) 'Handle with care'. *Nursing Times* **90**(13): 45–6.

Further reading and information sources

Medical Devices Agency (1996) *Sterilisation, Disinfection and Cleaning of Medical Equipment.* Medical Devices Agency, London.

Philpott-Howard J and Casewell M (1995) *Hospital Infection Control.* WB Saunders, London.

Rogers R, Salvage J and Cowell R (1999) 'Infection and infection risks' in *Nurses at Risk: A Guide to Health and Safety at Work,* 2nd edn. Macmillan, Basingstoke, pp. 142–76.

Royal College of Nursing (1994) *Guidelines on Infection Control in Hospital.* RCN, London.

Scoule B and Larson EL (1994) *Infections and Nursing Practice. Prevention and Control.* CV Mosby, London.

Visit the Health and Safety Executive Web Site at http://www.open.gov.uk/hse/hsehome.htm for up-to-date advice and guidelines on the use of disinfectants.

6 Preventing infection in hospital

CHAPTER OUTCOMES

After reading this chapter you should be able to:

■ Explain what is meant by the term 'nosocomial'

■ Discuss the problem of nosocomial infection both for the NHS and from the patient's perspective

■ State which infections occur most commonly in hospital

■ Discuss the approaches taken to monitor and control infection in hospital

■ List the main groups of bacteria responsible for infection in hospital and suggest the most effective control methods in each case

■ Outline the role of the infection control team and committee

---

Introduction – historical aspects of hospital infection

Hospital-acquired (nosocomial) infection is infection not present or incubating at the time of admission (Bennett and Brachman, 1979). It is not a new phenomenon, but the types of infection that commonly occur in hospital have changed dramatically since the second half of the 18th century when nosocomial infection first attracted the attention of scientists and medical staff (Selwyn, 1991). At this time, 'hospital fever' (typhus), dysentery and 'the itch' (scabies) were rife in hospitals.

However, even before the 'germ theory of infection' became widely accepted, the way in which it was transmitted was a cause of speculation, and in the 1830s the role played by staff in cross-infection became apparent with the work of Semmelweiss, Lister, Nightingale and Simpson.

The significance of nosocomial infection

The cost of nosocomial infection in financial terms is today considerable – to the government, to tax-payers and to patients. Hospital stay is usually increased, so 'hotel' costs often represent a substantial proportion of the additional expenditure. However, patients with infections require more drugs (antibiotics and analgesia), more dressings and more nursing time, whether they are in hospital or have returned to the community. In addition, patients face major inconvenience and distress while the waiting lists for elective procedures build up (Davey *et al.,* 1991). Thus, the need to develop effective control measures is now fully acknowledged by health service policy-makers, and in recent years a number of attempts have been made to quantify the risk of developing nosocomial infection as the first step towards preventing it. Hospital infection rates can be regarded as a marker of quality and can be used for the purposes of auditing and contract specification (RCN, 1994).

The extent of nosocomial infection

The extent of the problem can be estimated by prevalence or incidence surveys (Chapter 14).

Prevalence surveys

The first National Prevalence Survey conducted in the early 1980s showed that 9 per cent of hospital inpatients developed nosocomial infections, the most common being urinary tract infections. Surgical wound infections and infections of the lower respiratory tract were the second and third most common causes respectively (Meers *et al.,* 1981).

The second National Prevalence Survey (1993–94) was conducted in 157 centres in the UK and the Republic of Ireland by the Hospital Infection Society and the Infection Control Nurses Association (Emmerson *et al.,* 1996). Results again showed an overall rate of 9 per cent, infections falling into four major groups: urinary tract infections (23.2 per cent), lower respiratory tract infections (22.9 per cent), surgical wound infections (10.7 per cent) and skin infections (9.6 per cent). Urinary infections were most common in urosurgical and gynaecology patients, especially those over 75 years of age. Lower respiratory tract infections were seen most commonly in critical care units, especially in male patients aged over 75 years. The decline in the prevalence of surgical wound infection since 1981 is probably explained by a number of factors, including improvements in surgical technique, better bowel preparation and an increased use of antibiotic prophylaxis.

Incidence surveys

Incidence studies are more expensive and difficult to conduct than prevalence studies, and there has to date been no national study of this kind. Smaller-scale incidence studies indicate that, overall, the rate of nosocomial infection is 6 per cent. This figure is probably more accurate than statistics derived from prevalence data because patients who have developed infection generally stay in hospital longer, overestimating the true rate.

Monitoring nosocomial infection

Nosocomial infection can be monitored by surveillance or audit.

Surveillance

Surveillance consists of the routine collection and analysis of nosocomial infection rates with feedback to staff (DoH and PHLS, 1995). It gives infection control teams greater insight into the patterns of infection in hospital, drawing early attention to potential outbreaks. Feedback helps to reduce infection by stimulating the examination of local practices to identify areas in which remedial action should be taken and encouraging the most appropriate use of resources. The value of surveillance was first demonstrated in the USA, where hospitals cannot be licensed without evidence that effective infection control policies are operating. A major study involving 338 hospitals, the Study of the Efficacy of Nosocomial Infection Control (SENIC) project, revealed that surveillance with feedback to clinical staff could reduce nosocomial infection by 32 per cent; in hospitals without surveillance, the infection rate was higher (Haley et al., 1985).

Infection control experts and policy-makers in the UK have been slower to accept the potential of surveillance in the control of nosocomial infection. However, this situation is changing. The Public Health Laboratory Service (PHLS) in England and Wales has scrutinised the effectiveness of different methods of surveillance and used the most promising to look at nosocomial urinary, blood and lower respiratory infections (Glennister et al., 1992). In 1995, the PHLS established a Nosocomial Infection Surveillance Unit, and in 1996, the unit launched the Nosocomial Infection National Surveillance Scheme (NINSS). The function of the NINSS is to provide confidential data to hospitals so that infection control teams and clinicians can compare their own infection rates from year to year with anonymous data from other hospitals. This will enable each hospital to undertake surveillance targeted at a specific area or patient group. For example, it may be found advisable to monitor urinary infections or patients in critical care units. The success of an infection control activity can be examined by comparing the numbers of cases before and after the intervention.

Audit

Audit is another approach to infection control, often introduced at a local level. The audit cycle involves making systematic quantifiable comparisons between existing practice and explicit, agreed standards in order to highlight areas in which improvement could be made (Glover, 1992; Figure 6.1). It involves the systematic critical analysis of the quality of care and should include:

■ Procedures used to diagnose and treat patients
■ The use of resources
■ The resulting outcome and quality of life for the patient.

Nosocomial infection is a prime target for audit because is affects all three selection criteria (French, 1993). Effective methods of auditing using this approach have been developed (Millward *et al.*, 1993).

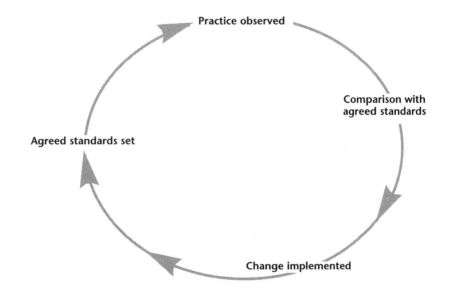

Figure 6.1   The audit cycle

Auditing infection control initiatives can be expensive and time-consuming if it involves obtaining and processing microbiological samples. An alternative approach is to audit the documentation concerned with infection prevention (French, 1993). Factors to be taken into consideration include:

■ Whether written documents exist for a given procedure (Table 6.1)
■ Their acceptability
■ Whether hospital practice adheres to the guidelines

■ Whether there is any demonstrable alteration in the nosocomial infection rate after introducing the new guideline or following a training programme to increase staff awareness of the established documentation.

In addition, many infection control teams are concerned about the distribution and behaviour of particular pathogens responsible for a high proportion of all infections occurring in hospital.

Table 6.1   Suggested documentation for infection control audit (adapted from French, 1993)

■ Care of urinary catheters

■ Care of intravenous lines

■ Staff occupational health policies (immunisation programmes for hepatitis B and rubella, and screening after exposure to patients with tuberculosis)

■ Disposal of contaminated waste

■ Disinfectant policies

■ Prevention of Legionnaire's disease

■ Antibiotic policies

■ Control of methicillin-resistant *Staphylococcus aureus*

■ Control of outbreaks of chickenpox

■ Isolation policies

Pathogens causing nosocomial infection

This section aims to cover nosocomial infections caused by staphylococci, streptococci and Gram-negative organisms.

Staphylococcal infection

Staphylococcal infections may be caused by organisms producing the enzyme coagulase, which clots plasma when the bacteria are grown on solid culture media. The bacterium known as *Staphylococcus aureus* may also be methicillin resistant. Other staphylococci causing infection, for example *Staphylococcus epidermidis*, are not coagulase producers.

Staphylococcus aureus

Staphylococcus aureus is a Gram-positive bacterium that produces the enzyme coagulase. It is carried in the nose, throat, axillae, toe webs and perineum of 30–50 per cent of healthy people without causing clinical infection. Asymptomatic carriage is clinically significant because the bacteria can be transferred to susceptible sites (for example, from the nose to a wound) or from a fit asymptomatic individual to someone less healthy who will succumb to clinical infection.

Staphylococcus aureus is the most common cause of pyogenic (pus-forming) infection, causing a range of infections that includes boils, abscesses, septic fingers, styes, impetigo, and sticky eyes in neonates. Transmission is through contact, mainly via hands. In hospital, *Staphylococcus aureus* causes serious wound infections, bronchopneumonia, osteomyelitis and endocarditis. Some strains produce toxins that cause extensive cellular damage. For example, the toxic shock syndrome associated with the use of vaginal tampons is caused by staphylococcal toxins. The main method of epidemiological typing used to identify whether a cluster of staphylococcal infections originate from a common source is phage typing. This has revealed outbreaks in intensive care and burns units.

Methicillin-resistant staphylococcal infection

Staphylococcus aureus first became significant as a hospital pathogen in the 1940s, a penicillin-resistant strain emerging during the next decade. Initially, two factors contributed to successful control: the development of new synthetic penicillins during the 1960s, and a flurry of research activity stimulated by the growing problems of nosocomial wound infection. Many hospital infection control policies date from the 1960s, and lessons learned at this time have contributed to the control of hospital infection in the UK. At first, improvement was dramatic and methicillin-resistant *Staphylococcus aureus* (MRSA) disappeared, only to be followed by its resurgence throughout the 1980s and 90s in many countries, including the UK.

Clinical Application

Methicillin

Methicillin, a modified penicillin, was introduced during the 1960s. It is no longer used therapeutically because more modern penicillin derivatives are better absorbed, but a bacterial strain that is resistant to methicillin will also be resistant to all penicillin derivatives and to cephalosporins, some also being resistant to aminoglycosides and macrolides. This means that a patient presenting with an infection that needs treatment before the results of sensitivity testing can be treated 'blind' only with vancomycin, which has the potential disadvantage of severe haemotoxicity and nephrotoxicity.

MRSA causes the same range of infections as methicillin-sensitive *Staphylococcus aureus*, is disseminated in the same way and is no more virulent. Most people become asymptomatic carriers and never develop clinical infection, especially if they are healthy. However, they operate as reservoirs and are therefore a risk to seriously ill patients. MRSA has become a cause for concern because it is extremely difficult to eradicate (Keane *et al.*, 1991). Skin lesions such as chronic wounds or cannula insertion points can become heavily colonised, so are particularly likely to operate as reservoirs. The risk of developing clinical MRSA infection is greater among older, more debilitated patients. Factors that encourage the dissemination of MRSA through a population of hospital patients include the prescription of two or more antibiotics to individual patients and poor infection control precautions, such as substandard handwashing (Casewell, 1986). MRSA has spread between hospitals when staff and patients have moved between sites (Boyce, 1991).

Epidemic methicillin-resistant *Staphylococcus aureus* (EMRSA) spreads more easily than other strains of MRSA and appears to colonise skin and mucous membranes more readily (French *et al.*, 1990). The first strain, EMRSA-1, was isolated in 1984 (Marples *et al.*, 1985), 16 strains now having been reported in the UK. EMRSA-1 and EMRSA-3 caused large outbreaks in the 1980s and contributed to a number of deaths, but they seldom affected healthy people and never spread beyond one or two NHS regions (Marples and Reith, 1992). The other strains caused fewer problems and are now seldom a source of infection, with the exception of EMRSA-14 and EMRSA-16, first isolated in 1991–1992. These have become widely disseminated in hospitals and have been detected in the community, particularly in residents in nursing homes (Cox *et al.*, 1995).

Guidelines for controlling MRSA

Guidelines for controlling MRSA have been developed and revised by the Combined Working Party of the British Society for Antimicrobial Chemotherapy, the Hospital Infection Society and the Infection Control Nurses Association (1998; see also Tables 6.2 and 6.3). Success depends on reducing transmission by detecting, treating and isolating all infected and colonised patients (Beedle, 1993). The unnecessary use of antibiotics should be avoided, and infection control precautions, especially handwashing, patient isolation and cohorting, and adequate cleaning (Combined Working Party, 1998), need to be rigorously performed. Programmes for community control involve treating MRSA-positive patients discharged from hospital (Cox *et al.*, 1995).

Treatment of MRSA

The drug of choice against MRSA is vancomycin, patients who experience toxic effects being given teicoplanin (Daum *et al.*, 1990). Combined therapy may be tried if single therapy has not been effective. Rifampicin and sodium fusidate may be effective together. Other drug combinations include rifampicin with a fluoroquinolone such as ciprofloxacin. Topical mupirocin is used to eradicate skin and nasal carriage.

Table 6.2 **Protocol for the ward screening of staff and patients for methicillin-resistant** *Staphylococcus aureus* **(MRSA)**

When	Sample site
New staff	Nose
	Lesions
Staff with positive nasal swabs	Nose
Admissions	Lesions
Existing patients	Groin/perineum
	Any manipulated sites – intravascular catheters, catheter specimens of urine, sputum
Other sites for sampling may be indicated in certain situations	Urine, faeces, vagina, axillae, throat (long-term positive swabs from the nose and people with dentures)
	In infants, a swab is obtained from the umbilicus

Based on guidelines produced by the Combined Working Party of the British Society for Antimicrobial Chemotherapy, the Hospital Infection Society and the Infection Control Nurses Association (1998)

NB. Action will differ between minimal-risk (for example psychiatric units), low-risk (for example most general medical wards), moderate-risk (for example general surgical wards) and high-risk (for example orthopaedic wards and intensive care wards and units) – always check the local protocols for your area.

It is important to keep MRSA in perspective, remembering that most carriers never develop clinical infection. Nevertheless, the control of this organism is likely to remain an infection control challenge for some time. For example, strains of mupirocin-resistant MRSA have emerged and are becoming more widespread (Dawson *et al.*, 1994). The topical application of fucidin is effective for patients carrying these strains.

Coagulase-negative staphylococci

Numerous species of staphylococci are unable to produce coagulase and are therefore described as coagulase-negative staphylococci (CNSs). The most well-known example of this group is *Staphylococcus epidermidis*, which is a skin commensal. As the ability to secrete coagulase is one of the factors contributing to the pathogenic potential of *Staphylococcus aureus*, CNSs were once believed to have low pathogenicity. However, these bacteria produce extracellular slime that enables them to adhere to plastic and metal surfaces. Once they become covered with slime, they are protected from the host defences and multiply, establishing a focus of infection. CNSs are associated with an increasing incidence of infections involving peritoneal dialysis catheters, prosthetic valves and orthopaedic implants. If they gain access to the bloodstream via intravascular devices, they cause septicaemia. Infections are difficult to eradicate because CNSs are naturally resistant to many antibiotics

(Harmory and Parisi, 1987). In some cases, it can be difficult to determine whether CNSs are behaving as contaminants or are clinically significant (Martin de Nicolas *et al.*, 1995).

Table 6.3   **Protocol for treating methicillin-resistant *Staphylococcus aureus* (MRSA) carriage, colonisation and infection**

- Bath patients daily (for 5 days) using an antiseptic detergent, for example chlorhexidine 4%. Observe for and report any skin irritation to the infection control team (other antiseptics or ones with emollients may be suggested). Staff carriers should follow this hygiene regimen

- Wash the hair twice weekly with antiseptic shampoo in patients who are skin carriers

- Apply hexachlorophane powder to the axillae and groins (contraindicated where open lesions exist and in small babies) in patients who are skin carriers

- Supply clean clothes, bedding and items for hygiene on completion of the treatment

- Apply mupirocin 2% three times a day for 5 days to treat nasal carriage (in patients and staff), and repeat nasal swab 2 days after finishing treatment. Where the nasal swabs remain positive, swab the throat to check for colonisation and give a repeat course of mupirocin. Other antibiotics, for example neomycin 0.5% with chlorhexidine 0.1%, will be needed if nasal swabs remain positive or mupirocin-resistant strains are isolated

- Administer oral treatment, for example 5 days of rifampicin with sodium fusidate or ciprofloxacin, for throat carriage. Repeat courses are not generally given as side-effects and bacterial resistance is increased where treatment is prolonged

- Apply mupirocin 0.5% to small skin lesions (not for use with large open areas or where plastic devices are in use) for up to a maximum of 10 days. Staff carriers should cover any lesions with an appropriate impermeable dressing

- Staff carriers may need to go off duty in high/moderate-risk areas. Those staff who do not respond to initial treatment courses may need systemic antibiotics. In extreme cases, a transfer to a lower-risk area may need to be considered

- Carriers should have three negative swabs (taken at weekly intervals) before MRSA clearance can be confirmed

- Vancomycin or teicoplanin (sometimes with rifampicin) is used to treat serious infections. Other drugs in use include rifampicin with sodium fusidate, ciprofloxacin and trimethoprim

- Patients previously affected by MRSA should have swabs taken on any readmission. This is especially important where antibiotics were prescribed. Their medical and nursing notes should carry an identifying label stating the history of MRSA carriage, colonisation or infection

Based on guidelines produced by the Combined Working Party of the British Society for Antimicrobial Chemotherapy, the Hospital Infection Society and the Infection Control Nurses Association (1998)

NB. Antibiotics that are used for systemic use, for example vancomycin, should not be applied topically.

Streptococcal infection

Streptococci are Gram-positive, chain-forming cocci classified into Lancefield groups A–S.

Group A beta-haemolytic streptococcus

Group A beta-haemolytic streptococcus (*Streptococcus pyogenes*) is responsible for serious infections – pharyngitis, skin infections and puerperal fever (Ayton, 1981). The bacteria can spread through the tissues by releasing toxins, so generalised infection may result. Scarlet fever is pharyngitis with a rash induced by the release of toxin. The toxins may also induce hypersensitivity reactions, for example glomerulonephritis and rheumatic fever, that develop up to 4 weeks after the infection.

Group A haemolytic streptococci were the first bacteria identified as a source of nosocomial infection and were responsible for major outbreaks in burns units and maternity and surgical wards between 1930 and 1950. The development of serological typing techniques revealed that cross-infection was common. Person-to-person transmission has been well documented. The bacteria are carried in the nasopharynx of 6–8 per cent of the general population, mostly children, carriers dispersing them by coughing, sneezing and talking. The droplets dry out, heavily contaminating the environment.

Following the introduction of penicillin, the incidence of streptococcal infection declined. Most strains are still sensitive, and until recently Group A streptococci remained a comparatively rare cause of infection, although its incidence is now increasing in hospital and in the community. Older people, especially those with serious underlying medical conditions, are most at risk, and there appears to be substantial risk of transmission in hospitals as well as the community (Davies *et al.*, 1996). Screening staff to exclude carriers, isolating infected patients until antibiotic therapy has become effective and environmental cleaning to remove reservoirs are recommended to control outbreaks (Sarangi and Rowsell, 1995).

Clinical Application

Necrotising Fasciitis

Necrotising fasciitis is severe inflammation of the muscle sheath, leading to extensive and rapid destruction of soft tissues. Patients suffer acute pain and may need radical excision of the affected tissues or amputation. The mortality rate is high. In 1994, a cluster of five cases was reported in Gloucester, but this did not represent an outbreak as each was caused by a different strain of group A streptococcus and the geographic pattern appeared to be coincidental.

Group B streptococci

Group B streptococci are commensals in the gut and vagina but can cause meningitis and septicaemia in the newborn if contamination occurs during delivery.

Viridans group

The viridans group of streptococci are commensals but are well known for their ability to cause endocarditis in patients with previously damaged heart valves, gaining access to the bloodstream after dental treatment.

Pneumococcus

The pneumococcus (*Streptococcus pneumoniae*) is a commensal in the respiratory tract. It causes a range of serious infections, including otitis media, pneumonia and meningitis. Some strains have become resistant to penicillin, and cross-infection has been attributed to a failure to identify and isolate infected patients and carriers.

Gram-negative infections

The initial conquest of nosocomial staphylococcal infection in the 1960s was followed by increasing colonisation and infection by coliform bacteria:

- *Pseudomonas*
- *Klebsiella*
- *Escherichia coli*
- *Proteus*

The coliforms

Coliforms survive in minute traces of moisture – on the hands (Burke *et al.,* 1971), on patients' skin (Montgommerie and Morrow, 1980) and on articles that come into direct contact with patients (Sanderson and Weissler, 1992). Coliforms had previously been considered to have very low pathogenic potential, but it soon became apparent that cross-infection could readily occur in acute and long-stay wards, contributing significantly to morbidity and mortality, especially among the critically ill (Swiatlo *et al.,* 1987). Coliforms are naturally resistant to many antibiotics, and the prevention of infection depends on adhering to the fundamental principles of infection control, especially handwashing, as environmental contamination readily occurs and reservoirs of infection may develop (Garland *et al.,* 1996). The bacteria may ascend to the bladder, colonise the gut and appear in the faeces, and can be transferred from the oropharynx to the lower respiratory passages, causing pneumonia.

Vancomycin-resistant enterococcal infection

Enterococcus faecalis and *Enterococcus faecium* are normal commensals in the human bowel but can cause urinary and wound infections in seriously ill patients. Enterococci are becoming a leading cause of nosocomial infection (Chadwick *et al.,*

1996), their emergence being associated with the widespread use of antibiotics, particularly cefotaxime (Quale *et al.*, 1996). Vancomycin-resistant enterococci (VRE) are readily disseminated within hospital, but much remains to be learned about their behaviour (Chadwick and Oppenheim, 1994). Hands probably operate as vectors, and environmental contamination is an important source (Bonten *et al.*, 1996). Cross-infection appears to be possible via contaminated clinical equipment such as thermometers (Livornese *et al.*, 1992). Enterococci are difficult to destroy. They can withstand exposure to the temperature currently recommended for bedpan washer–disinfector machines (80 ^{0}C for 1 minute) and high concentrations of hypochlorites (Kearns *et al.*, 1995). Environmental control is therefore difficult. However, the patient's condition frequently improves without specific treatment providing that the focus of infection (for example, a catheter) is removed. The withdrawal of all antibiotic therapy appears to be beneficial because it allows the bowel to recolonise with the patient's normal flora. There is still some debate concerning the value of isolation.

The infection control team in hospital

The Cooke Report (DHSS, 1988) recommended the provision of an infection control committee, an infection control nurse in all hospitals providing acute services, and the management of infection outbreaks. This was updated in 1995 to include guidance on routine surveillance and information for purchasers (DoH and PHLS, 1995).

The role of the infection control team

The infection control team is responsible for, and reports to the Chief Executive on, all aspects of the surveillance, prevention and control of infection in hospital. Its role is to implement an annual programme and policies of infection control, and to offer a 24-hour service to prevent and control infection, providing advice and education to all staff. The infection control doctor and nurse are key members of the team.

The infection control nurse

The infection control nurse is responsible for implementing the recommendations of the infection control team on a day-to-day basis. This involves liaison with staff at all levels and establishing educational programmes in addition to collecting surveillance data and ensuring that the annual programme is implemented. Some Trusts have established infection control link nurses at ward level to facilitate liaison between the clinical areas and the infection control team. They have an important role in providing early information to curtail possible outbreaks, and in drawing attention to changes in practice or equipment that may have implications for infection (Teare and Peacock, 1996).

The infection control committee

The infection control committee should cover every hospital. Membership should include the infection control doctor and nurse, the Chief Executive, the consultant in communicable disease control (CCDC) for the Health Authority in whose area the hospital is situated, the occupational doctor or nurse, the infectious diseases physician if there is one, senior clinical doctors and a senior clinical nurse. Other staff may be co-opted as necessary. The committee should meet at least twice a year. Its function is to collaborate with other staff in the prevention and control of infection (Table 6.4).

Table 6.4   Functions of the infection control committee

- To advise and support the infection control team
- To consider reports on infection and infection control problems
- To develop plans for managing outbreaks
- To plan, review and present the results of annual infection prevention and control programmes
- To advise on the most effective use of resources to control infection
- To advise on staff education programmes

Hospital infection control policies, guidelines and standards

In the UK, the Department of Health publishes a range of policy documents on issues related to hospital infection. These take the form of reports, safety bulletins, codes of practice and health notices sent as recommendations. Guidance is sought from an expert panel of medical microbiologists and pharmacists comprising the Microbiology Advisory Committee before publication and in response to specific enquiries from manufacturers. The information is implemented locally according to requirements.

Standards

Standards can be given for marketable products by an official body as independent confirmation that the equipment meets a required level of performance and safety, one example being the kite mark awarded by the British Standards Institute. Quality standards for healthcare products benefit manufacturers, patients and staff alike. If a fault develops during the manufacturing process, it is possible to determine from the manufacturer's detailed records the point at which it occurred and to recall all items from the same defective batch. Hospital purchasing policies usually demand British Standards Institute standards as the basis for informed

---

Clinical Application

Key Elements of an Effective Infection Control Policy

To be effective, a policy must fulfil the following criteria identified by Simpson (1991):

- The objectives should be clearly expressed
- The information should be easy to understand
- The information should be easy to find (for example, with adequate cross-referencing when necessary)
- The information should be practical as compliance with complicated, time-consuming procedures will be poor
- The necessary equipment must be readily available

---

selection. An example is the specification demanded for sharps disposal containers (BS 7320). There are, however, some exceptions for which no standard specifications have been developed and for which interest has only recently been registered, notably the bactericidal effectiveness of environmental and hand disinfectants (Simpson, 1991).

REVISION CHECKLIST: KEY AREAS

- ❏ Introduction – historical aspects of hospital infection

- ❏ The significance of nosocomial infection: The extent of nosocomial infection, Monitoring nosocomial infection

- ❏ Pathogens causing nosocomial infection: Staphylococcal infection, Streptococcal infection, Gram-negative infections

- ❏ The infection control team in hospital: The role of the infection control team, Hospital infection control policies, Guidelines and standards

Activities – linking knowledge to clinical practice

1 **Obtain** the infection control document used in your clinical setting. Select ONE section of particular interest or relevance (for example, the isolation policy or guidelines for decontaminating a particular piece of equipment) and critically evaluate it in terms of the recommendations suggested by Simpson (1991).

2 'Nosocomial infections are so widespread that efforts to control them are not worthwhile, especially as the most serious results occur mainly in the very elderly and sick, for whom the risk of mortality is already high.'

Debate this with either a group of students on your course or members of the nursing/medical team in your practice area.

3 Review the printed material available in your area for patients with MRSA:

(a) Is the information up to date?

(b) Is the information easy to understand?

(c) Does the material provide enough information?

(d) Does the material provide reassurance for patients and their families?

SELF-ASSESSMENT

1. Surgical wound infections are the most commonly acquired infections in hospital.   True? ☐ False? ☐

2. Surveillance of infection is conducted at national level in the UK.   True? ☐ False? ☐

3. Staphylococci are responsible for more nosocomial infections today than are streptococci.   True? ☐ False? ☐

4. Explain why MRSA is a particular infection control threat in hospitals.

5. Explain why EMRSA is a particular infection control threat in hospitals.

6. *Staphylococcus epidermidis* is coagulase positive.   True? ☐ False? ☐

7. VRE owes its pathogenicity to its ability to produce slime.   True? ☐ False? ☐

References

Ayton M (1981) 'An outbreak of streptococcal infection in a children's ward'. *Nursing Times* **77**(10): 13–15.

Beedle D (1993) 'Beating the bug'. *Nursing Times Journal of Infection Control* (Nursing Supplement) **89**(45): i–iv.

Bennett JV and Brachman PS (1979) *Hospital Infections*. Little, Brown, Boston.

Bonten M, Hayden MK, Nathan C et al. (1996) 'Epidemiology of colonisation of patients and environment with vancomycin-resistant enterococci'. Lancet 348: 1615–19.

Boyce JM (1991) 'Patterns of methicillin-resistant Staphylococcus aureus prevalence'. Infection Control and Hospital Epidemiology 12(2): 79–82.

Burke JP, Ingall D, Klein JO et al. (1971) 'Proteus mirabilis infections in a hospital nursery traced to a human carrier'. New England Journal of Medicine 284: 115–21.

Casewell MW (1986) 'Epidemiology and control of "modern" methicillin-resistant Staphylococcus aureus'. Journal of Hospital Infection (Supplement A) 7: 1–11.

Chadwick PR and Oppenheim BA (1994) 'Vancomycin-resistant enterococci and bedpan washer machines'. Lancet 344: 685.

Chadwick PR, Chadwick CD and Oppenheim BA (1996) 'Report of a meeting on the epidemiology and control of glycopeptide-resistant enterococci'. Journal of Hospital Infection 33: 89–92.

Combined Working Party of the British Society for Antimicrobial Chemotherapy, the Hospital Infection Society and the Infection Control Nurses Association (1998) 'Revised guidelines for the control of methicillin-resistant Staphylococcus aureus infection in hospital'. Journal of Hospital Infection 39: 259–90.

Cox RA, Mallaghan C, Conquest C et al. (1995) 'Epidemic methicillin-resistant Staphylococcus aureus: controlling the spread outside hospital'. Journal of Hospital Infection 29: 107–19.

Daum TE, Schaberg DR, Terpinning MS et al. (1990) 'Increasing resistance of Staphylococcus aureus to ciprofloxacin'. Antimicrobial Agents and Chemotherapy 34: 1862–3.

Davey P, Hernanz C, Lynch W et al. (1991) 'Human and non-financial costs of hospital acquired infection'. Journal of Hospital Infection (Supplement A) 18: 79–84.

Davies HD, McGeer A, Schwartz B et al. (1996) 'Invasive group A streptococcal infections in Ontario, Canada'. New England Journal of Medicine 335: 547–54.

Dawson SJ, Finn LF, McCulloch JE et al. (1994) 'Mupirocin-resistant MRSA'. Journal of Hospital Infection 28: 75–7.

Department of Health and Public Health Laboratory Service (1995) Hospital Infection Control. Guidance on the control of infection in hospitals. DoH/PHLS, London.

Department of Health and Social Security (1988) Hospital Infection Control. Guidance on the Control of Infection in Hospitals Prepared by the Joint DHSS/PHLS Hospital Infection Working Group (Cooke Report). HMSO, London.

Emmerson AM, Enstone JE, Griffin M et al. (1996) The second National Prevalence Survey of Infection in Hospitals – overview of the results'. Journal of Hospital Infection 32: 175–90.

French GL (1993) 'Closing the loop: audit in infection control'. Journal of Hospital Infection 24: 301–8.

French GL, Cheng AFB, Ling JL et al. (1990) 'Hong Kong strains of methicillin-resistant and methicillin-sensitive Staphylococcus aureus have similar virulence'. Journal of Hospital Infection 15: 117–25.

Garland SM, Mackay S, Tabrizi S et al. (1996) 'Pseudomonas outbreak associated with a contaminated blood gas analyser in a neonatal intensive care unit'. Journal of Hospital Infection 33: 145–51.

Glenister HM, Taylor LJ, Cooke EM et al. (1992) A Study of Surveillance Methods for Detecting Hospital Infection. PHLS, Colindale, London.

Glover S (1992) Making Medical Audit more Effective. Joint Centre for Education in Medicine, London.

Haley RW, Cuylver DH and White JW (1985) 'The efficacy of infection surveillance and control programs in preventing nosocomial infection in US hospitals'. American Journal of Epidemiology 121: 182–205.

Harmory BH and Parisi JT (1987) 'Staphylococcus epidermidis: a significant nosocomial pathogen'. Journal of Hospital Infection 15: 59–74.

Keane CT, Coleman DC and Cafferkey M (1991) 'Methicillin-resistant Staphylococcus aureus: a reappraisal'. Journal of Hospital Infection 19: 147–52.

Kearns AM, Freeman R and Lightfoot NF (1995) 'Nosocomial enterococci: resistance to heat and sodium hypochlorite'. *Journal of Hospital Infection* **30**: 193–9.

Livornese LL, Dias S, Samel C *et al.* (1992) 'Hospital-acquired infection with vancomycin-resistant *Enterococcus faecium* transmitted by electronic thermometers'. *Annals of Internal Medicine* **117**: 112–16.

Marples RR and Reith S (1992) 'Methicillin-resistant *Staphylococcus aureus* in England and Wales'. *Communicable Disease Report* **2**(3): R25–R29.

Marples RR, Richardson JF and de Saxe MJ (1985) 'Bacteriological characters of strains of *Staphylococcus aureus* submitted to a reference laboratory related to methicillin-resistance'. *Journal of Hygiene* **96**: 217–23.

Martin de Nicolas MM, Vindel A and Saez-Nieto JA (1995) 'Epidemiological typing of clinically significant strains of coagulase-negative staphylococci'. *Journal of Hospital Infection* **29**: 35–43.

Meers PD, Ayliffe GAJ, Emmerson AM *et al.* (1981) 'Report of the National Survey of Infection in Hospitals'. *Journal of Hospital Infection* **2**: 23–8.

Millward S, Barnett J and Thomlinson DA (1993) 'Clinical infection audit programme: evaluation of an audit tool used by infection control nurses to monitor standards and assess staff training'. *Journal of Hospital Infection* **24**: 219–32.

Montgommerie JZ and Morrow JW (1980) 'Long-term pseudomonas colonisation in spinal injury patients'. *American Journal of Epidemiology* **112**: 508–17.

Quale J, Landman D, Atwood E *et al.* (1996) 'Experience with a hospital wide outbreak of vancomycin-resistant enterococci'. *American Journal of Infection Control* **24**: 372–9.

Royal College of Nursing (1994) *Guidelines on Infection Control in Hospital.* RCN, London.

Sanderson PJ and Weissler S (1992) 'Recovery of coliforms from the hands of nurses and patients: activities leading to contamination'. *Journal of Hospital Infection* **21**: 85–93.

Sarangi J and Rowsell R (1995) 'A nursing home outbreak of Group A streptococcal infection: case control study of environmental contamination'. *Journal of Hospital Infection* **30**: 162–4.

Selwyn S (1991) 'Hospital infection: the first 2500 years'. *Journal of Hospital Infection* (Supplement A) **18**: 5–64.

Simpson RA (1991) 'Using guidelines , policies and standards. Are we in control?' *Journal of Hospital Infection* (Supplement A) **18**: 99–105.

Swiatlo E, Kocka C, Chittom AL *et al.* (1987) 'Survey of multiply resistant *Providenti stuartii* in a chronic care unit'. *Journal of Hospital Infection* **9**: 182–90.

Teare EL and Peacock A (1996) 'The development of an infection control link-nurse programme in a district general hospital'. *Journal of Hospital Infection* **34**: 267–78.

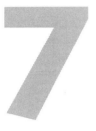

Urinary infections

CHAPTER OUTCOMES

After reading this chapter you should be able to:

- Define the terms 'bacteriuria', 'biofilm' and 'encrustation' and explain how these occur
- State the usual reasons for urinary catheterisation and justify why they are necessary in particular circumstances
- Suggest feasible alternatives to urinary catheterisation
- List the organisms commonly responsible for urinary infection
- State the complications associated with urinary catheterisation and urinary infection, explain how they arise and make recommendations for clinical practice (in the light of current research findings)
- Describe different methods for auditing the management of patients with indwelling urinary catheters

---

Introduction – urinary infection and catheterisation

Urinary infection accounts for nearly a quarter of all nosocomial infections. To understand the relative importance of urinary infection, it should be remembered that wound infection, which receives substantial publicity, represents some 10 per cent of nosocomial infection. Urinary infection is usually associated with catheterisation. Apart from the considerable discomfort to patients and the cost implications, urinary infection can cause serious side-effects, including septicaemia and death.

The use of urinary catheters

In a typical district general hospital within the UK, 10 per cent of inpatients are catheterised at some point during their admission (Mulhall *et al.,* 1988). This may be:

- Short term (1–7 days)

- Medium term (8–28 days)

- Long term (more than 28 days)

- Intermittently to relieve urinary retention in the patient with an atonic bladder or paraplegia. Self-catheterisation as a clean procedure is often performed by this client group, both in hospital and at home.

The average length of time for a catheter to remain in situ during short-term hospital use is 4 days (Crow *et al.,* 1986). Four per cent of patients nursed at home use catheters (Roe, 1989), the average period of catheterisation for this client group being 4 years, although catheterisation for up to 17 years has been recorded (Roe and Brocklehurst, 1987).

The complications of urinary catheterisation

Complications arising from urethral catheterisation represent a considerable nursing challenge. Infection is a major complication, significant because of its frequency and associated side-effects.

Urinary infection may result from a small inoculum of bacteria since the bladder has little defence against invading pathogens (Stickler and Chawla, 1987). Risk is increased by the presence of an indwelling urethral catheter because it operates as a foreign body, interfering with the normal process of the flushing effect that eliminates bacteria from the healthy bladder (Falkiner, 1993). Infections developing through catheterisation represent the most frequent and intractable infection control problem in hospital, likely to increase as the population ages (Kunin *et al.,* 1987a). The bacterial strains responsible are frequently antibiotic resistant. The move toward community care will not necessarily reduce the emergence of antibiotic resistance as many people nursed at home require intermittent admission for respite care or to undergo particular procedures, exposing them to hospital pathogens.

The risk of catheter-associated urinary infection is greatest for those with severe underlying illness and increases with the length of use. Up to half of all catheterised patients develop bacteriuria (the presence of bacteria in the urine) 100 000 pathogens in 1 ml of freshly voided urine representing an infection (Trilla *et al.,* 1991), inevitably appearing within 4 weeks (Slade and Gillespie, 1985). Catheter-associated urinary infection contributes directly to further morbidity and may result in mortality. Clifford (1982) estimated that 40 000–50 000 patients develop septicaemia as a result of ascending urinary infection every year in the UK, and that for a small but significant number (approximately 500), the consequences are fatal. This is supported by more recent data (Platt *et al.*, 1983; Kunin *et al.*, 1992). The best way to prevent urinary infection is to avoid catheterisation or, if it is inevitable, to remove the catheter as soon as possible (Jepson *et al.*, 1982).

Clinical Application

Alternatives to Indwelling Urinary Catheters

Possible alternatives include intermittent catheterisation, condom drainage systems and incontinence aids and garments. A careful assessment of individual patient/client need, coupled with a choice of appropriate equipment from the wide range now commercially available, enhances quality of care. Such alternatives may not, however, necessarily be associated with a reduction in infection rates: urinary tract infection may still occur with condom drainage systems (Montgommerie and Morrow, 1978). For individuals for whom no alternative to long-term catheterisation currently exists, it is worth trying newer products such as the conformable catheter, which conforms to the shape of the urethra and allows partial bladder filling (Brocklehurst *et al.,* 1988). The bladder no longer collapses, thus reducing the likelihood of irritation, bypassing and leakage.

Organisms responsible for urinary infection

Organisms responsible for urinary infection are mainly Gram-negative bacilli and *Staphylococcus epidermidis*. The ability to attach to the mucosal surface of the urinary tract enhances virulence. Most *Escherichia coli* urinary infections are caused by a few serotypes carrying a particular surface antigen (antigen K), which appears to offer protection against phagocytes. Certain strains of *Proteus* are particularly successful as urinary pathogens because pili enable them to attach to the host's epithelium. They are thus less easily dislodged, ascend the ureters and cause pyelonephritis. It may in future be possible to avoid infection by reducing their adherence to the bladder epithelium. Cranberry juice reduces adherence but its success in preventing infection has not yet been tested in controlled trials (Beachy, 1981; Sobota, 1984). The success of *Staphylococcus epidermidis* as a urinary pathogen is related to its ability to adhere to plastic surfaces (Pascual *et al.*, 1993).

Some bacteria contaminating urine float freely in suspension. Others adhere to surfaces, where they deposit extracellular secretions forming a biofilm (a layer of micro-organisms and proteins) on the sides of the catheter and drainage apparatus (Mulhall, 1991). This eventually forms a glycocalyx (protein and sugar coating), which becomes cemented into position, contributing to the problem of encrustation discussed below.

The closed urinary drainage system: portals of entry

The earliest indwelling catheters emptied into glass-stoppered bottles. The closed system of drainage was introduced by Dukes in 1928, but its value in preventing infection was not appreciated until the 1960s, when two independent teams established that it could reduce the development of sepsis from 80 per cent to 10 per cent (Gillespie, 1960; Sandford, 1964). The term 'closed drainage' is, however, not strictly accurate as there are numerous portals of entry for pathogens (Figure 7.1) and the system must be opened to allow emptying and be disconnected when the drainage bag is changed.

There is some debate concerning the source of pathogens responsible for catheter-associated urinary infection. Possible routes are indicated in Table 7.1, but there is disagreement over the most important. According to one school of thought, migration from the contaminated bag constitutes a major factor (Maizels and Shaeffer, 1980), contamination of the catheter from the drainage bag occurring within 24 hours (Rogers *et al.*, 1996). Another view holds that access via the periurethral space (that between the walls of the catheter and the urethra) is of greater importance (Garibaldi *et al.*, 1980). A resolution of this debate would be welcome in view of the associated clinical implications. Endemic and epidemic infections have been associated with contamination of the environment and nurses' hands by bacteria of the same strain (Shaberg *et al.*, 1976; Sanderson and Weissler, 1992). This does not, however, prove that they are exogenously acquired: organisms from the perianal region may first contaminate the immediate patient environment, colonise the hands of patients and nurses, and then gain access to the bladder when the catheter is manipulated. Whatever the source, a strict regimen of hand hygiene on the part of both patient and nurse is necessary before and after the system is handled.

Table 7.1   Access of pathogens to the 'closed system' of drainage

- On the catheter tip during insertion

- During disconnection of drainage bag and tubing (accidental or planned change)

- Migration along the lumen of the catheter from a contaminated drainage system

- Migration via the periurethral space in the film of moisture between the outside of the catheter and the urethra

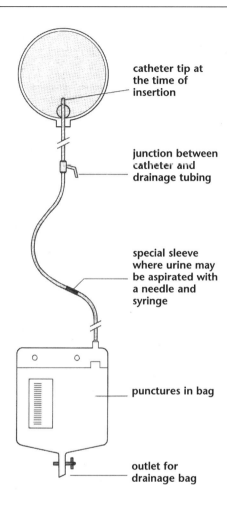

catheter tip at
the time of
insertion

junction between
catheter and
drainage tubing

special sleeve
where urine may
be aspirated with
a needle and
syringe

punctures in bag

outlet for
drainage bag

Figure 7.1   The 'closed system' of catheter drainage: portals of entry

Complications secondary to urinary infection in catheterised patients

Complications secondary to urinary infection include:

- Encrustation
- Blockage
- Leakage
- Pain and discomfort

All are related to infection and to each other (Ferrie, 1979).

Encrustation

Encrustation affects 16–28 per cent of catheterised patients. Bacteria collecting on the surfaces of the catheter and drainage apparatus secrete extracellular products to form a biofilm (Mulhall *et al.*, 1993). Surfaces in direct contact with the urethral and bladder epithelia are protected by a mucus layer that prevents the deposits of adherence (Kunin *et al.*, 1987b). Encrustations consist of calcium and magnesium salts precipitated as large crystals and smaller, powdery deposits. Infection with *Proteus* is particularly likely to cause encrustation because members of this genus secrete an enzyme, urease, that catabolises urea to produce ammonium ions. The resulting highly alkaline urine favours the formation of insoluble salts, which precipitate from solution.

Blockage

Blockages develop when the eyes of the catheter become occluded as the sequel to encrustation.

Leakage

Leakage around the outside of the catheter follows blockage.

Pain and discomfort

Pain and discomfort are experienced if rigid or irritant catheters remain in the bladder. If a leaking catheter is replaced with a larger one, the problem is exacerbated and discomfort increases.

Recommendations for clinical practice: reducing the problems of catheterisation

Recommendations for clinical practice are possible, although, as indicated above, some questions remain unanswered and more research is needed.

Choice of catheter material

Many catheters are made of plastic or latex. These substances are inexpensive but not suitable for long-term indwelling catheters because they are particularly irritant (Belfield, 1988). Teflon, silicone, silicone–teflon combinations, elastomers and hydrogels are newer, more suitable materials, their smooth finish being less likely to result in encrustation or irritation (Cox *et al.*, 1988). Some patients are more likely to develop encrustations than others, suggesting that the formation of deposits is not simply a reaction between alkaline urine and the catheter. It is possible to identify patients particularly at risk of developing encrustations (Kunin *et al.*, 1987b) and to plan their care accordingly.

Catheter length

Catheter length should be determined by the length of the urethra. The standard catheter length for males is 40 cm. For females in whom the urethra is on average 15 cm shorter, the standard length is 25 cm. Women should not be given male-length catheters because this increases the risk of kinking and dragging, leading to accidental disconnection. An excessively long catheter is also more difficult to conceal beneath clothing if the individual is mobile.

Clinical Application

Indicators of Catheter Blockage

It is possible to identify patients at risk of recurrent catheter blockage. The results of a prospective longitudinal study with 47 catheterised patients nursed in the community provided firm evidence that catheter blockage was strongly related to problems of leakage and urinary retention but not to the length of time the catheter had been *in situ*, to fluid intake or to the type of drainage bag employed. The 18 patients for whom blockage was a problem needed recatheterisation at least every 6 weeks, had a higher urinary pH than others in the sample and showed a higher concentration of ammonium ions. These characteristics could be used to identify patients more likely to develop a blocked catheter, enabling nurses to plan care rather than resorting to crisis management, as so often happens at present (Getliffe, 1994).

Catheter gauge

Catheter gauge is measured using a unit called a Charrière (Ch), 1 Ch measuring 0.33 mm. The optimal gauge is 12–16 Ch for males and 12–14 Ch for females. Larger gauges are not usually justified because a 12 Ch catheter is capable of draining 100 litres of fluid over 24 hours, a capacity far greater than the actual requirement. Larger dimensions are necessary only when problems are anticipated. For example, experience may show that particular patients produce urine containing considerable amounts of debris, and these may fare better with 18 Ch catheters. Following transurethral prostatectomy, a 22 Ch gauge catheter is essential to drain blood clots. There is no justification for fitting a larger gauge catheter than that required: it will irritate the urethral mucosa, promoting bypassing and leakage, and will be painful (Crow *et al.*, 1986).

Balloons

Balloons are available in two standard sizes, 10 ml and 30 ml, with smaller and larger ones intended for special purposes. A larger size might be required for a

---

Clinical Application

Summary Checklist for Safer Catheterisation

The decisions taken by nurses prior to inserting a urinary catheter can have far-reaching consequences for the patient. Making the correct choices can reduce the incidence of catheter-related complications, especially infection.

Checklist

- Does this patient really need a urinary catheter or is there a viable alternative?
- Does the patient and his or her carer possess sufficient information to understand and accept the need for urinary catheterisation?
- Do I need to consult another professional?
- Choose a catheter of the correct size – usually 12–14 Ch for females and 12–16 Ch for males.
- Choose a catheter length to suit the gender – 25 cm for females and 40 cm for males.
- Choose the most appropriate catheter material for the length of time the patient is likely to be catheterised and for particular personal characteristics.
- Choose an indwelling catheter with a 10 ml balloon for routine use.
- Choose the most appropriate bag and drainage system.
- Use aseptic technique with sterile gloves for catheter insertion.
- Instil anaesthetic lubricating gel into the urethra prior to catheterisation.
- Choose non-irritant antiseptic solutions for perineal cleansing.
- Ask again whether catheterisation is the only option for this patient.

---

woman with weak pelvic muscles catheterised in the long term, or to prevent bleeding from the prostate bed following surgery. The 10 ml size is recommended for routine use. The catheterised bladder is always fully drained and thus permanently collapsed. A larger balloon would be in greater contact with the bladder wall and would therefore be more likely to cause irritation. Larger balloons induce leakage (Kennedy *et al.*, 1983) and can damage the bladder neck (Kristiansen *et al.*, 1983). Balloons should be filled with sterile water because saline may crystallise, blocking the inflation channel. Deflation and removal are then difficult.

Insertion

Insertion should be performed with an aseptic technique using sterile gloves and equipment, anaesthetic gel being used before the catheter is inserted. Some authors recommend cleansing the perineum with chlorhexidine (Cohen, 1985) or povidone iodine (Flynn and Blandy, 1980) immediately before insertion in order to reduce sepsis. However, these irritate delicate tissue if contact is prolonged, and caution must be exercised if they are used for this purpose.

Management and choice of drainage system

Management and choice of drainage system also merit consideration in view of their possible contribution to infection.

Choice of bag

The following features for the bag are highly desirable: a self sealing sleeve to allow the aspiration of specimens without breaking the system. This should be disinfected with alcohol before a sample is collected (Simpson *et al.*, 1995). The system should have non-return valves and a sufficient length of tubing for the bag to hang free. The outlet should never touch the floor and the bag should always be positioned lower than the bladder so that the urine drains under gravity.

Emptying

Emptying disrupts the closed system of drainage. Frequent emptying is sometimes avoided because it may increase risk of contamination (Platt *et al.*, 1983; Crow *et al.*, 1986). However, a full bag becomes heavy and drags uncomfortably, especially in mobile patients. It looks unsightly and the contents develop an odour. The decision of when to empty is thus a judgement made according to individual circumstance. Hands and the environment can become contaminated during emptying (Glenister, 1987), so gloves should be worn and the hands should be decontaminated before and afterwards. 'Catheter rounds', in which one pair of gloves is worn and one receptacle used to empty a number of bags in sequence, are not considered good practice because they offer so many opportunities for contamination, although Mulhall *et al.* (1993) report satisfactory decontamination of gloved hands using an alcoholic rub between patients. Cross-infection can be avoided by using sterile receptacles. This may not be possible on the grounds of expense, but disposables provide an acceptable alternative (Roe, 1993). Failing this, the receptacle can be put through the bedpan washer between uses.

Bag changes

Bag changes involve disconnection of the closed system and may be avoided to reduce this situation. The Department of Health recommends a change after 5–7 days, a figure supported by research findings (Rogers *et al.*, 1996). Prompt disposal is essential in hospital to prevent cross-infection. Suggestions that bags could be reused in the community may be impractical as people at home may lack the facilities to decontaminate bags adequately, or may be unable to do so through lack of manual dexterity if they are disabled or infirm (Roe, 1993).

Additives to the drainage system

Additives to the drainage system are no longer thought to offer any advantage in preventing infection and are ineffective once infection has become established (Stickler *et al.*, 1987).

Meatal care

Meatal care remains an area in which firm recommendations cannot currently be made. The results of trials involving the use of disinfectants such as chlorhexidine and povidone iodine have produced mixed results (Falkiner, 1993). Until more research becomes available, the aim of meatal care should be to keep the patient clean and comfortable by washing the area at least twice daily with soap and water. Harsh disinfectants may damage the surrounding epithelium, leading to inflammation and discomfort.

Irrigation

Irrigation is essential after transurethral prostatectomy to relieve physical blockage by blood clots and may be necessary for patients catheterised in the long term if encrustations form. It is possible to anticipate problems and employ catheters with three-way taps so that irrigation can be performed without disconnecting the drainage system. Proprietary solutions intended for instillation in order to reduce encrustation are available. Most are weakly acidic and may help by reducing pH, thus decreasing urease activity as well as exerting mechanical action, but their value in controlled trials has yet to be established.

Patient education

Patient education in relation to catheter care has traditionally been poor (Roe and Brocklehurst, 1987). In an experimental study, subjects receiving an educational intervention and an information booklet proved more knowledgeable about the function of the catheter and its associated risks as well as demonstrating better handwashing performance, although this was not sustained over time (Roe, 1989). The author concluded that it is worth educating patients about their catheters, that teaching should begin as soon as the need for catheterisation is apparent and that it should be reinforced at regular intervals.

Auditing the use of urinary catheters

Urinary infections were the most common nosocomial infection reported during the second National Prevalence Survey, occurring in 23 per cent of patients, mainly those with catheters. They were especially common in urosurgical and gynaecology patients over 75 years of age (Emmerson *et al.*, 1996). A study by Crow *et al.* (1986) revealed that 44 per cent of patients developed significant bacteriuria within 72 hours, this figure rising to 90 per cent 17 days later. Preventing catheter-associated urinary infection and its attendant problems remains an important challenge, and an audit of guidelines has been suggested as one of the ways forward (French, 1993). Process and outcome measures are available (Curran, 1993; Table 7.2).

Table 7.2   Auditing the use of urinary catheters

Process

- ▪ To determine the incidence of urinary tract infections among catheterised patients
- ▪ To assess whether the use of indwelling urethral catheters is appropriate
- ▪ To determine whether the choice of catheter is appropriate (according to research findings)
- ▪ To determine whether catheter care is appropriate (according to research findings)
- ▪ To identify catheter-associated procedures that could be avoided if their use were abandoned
- ▪ To target infection control and other resources to clinical settings with a high incidence of catheter-associated problems
- ▪ To ensure that nursing and medical staff have the knowledge and resources to select, insert and maintain catheters and give appropriate care to patients

Outcome

- ▪ To reduce the incidence of urinary tract infection in catheterised patients
- ▪ To reduce patients' discomfort and inconvenience
- ▪ To reduce costs through the appropriate use of resources

REVISION CHECKLIST: KEY AREAS

- ❏ Introduction – urinary infection and catheterisation: The use of urinary catheters, The complications of urinary catheterisation, Organisms responsible for urinary infection

- ❏ The closed urinary drainage system: portals of entry: Complications secondary to urinary infection in catheterised patients

- ❏ Recommendations for clinical practice: reducing the problems of catheterisation:

Choice of catheter material, Catheter length, Catheter gauge, Balloons, Insertion

- ❏ Management and choice of drainage system: Choice of bag, Emptying, Bag changes, Additives to the drainage system, Meatal care, Irrigation, Patient education

- ❏ Auditing the use of urinary catheters

Activities – linking knowledge to clinical practice

1 **Find** out whether routine statistics for urinary infection are maintained in your clinical area. (This could be an entire hospital, a particular ward or department, or a community nursing caseload.) Establish who is responsible for compiling the records and the criteria used to determine whether a patient has a clinical infection. If appropriate, examine the figures to see how they compare with the results of the Second National Prevalence Survey findings (Emmerson *et al.*, 1996).

2 **Is there** a system of audit to monitor the rate of urinary infection or the use of catheters within your clinical setting? Is it satisfactory? What criteria would you employ to set up a more valid and reliable system? How would you communicate your findings?

SELF-ASSESSMENT

1. Bacteriuria is:
   (a) the presence of 100 000 or more pathogens per ml of urine ☐
   (b) the presence of sufficient bacteria in the urine to give rise to clinical infection ☐
   (c) the presence of sufficient bacteria in the urine to give rise to the signs and symptoms of urinary infection ☐
   (d) the presence of neutrophils in urine ☐

2. A biofilm is:
   (a) a collection of mineral salts bound to a solid surface ☐
   (b) a collection of micro-organisms and their extracellular products bound to a solid surface ☐
   (c) a collection of mineral salts bound to a catheter ☐
   (d) calcium and magnesium salts bound to a solid surface ☐

3. The size of the inoculating dose necessary to result in a urinary infection is small since the bladder has few defences against invading pathogens. True? ☐ False? ☐

4. The size of the inoculating dose necessary to result in a urinary infection is small since the bacteria responsible are highly virulent. True? ☐ False? ☐

5. Which of the following are common urinary pathogens?
   (a) *Staphylococcus epidermidis* ☐
   (b) *Escherichia coli* ☐
   (c) *Mycobacterium tuberculosis* ☐
   (d) *Bacteroides* ☐
   (e) *Mycobacterium leprae* ☐
   (f) *Proteus* ☐

6. Complications secondary to urinary infection include ....

References

Beachy EH (1981) 'Bacterial adherence: adhesion receptor interactions mediating the attachment of bacteria to mucosal surfaces'. *Journal of Infectious Diseases* **143**: 325–45.

Belfield PW (1988) 'Urinary catheters'. *British Medical Journal* **296**: 836–7.

Brocklehurst JC, Hickley DS, Davies I *et al.* (1988) 'A new urethral catheter'. *British Medical Journal* **296**: 1691–3.

Clifford CM (1982) 'Urinary tract infection: a brief selective review'. *International Journal of Nursing Studies* **19**: 213–22.

Cohen A (1985) 'A microbiological comparison of a povidone iodine lubricating gel and a control as catheter lubricants'. *Journal of Hospital Infection* (Supplement) **6**: 155–61.

Cox AJ, Hukins DWL and Sutton TM (1988) 'Comparison of in vitro encrustation on silicone and hydrogel coated latex catheters'. *British Journal of Urology* **61**: 156–61.

Crow R, Chapman R, Roe B *et al.* (1986) *Study of Patients with an Indwelling Urinary Catheter and Related Nursing Practice.* Nursing Practice Research Unit, University of Surrey.

Curran E (1993) 'A programme to audit the use of urinary catheters'. *Journal of Clinical Nursing* **1**: 329–34.

Emmerson AM, Enstone JE, Griffin M *et al.* (1996) 'The Second National Prevalence Survey of Infection in Hospitals – overview of the results'. *Journal of Hospital Infection* **32**: 175–90.

Falkiner FR (1993) 'The insertion and management of indwelling urethral catheters – minimising the risk of infection'. *Journal of Hospital Infection* **25**: 79–90.

Ferrie BCT (1979) 'Long term catheter drainage'. *British Medical Journal* **2**: 1946–7.

Flynn JT and Blandy JP (1980) 'Urethral catheterisation'. *British Medical Journal* **281**: 928–30.

French GL (1993) 'Closing the loop: audit in infection control'. *Journal of Hospital Infection* **24**: 301–8.

Garibaldi RA, Burke JP, Britt A *et al.* (1980) 'Meatal colonisation and catheter-associated bacteriuria'. *New England Journal of Medicine* **303**: 316–18.

Getliffe KA (1994) 'The characteristics and management of patients with recurrent blockage of long-term urinary catheters'. *Journal of Advanced Nursing* **20**: 140–9.

Gillespie WA (1960) 'The diagnosis, epidemiology and control of urinary tract infection in urology and gynaecology'. *Journal of Clinical Pathology* **13**: 187–94.

Glenister H (1987) 'The passage of infection'. *Nursing Times* **83**(22): 68–73.

Jepson OB, Olesen Larsen S and Dankert J (1982) 'Urinary tract infection and bacteriuria in hospitalised medical patients – a European multicentre prevalence survey of nosocomial infection'. *Journal of Hospital Infection* **3**: 241–52.

Kennedy AP, Brocklehurst JC and Lye M (1983) 'Factors related to the problems of long-term catheterisation'. *Journal of Advanced Nursing* **8**: 207–12.

Kristiansen P, Pompeius R and Wadstrom LB (1983) 'Long-term urethral catheter drainage and bladder capacity'. *Neurology and Urodynamics* **2**: 135–43.

Kunin CM, Chin QF and Chambers A (1987a) 'Indwelling urinary catheters in the elderly'. *American Journal of Medicine* **82**: 405–11.

Kunin CM, Chin QF and Chambers A (1987b) 'Formation of encrustations on indwelling urinary catheters in the elderly'. *Journal of Urology* **138**: 899–902.

Kunin CM, Douthitt S, Daning J *et al.* (1992) 'The association between the use of urinary catheters and morbidity and mortality among elderly patients in nursing homes'. *American Journal of Epidemiology* **135**: 291–301.

Maizels M and Schaeffer AJ (1980) 'Decreased incidence of bacteriuria associated with instillation of hydrogen peroxide into the urethra catheter drainage bag'. *Journal of Urology* **123**: 841–5.

Montgommerie JZ and Morrow JW (1978) 'Pseudomonas colonisation in patients with spinal cord injury'. *American Journal of Epidemiology* **108**: 328–36.

Mulhall A (1991) 'Biofilms and urethral catheter infections'. *Nursing Standard* **5**(18): 26–8.

Mulhall A, Chapman RG and Crow RA (1988) 'Bacteriuria during indwelling catheterisation'. *Journal of Hospital Infection* **11**: 235–62.

Mulhall A, King S, Lee K *et al.* (1993) 'Maintenance of closed urinary drainage systems: are practitioners more aware of the dangers?' *Journal of Clinical Nursing* **2**: 135–40.

Pascual A, Ramirez de Arellano E, Martinez-Martinez L *et al.* (1993) 'Effect of polyurethane catheters and bacterial biofilms on the in vitro activity of antimicrobials against *Staphylococcus epidermidis. Journal of Hospital Infection* **24**: 211–18.

Platt R, Polk BF, Murdoch B *et al.* (1983) 'Reduction of mortality associated with nosocomial urinary tract infection'. *Lancet* **1**: 893–7.

Roe B (1989) 'Long-term catheter care in the community'. *Nursing Times* **85**(36): 43–4.

Roe B (1993) 'Catheter-associated urinary tract infection: a review'. *Journal of Clinical Nursing* **2**: 197–203.

Roe B and Brocklehurst JC (1987) 'Study of patients with indwelling catheters'. *Journal of Advanced Nursing* **12**: 713–18.

Rogers J, Norkett DI, Bracegirdle P *et al.* (1996) 'Examination of biofilm formation and risk of infection associated with the use of urinary catheters with leg bags'. *Journal of Hospital Infection* **32**: 105–15.

Sanderson PJ and Weissler S (1992) 'Recovery of coliforms from the hands of nurses and patients: activities leading to contamination'. *Journal of Hospital Infection* **21**: 85–94.

Sandford JP (1964) 'Hospital acquired urinary tract infection'. *Annals of Internal Medicine* **60**: 903–14.

Shaberg DR, Weinstein RA and Stamm WE (1976) 'Epidemics of nosocomial urinary tract infection caused by multiply-resistant Gram-negative bacilli: epidemiology and control of infection'. *Journal of Infectious Diseases* **133**: 363–6.

Simpson LR, Babb JR and Fraise AP (1995) 'Infection risk and potential contamination of urine specimens associated with sample port design of catheter leg bags'. *Journal of Hospital Infection* **30**: 95–102.

Slade N and Gillespie WA (1985) *The Urinary Tract and the Catheter: Infection and Other Problems.* John Wiley & Sons, Chichester.

Sobota AE (1984) 'Inhibition of bacterial adherence by cranberry juice: potential use for urinary tract infections'. *Journal of Urology* **131**: 1013–16.

Stickler DJ and Chawla JC (1987) 'The role of antiseptics in the management of patients with long term indwelling bladder catheters'. *Journal of Hospital Infection* **10**: 219–28.

Stickler DJ, Clayton CL and Chawla JC (1987) 'The resistance of urinary tract pathogens to chlorhexidine bladder washouts'. *Journal of Hospital Infection* **10**: 28–39.

Trilla A, Gatell M, Mensa J *et al.* (1991) 'Risk factors for nosocomial bacteraemia in a large Spanish teaching hospital: a case control study'. *Infection Control and Hospital Epidemiology* **12**: 150–6.

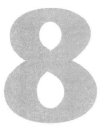

Wound infections

CHAPTER OUTCOMES

After reading this chapter you should be able to:

■ Explain the terms 'collagen', 'fibroblast', 'connective tissue' and 'granulation'

■ Explain what is meant by healing by first and secondary intention, and primary and secondary wound closure

■ Name the four categories of wound described by the National Research Council (1964) and state their significance when calculating wound infection rates

■ Discuss the criteria used to determine wound infection

■ Describe each of the stages of tissue repair

■ State the factors that contribute to the development of wound infection

■ Describe the ideal wound healing environment

■ Debate the role of the aseptic dressing techniques in the treatment of surgical and chronic wounds

---

Introduction to wounds and wound healing

The ability of tissues to undergo repair depends on:

■ **The condition of the wound** (the specific microenvironment), which is influenced by the wound dressing. As shown in Figure 8.1, healing proceeds better in a wound that has been covered as a moist environment encourages cells to multiply and migrate more easily across the wound surface (Winter, 1962). A second important function of the dressing is occlusion: extraneous pathogens are prevented from contaminating the wound while organisms already present are unable to escape, preventing cross-infection.

■ **The patient's general health**: nutritional status, metabolic disturbance and genetically inherited traits (for example, haemophilia) are important.

A holistic approach is therefore appropriate in order to promote healing and prevent infection, taking both the above factors into consideration.

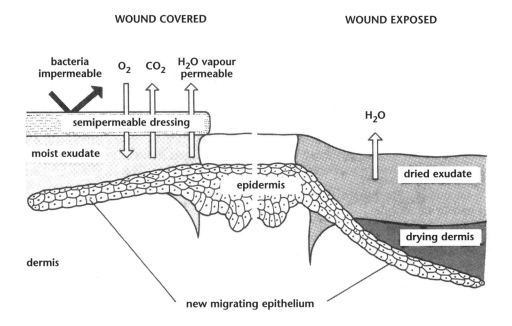

Figure 8.1   Difference between a covered and an exposed wound

There is still considerable ignorance about the ideal wound healing environment. Until the 1960s, the most effective healing environment was considered to be a dry wound covered by a scab. This view was challenged by Winter (1962), who undertook trials to measure the rate of epithelialisation (the process by which epidermal cells regenerate and move from the wound edges to grow across the raw area) of superficial wounds in the skin of young pigs. Half of the wounds were exposed to air so that they would dry out. The other half were occluded with a polythene film dressing to create a moist environment at the wound surface. The covered wounds healed twice as fast as those which had been exposed. Today, it is accepted that dressings that create a moist environment promote healing (Table 8.1), but nurses have been slow to acknowledge these findings (Murray, 1988).

Table 8.1   Characteristics of the ideal wound dressing

- Absorbs excess exudate and toxins
- Maintains a moist environment over the wound surface
- Permits gaseous exchange
- Presents an occlusive barrier to micro-organisms
- Provides thermal insulation
- Does not contain particulate contaminants
- Is non-adherent

The skin is the body's major barrier against invading pathogens; when it is no longer intact, infection becomes a major risk. In the case of surgical wounds, infection usually originates in theatre (Pollock and Evans, 1983). The surfaces of chronic wounds (pressure sores and leg ulcers, for example) are frequently covered in micro-organisms, some of which are capable of operating as pathogens (Leaper, 1995), but there is no evidence that they interfere with healing in normal circumstances (Brennan *et al.*, 1985). The presence of foreign material is, however, known to slow healing and increase the risk of infection in all types of wound (Johnson, 1988).

Historical aspects of wound care

In the past, the development of sepsis with the formation of pus was considered not only normal, but also desirable. Many different substances were applied to secure it. One of the earliest records from a Mesopotamian clay tablet from 2500 BC advocated the use of honey and resin, which have antiseptic properties (Forrest, 1982). Some people remain enthusiastic about these 'natural' remedies, but the modern approach to wound healing, with its emphasis on occlusion and providing a moist environment, is more effective than folk cures.

During the 16th century, air was considered particularly injurious to healing tissues, so wounds were kept warm, dark and moist until the 1860s, when Lister discovered that applying carbolic spray to surgical dressings reduced infection. His discovery was possible because major advances were made in chemistry throughout the 1800s, notably the isolation of chlorine and iodine, which have disinfectant properties. Through Lister's work and the increasing sophistication of anaesthesia, longer operations became possible, and a higher proportion of patients survived. Today, the care of patients undergoing surgery remains an important nursing responsibility. However, the prevention of surgical sepsis also depends on the patient's general health and the surgeon's skill. The care of patients with other types of wound, for example leg ulcers, is a major and growing nursing challenge.

Classifying wounds

Numerous categories of wound classification exist. The amount of tissue lost and the extent of contamination are among those most commonly employed. Both influence the risk of infection.

Amount of tissue lost

There are two categories here:

- Wounds in which there is minimal tissue loss (a cut with a knife or a surgical incision) and healing occurs by first intention (see below).

- Wounds where extensive tissue is lost and healing is by secondary intention (see below), with more extensive tissue replacement and regeneration (as seen, for example, with pressure sores, varicose ulcers and burns). This type of wound is more often contaminated and heals more slowly so there is greater scope for infection to supervene. In the case of non-surgical wounds, the patient's underlying poor health may have contributed to the development of the lesion in the first place: unless attention is paid to factors such as nutrition and hydration, healing may not occur at all. The choice of an appropriate dressing plays a key role in the healing of wounds in this category (Westaby, 1985).

Table 8.2   Wound classification (adapted from the National Research Council system of wound classification, 1964)

- **Clean wounds**: no inflammation, no lapse in aseptic technique during surgery and no entry into the respiratory and gastrointestinal tracts. Cholecystectomy, hysterectomy and appendicectomy without evidence of inflammation are placed in the clean category

- **Clean contaminated wounds**: those generated by surgical procedures that involve entry into the respiratory or gastrointestinal tract, but where no significant spillage has occurred

- **Contaminated wounds**: evidence of acute inflammation without the formation of pus, or where gross spillage has occurred from a hollow internal organ. An otherwise clean operation in which there has been a major breach of aseptic technique and recent traumatic wounds are considered to be contaminated

- **Dirty wounds**: pus or a perforated internal organ is encountered. Traumatic wounds not of recent origin are also placed in this category

Extent of wound contamination

This system was developed by the National Research Council (1964) to allow a direct comparison of infection rates between wounds likely to share similar degrees of contamination. Operations performed at anatomical locations that are normally sterile and those in parts of the body where bacteria are present clearly cannot be expected to show a similar rate of sepsis.

The stages of wound healing are outlined below, drawing attention to factors that may influence the development of sepsis. The process of healing is divided into numerous stages for convenience, but in reality they overlap and the process is continuous.

Stages of wound healing

There are two main phases:

1. The **proliferative** phase, when most tissue regeneration takes place
2. The phase of **maturation**, when the new tissues become stronger.

Proliferative phase

The proliferative phase encompasses (Figures 8.2 and 8.3):

■ The inflammatory response
■ Collagen synthesis: tissue regeneration and the replacement of cells lost through trauma
■ Angiogenesis: the formation of new blood vessels
■ Epithelialisation to cover the raw, wounded surface.

Healing by first intention

The inflammatory response

The inflammatory response continues for approximately 3 days (see Chapter 2). Heavy contamination (with bacteria or cellular debris) prolongs inflammation and interferes with healing and the cosmetic result. Surgical debridement may be necessary to prevent complications.

Collagen synthesis

Collagen synthesis commences as inflammation subsides and the macrophages responsible for ingesting debris in the wound attract fibroblast cells to the local area. Fibroblasts are connective tissue cells producing collagen, a tough protein that gives strength to skin, bone and tendons. Collagen forms a meshwork to support the granulation tissue that will eventually fill the cleft of the wound. Collagen synthesis reaches a peak between the fifth and seventh postoperative day and proceeds more effectively in moist, occluded wounds. Infection disrupts healing; many pathogens release an enzyme called collagenase, which digests collagen fibres, reducing the strength of the new tissue. Collagen synthesis is promoted at low pH in an environment where high concentrations of lactate ions and vitamin C are present. These conditions are most prevalent deep within the tissues, where cells that are still viable undergo metabolism to release lactate. Thus, collagen formation begins deep within the undamaged areas and works outwards.

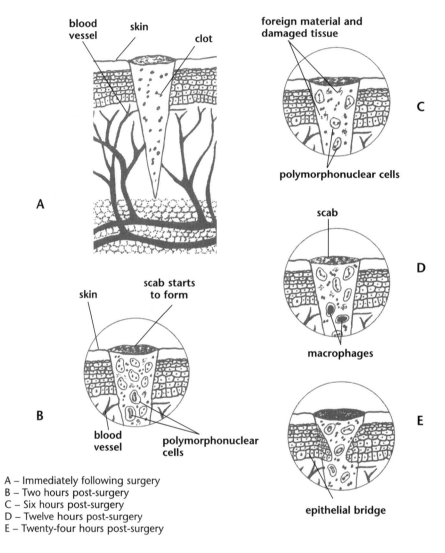

A – Immediately following surgery
B – Two hours post-surgery
C – Six hours post-surgery
D – Twelve hours post-surgery
E – Twenty-four hours post-surgery

Figure 8.2   Hour-by-hour view of the wound healing process I (adapted from Westaby, 1985)

Angiogenesis

Angiogenesis commences deep in the tissues, just as collagen formation is occurring. New capillaries are stimulated by low oxygen tension to grow from the healthy margins of the wound and invade the area of regeneration.

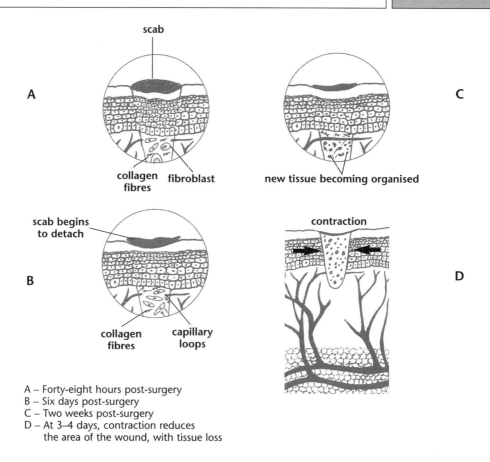

A – Forty-eight hours post-surgery
B – Six days post-surgery
C – Two weeks post-surgery
D – At 3–4 days, contraction reduces
    the area of the wound, with tissue loss

Figure 8.3　Hour-by-hour view of the wound healing process II (adapted from Westaby, 1985)

Epithelialisation

Epithelialisation commences within 24 hours in a clean wound with minimal tissue loss. Healthy epidermal cells at the edges of the wound multiply and then move in a sheet across the surface until the raw area is completely covered by a new, intact layer, several cells thick (Figure 8.3). In dry wounds, new epithelial cells cannot migrate as effectively as they would in a moist environment because their progress is impeded by collagen fibres attaching the hard scab to the underlying dermis. Where the cells meet at the middle of the damaged area, further movement is inhibited. Once epithelialisation is complete, a protein called keratin is deposited in skin cells, making them tough and waterproof. Cells lining the sebaceous glands and hair follicles present in the skin also multiply and migrate first upwards and then over the wound surface, contributing to epithelialisation. Severely damaged tissues (such as full-thickness burns) take longer to undergo epithelialisation because the sebaceous glands and hair follicles are lost: skin grafting may be necessary.

Epithelial cells retain the ability to multiply throughout the life of the individual because they are undifferentiated (that is, they have not undergone specialisation). Highly differentiated tissues (for example, neurones and muscle cells) are unable to multiply after embryonic life, and when irrevocably damaged can be replaced only by non-functional scar tissue. Epithelialisation seals the wound from pathogenic invasion, but the new cells are delicate so the tissue must be handled gently. The epithelialisation of a clean surgical wound is generally complete by the third post-operative day; this is why dressings applied in the operating theatre are usually kept intact until this time. Once an intact layer of cells has formed, the protective scab from the blood clot previously covering the damaged area is able to slough away. At one time, it was common to swab clean wounds with normal saline or other solutions. This practice is now discouraged, being a waste of time and resources. Unnecessary interference may also traumatise the fragile new tissue and increases the possibility of contamination (Johnson, 1988). A scab visible over a wound is indicative of underlying repair and should not be removed.

Healing by secondary intention

Healing by secondary intention occurs when there has been greater tissue loss and more granulation tissue is needed to occupy the resulting space. Healing occurs mainly by contraction effected by specialised cells in the granulation tissue, called myofibroblasts; epithelialisation is of less importance than in lesions where tissue loss has been slight (Leaper, 1995). Tissue repair is often prolonged, with repeated episodes of inflammation, fibroblast activity, excessive formation of collagen and renewed damage. Scarring can be pronounced because of the formation of excess granulation tissue. However, scarring from exuberant granulation can result in poorly managed surgical wounds, and there may be hypertrophy in chronic or surgical wounds that have become infected: the inflammatory response is prolonged and necrotic tissue, foreign bodies or excess suture material may be retained.

Phase of maturation

The signs and symptoms of inflammation gradually subside during the proliferative phase of healing in surgical and properly managed non-surgical lesions, but the wound retains its red, raised appearance and may feel itchy for several months. The collagen fibres are haphazardly arranged. Throughout the phase of maturation, which may take up to a year, they realign at right angles to the direction of wounding. This laces the edges together in a tight three-dimensional weave. As maturation progresses, the wound becomes less vascular, the fibroblasts shrink and the tissue becomes stronger, although this varies between tissues of different types. Intestinal anastomoses may regain the strength of the original tissue within 7 days. Skin and fascia slowly regain strength.

Surgical intervention and approaches to wound repair

Minor wounds heal spontaneously. When damage is more extensive, surgical intervention is required to speed tissue repair, avoid infection and help to reduce deformity. The approach chosen will depend on the amount of tissue lost. The edges of a clean wound can be sutured together if there has been minimal tissue loss. When extensive areas of tissue have been removed, plastic surgery is necessary, employing flaps or skin grafts. The method of closure is dictated by the estimated risk of infection. Experience with traumatic wounds sustained during warfare have illustrated the dangers associated with the immediate closure of heavily contaminated wounds: abscess formation, septicaemia and dehiscence. Three approaches to wound repair are possible (Figure 8.4):

- Primary closure
- Delayed primary closure
- Secondary intention.

Primary closure

Primary closure is appropriate for clean wounds, clean contaminated wounds and traumatic wounds where thorough debridement has been possible.

Delayed primary closure

Delayed primary closure is the method of choice for large, heavily contaminated wounds, usually traumatic in origin (Whiteside and Moorhead, 1994). The wound is left open or loosely packed and covered with a sterile, non-adherent dressing. Suturing or grafting is not undertaken until 4–5 days after injury, when the development of infection appears to be reduced. By this stage, the inflammatory response is well developed and may boost the immune reaction.

Mechanical cleansing is necessary to remove debris from heavily contaminated wounds (for example, traumatic wounds or infected joints after orthopaedic surgery). It may be undertaken in theatre before the tissues are closed or be performed in conjunction with delayed wound closure. A stream of sterile irrigating fluid is driven across the surface by hydrostatic pressure to remove contaminants physically. The high pressure of the fluid required to maintain continuous irrigation may be damaging, so intermittent irrigation via a syringe, with frequent dressing changes, may be used instead.

Secondary intention

In secondary intention, the wound is allowed to close through contraction, granulation and epithelialisation. Granulation occurs upwards from the base until the cavity is filled. It is appropriate to allow healing by secondary intention when there has been considerable tissue loss. It is also appropriate for superficial burns and donor sites where skin has been lost over a wide surface area but the wound is not deep. Disadvantages of this method include scarring, contracture and distortion.

These effects are most marked around bones and joints where the tissues become constricted during movement.

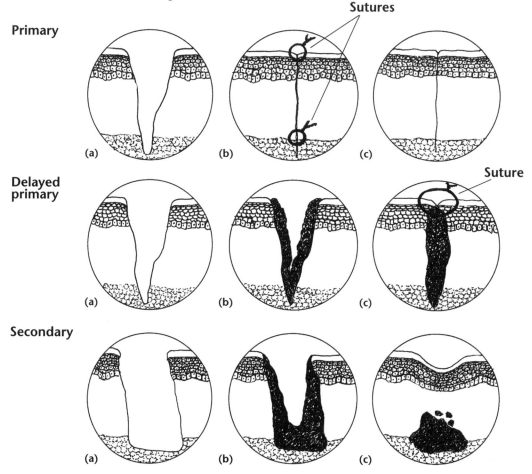

Figure 8.4   Approaches to wound repair (adapted from Westaby, 1985)

Wound infection

As with any nosocomial infection, wound infection adds to the cost of personal and health care, interferes with recovery, detracts from quality of life and in severe cases contributes to mortality. In the past, surgical wound infection contributed directly to the length of hospitalisation (Coello *et al.*, 1993), but this is becoming less likely as people are discharged into the care of the community nurse. The effect may be to reduce the hotel costs associated with hospital stay, but it will not diminish the expense of dressings or antibiotics.

The first major research study to examine the surgical wound infection rate was performed by Cruse and Foord (1973) in Canada. The incidence of surgical wound sepsis was determined prospectively in an 850-bed hospital over a period of 5 years. A 10-year follow-up study has since been published (Cruse and Foord, 1980). All wounds were examined daily until the twenty-eighth postoperative day, excluding patients with burns and those who had undergone gynaecological, rectal and oral procedures. Initially, 23 649 wounds were examined, 1124 becoming infected, which gave an overall sepsis rate of 4.8 per cent. However, rates differed according to wound category, dirty wounds being over 20 times more likely to become infected (Table 8.3).

Table 8.3   Infection rates for different wound categories

	Percentage
Clean	1.8
Clean–contaminated	8.9
Contaminated	21.5
Dirty	28.3

(*Source*: Cruse and Foord, 1973)

Overall, the results suggest that surgical wound infection is most closely associated with the type of procedure undertaken. Standards are best judged according to the rates obtained for clean wounds, the development of sepsis then being independent of extraneous factors such as the degree of contamination and the presence of necrotic tissue. Most hospital infection control teams today would consider a clean wound infection rate of 1 per cent to be exemplary, one of 1–2 per cent to be acceptable and a higher level to be indicative that investigation should be undertaken to review and improve current practice. Surgery is increasingly being performed on a day-care basis, and unless special provision is made to follow patients up in the community, infection may not be reported. In areas where purchasers demand this type of information before placing contracts, initiatives to follow patients up at home are being instituted (Holmes and Readman, 1994).

In the 1993–94 second National Prevalence Survey, wound infections accounted for 10.7 per cent of all nosocomial infections. They were less common than urinary or lower respiratory tract infections (Emmerson *et al.*, 1996). The organisms responsible are shown in Table 8.4.

Table 8.4   Bacteria associated with surgical wound infection

Bacteria	Postoperative day of onset
Staphylococcus	3–5 days
Gram-negative rods	5 days
Streptococcus	2–3 days
Clostridium perfringens (very rare, causes gas gangrene)	1–3 days

Auditing wound infection

Surgical wound infection is a key area for clinical audit because the information yielded (Glenister, 1993):

■ Can be used to help to evaluate changes in practice
■ Is useful in studying the epidemiology of wound infection
■ Provides data on the quality of health care required by purchasers.

During the audit cycle, the level of surgical infection can be taken as the standard. The collection, analysis and interpretation of data are used to obtain and measure this agreed standard. Data collection is the most time-consuming and difficult part of the exercise. It requires careful planning, tight criteria for the inclusion of subjects and a clear definition of the criteria used to determine the existence of infection if the results are to be considered reliable and the resulting decisions are to be sound. The best use of surgical wound audit involves a re-examination of the same clinical area on repeated occasions, especially after the implementation of change, rather than the production of league tables (Humphreys and Emmerson, 1993). The findings must be interpreted with caution as comparisons are only meaningful between areas with similar patient profiles. Following up patients in the community may be difficult and time-consuming, but without this information data are incomplete because of today's shorter hospital stays and day surgery (Wilson, 1995).

Identifying wound infection

The inflammatory response to infection and tissue damage is similar, so confusion inevitably arises when identifying wounds that are clinically infected and those which are merely colonised with commensal flora not invading the tissues (Hutchinson and Lawrence, 1991). Some authors suggest that clinical infection should be diagnosed in the presence of bacterial counts greater than 10^5 colony-forming units per gram of tissue (Borneside and Borneside, 1979). There is, however, evidence that burns continue to heal in the presence of higher bacterial counts, although the risks of graft rejection are increased (Pruitt, 1984). Micro-organisms present in wound exudate may not necessarily be invading the tissues, and their presence should thus be regarded as indicative but not diagnostic of infection. The results of microbiological examination must therefore be evaluated in conjunction with other factors, which have been identified by Cutting and Harding (1994):

■ Abscess formation   ■ Friable granulation tissue, which bleeds easily
■ Cellulitis   ■ 'Pocketing' at the base of the wound
■ Discharge   ■ Throbbing pain
■ Delayed healing   ■ Odour
■ Discolouration   ■ Dehiscence

Abscess formation

Abscesses are localised collections of necrotic tissue, bacteria and phagocytic leucocytes (purulent material) contained within a fibrin network. They may exert considerable pressure, forcing bacteria into the surrounding tissues or the blood and lymphatic vessels, resulting in septicaemia. Wherever possible, an abscess should be incised and drained. Antibiotics cannot penetrate a mass of purulent tissue and will be ineffective. Staphylococci are the pyogenic bacteria most likely to cause abscesses.

Cellulitis

Cellulitis is diffuse inflammation of the connective tissue, usually occurring subcutaneously. The causative organism in most cases is the haemolytic streptococcus. The presence of cellulitis is indicated by the classic hallmarks of inflammation: erythema and local heat with accompanying pain and oedema. Vesicles may develop in severe cases, leading to ulceration and necrosis. The rare condition of necrotising fasciitis is caused by streptococci, although other bacteria may become involved as the condition progresses (Neal, 1994).

Discharge

Discharge (serum, leucocytes and debris) from a freshly created wound is normal but should diminish as healing progresses. The discharge contains growth factors, bactericides and nutrients, and promotes tissue repair (Ryan, 1985). A healthy wound is moist rather than wet. Excessive exudate can be avoided by applying occlusive dressings (hydrocolloids and hydrogels). The amount of exudate to be expected and therefore judged as 'normal' probably depends on the nature and extent of the wounding: considerable quantities of serum may escape from burns, necessitating fluid replacement therapy.

Clinical Application

Abnormal Wound Discharge

The following types of wound discharge should not be considered normal and suggest that infection has occurred:

- Serous exudate where there is evidence of severe inflammation
- Seropurulent and haemopurulent discharge
- Pus – this must be distinguished from slough (moist, devitalised tissue), which may be present without infection.

Delayed healing

The length of time that a wound of a given type should take to heal is a matter of clinical judgement. Factors other than infection (poor nutrition, pre-existing metabolic disorders, corticosteroid therapy and age, for example) may be operating and must be taken into consideration, especially if there is no other indication of sepsis.

Discolouration

Again, much depends on clinical judgement, especially familiarity with the expected appearance of inflamed tissues responding to trauma in the normal way and the effect of different dressing materials. Sepsis is sometimes mistakenly attributed to the effect of a wound care product (Leaper, 1996). Healthy granulation tissue appears moist (rather than wet) and red or pink, discolouration suggesting infection. A yellow membrane developing over the surface of a wound represents fibrin. If removed, it will return within a few days.

Friable granulation tissue

Friable granulation tissue that bleeds spontaneously or in response to light pressure suggests infection. It looks raw and is tender (Marks *et al.*, 1985).

Pockets of infection

'Pockets' of infection may develop in the deepest part of a granulating wound. They must be drained to allow the new, healthy tissue to develop (Marks *et al.*, 1985). The traditional method of avoiding this complication is packing, but care must be taken: overzealously forcing large quantities of dressing material into a wound cavity may damage the tissue, especially if metal forceps are used. Silicone and elastomer dressings to fill the cavity are more effective.

Throbbing pain

Throbbing pain is an indication of severe inflammation, the resulting oedema exerting pressure on adjacent tissues. Chemicals released as part of the inflammatory response (bradykinins and prostaglandins) further contribute to the pain.

Odour

Odour may be detectable in healthy wounds but should not be pervasive or unpleasant. It is caused by putrefaction of the tissues with the activity of Gram-negative and anaerobic bacteria. Streptococcal and staphylococcal infections do not usually produce a noticeable odour, an offensive putrid smell indicating the presence of anaerobes (Jones *et al.*, 1978; Neal, 1994). Odour is among the most distressing problems experienced by people with fungating wounds, severely reducing their quality of life and restricting their social activities (Thomlinson, 1980).

Dehiscence

Dehiscence occurs in severely infected wounds because the bacteria break down collagen, undermining the strength of the regenerating tissues.

Factors associated with surgical wound infection

Factors influencing the development of surgical sepsis fall into two categories (Cruse and Foord, 1973):

- The dose of contaminating bacteria
- The patient's resistance.

Dose of contaminating bacteria

Many factors affect the dose of contaminating bacteria including conditions in the operating theatre, the length of the operation and theatre attire (see Chapter 5). Other factors, such as skin preparation and prophylaxis with antibiotics, are also addressed in this section.

Conditions in the operating theatre

The conditions in theatre are also covered to some extent in Chapter 5, but their importance warrants further discussion. Postoperative infections in general surgery are mainly endogenous, but airborne organisms cause some cases, especially in orthopaedic patients when prostheses are inserted (Babb *et al.*, 1995).

Exogenous surgical infection is possible via the airborne route or by contact spread from hands or instruments. A single skin scale from a staphylococcal carrier may transport up to a hundred individual bacteria. Skin scales may become airborne, settle onto the hands of staff or the drapes and then become carried into the wound. The number of airborne particles in the operating room is proportional to the number of people present and their level of activity; this is because the friction of clothing against the skin releases skin squames. Special ventilation systems are used to filter out airborne bacteria and to prevent those in the corridors and theatre suite entering the operating room. Further precautions to reduce infection include:

- Restricting the number of people present in theatre during an operation and reducing the levels of activity of those who are present: spectators should use a viewing gallery

- Regularly maintaining the operating environment: dust should not be allowed to settle on any surface, and filters in the ventilation system should be checked.

Considerable research has been undertaken with orthopaedic patients because infection is so damaging and will ultimately reduce mobility to less than that present before surgery. Treatment with antibiotics is not always successful, and the removal of the prosthesis is in some cases inevitable.

Duration of operative procedures

The duration of the operation is related to the development of surgical sepsis as the exposure of the tissues is increased during longer procedures. Tissues are also likely

Clinical Application

Theatre Ventilation Systems

Ventilation systems in operating theatres are designed to filter airborne bacteria and to prevent the spread of bacteria from the theatre suite and corridors to the operating theatre.

Several points should be noted:

- Ventilation systems must undergo regular and properly planned maintenance.
- Airborne bacteria are removed by forcing air through filters before it enters the operating theatre.
- The higher air pressure in operating theatres prevents unfiltered air moving into the theatres from other areas of the theatre suite.
- Filtered air is continually being renewed in the operating theatre, most systems renewing the air about 20 times every hour.
- Specialised ventilation systems may be installed in some high-risk situations, for example orthopaedic surgery involving the use of prostheses.

to be manipulated more during long, complicated operations, introducing more opportunities for operator error and contamination by contact. After the first hour the infection rate tends to double for every additional hour that the operation is prolonged. Reducing the number of people present and the amount of movement in theatre helps to reduce the risk of infection – movement increases the number of airborne particles so that more are available to settle into the wound.

Preoperative hygiene

Preoperative showering with antiseptics reduced the rate of infection in the study by Cruse and Foord (1973). This finding has been highly publicised by pharmaceutical companies, but the results have not been supported by other large-scale, well-planned epidemiological studies (Byrne *et al.*, 1990; Lynch *et al.*, 1992).

Preoperative shaving

Shaving the operation site the day before surgery increases the risk of infection by creating abrasions that provide more crevices to harbour the bacteria (Cruse and Foord, 1980; Hallstrom and Beck, 1993). Depilatory creams reduce the incidence of infection when hair growing directly over the operating site must be removed (Seropian and Reynolds, 1971).

Wound site

The wound site appears to be a major factor influencing the development of sepsis. Wounds in well-vascularised regions fare better, as discussed below. Moist areas are difficult to manage, especially if dressings are difficult to apply and retain in position, for example over incisions in the inguinal, perianal and vulval areas. Tissue at other, unexpected anatomical locations may also be susceptible to contamination and infection. A high incidence of infection has been associated with coronary artery bypass graft operations when the veins have been harvested from the legs (Wells, 1983). The bacteria responsible were mainly faecal in origin, suggesting contamination from the perineum. The surgeon who harvests the veins should scrub again and put on a new gown and gloves before undertaking further clean activities.

Vascularisation

Vascularisation influences infection and tissue necrosis. The beneficial effects of inflammation depend on an adequate blood supply, excessive blood loss delaying healing. Non-surgical wounds tend to develop at anatomical locations where vascularisation is poor: minor trauma may trigger the formation of ulcers on the front of the leg, especially in older adults and others with impaired circulation.

Poor surgical technique

Delayed healing and sepsis are the products of poor surgical technique. Roughly handling the tissues, the excessive use of diathermy and tight suturing impair healing and promote infection (Leaper, 1995).

Length of pre- and postoperative stay

The longer the period spent in hospital before surgery, the higher the wound infection rate: Cruse and Foord (1973) reported a rate of 1.1 per cent for those admitted 1 day before surgery compared with 2 per cent for those present in hospital for a week before their operation. The present trend towards day-case surgery and the move towards GPs performing minor procedures are therefore to be welcomed. More work needs to be conducted to detect possible differences between the infection rate for day-case and outpatient surgery.

Antibiotic prophylaxis

Antibiotic prophylaxis given systemically to surgical patients has dramatically reduced the incidence of surgical wound infection. Nevertheless, antibiotics are not 'wonder drugs'. It is good practice to prescribe them only to protect a particular patient from bacteria known to represent a specific threat according to the type of procedure undertaken, and not as part of a blanket policy intended to 'destroy all known germs' (Easmon, 1984). For example, the patient undergoing abdominal or gynaecological surgery will benefit from prophylactic metronidazole because anaerobes in the gut or vagina may cause infection; the drug is of no value to the patient undergoing repair of a traumatic wound restricted to the surface tissues where anaerobes do not survive.

Presence of foreign bodies

Foreign bodies promote the development of infection. Sutures, especially multi-braided types, trap bacteria (Gristina *et al.*, 1985). For the normal, healthy adult patient, it has been estimated that 10^6 bacteria must be present for every gram of tissue to result in clinical infection: local and humoral immunological defence mechanisms are usually able to cope with a smaller number of bacteria but are more easily overwhelmed in the presence of foreign material: one silk suture dramatically reduces the threshold for clinical infection. Resistance to invading pathogens develops more rapidly in wounds held together with sterile adhesive tapes (for example, Steristrips) than in those which have been conventionally sutured. Particles from gauze and cotton dressings may leave contaminants in a wound and should thus be avoided. Capillary loops may grow up into the weave, leading to trauma when they are removed (Wood, 1976).

Wound drainage

Wound drainage is intended to prevent the accumulation of body fluids (blood, serous exudate and bile) within the tissues, which will operate as a nidus for infection and promote abscess formation. Closed suction drainage significantly reduces the incidence of postoperative sepsis. In the study by Cruse and Foord (1973), the infection rate for clean contaminated wounds without drainage was 2.2 per cent compared with 1.8 per cent for those treated by drainage without suction through a separate stab wound. With closed suction drains, the infection rate was 0.6 per cent. The rate of infection was substantially higher when the drain was inserted via the wound itself. When drains are manipulated, an aseptic technique must be adopted; skin bacteria have been isolated from the lumen of drains, indicating that they may move from the exterior towards the internal tissues as well as in the reverse direction (Nora, 1972). The presence of a haematoma also increases the risk of infection.

Bowel preparation

Bowel preparation is essential to reduce the risk of endogenous infection with Gram-negative bacilli in patients undergoing procedures involving the gastrointestinal tract (Bucknall, 1982). This preparation usually involves measures to empty the bowel and antibiotic prophylaxis.

Patient's resistance

For people admitted from a waiting list to undergo elective operations, it is possible to enhance resistance to infection through careful nursing and medical assessment and intervention. The following measures place the individual in a better position to withstand the challenge of surgery:

- Optimal fluid and electrolyte balance
- Optimal nutritional status, with the correction of any negative nitrogen balance
- The correction of a low haemoglobin level
- The control of any underlying metabolic disorder (for example, diabetes mellitus)
- The opportunity to learn and practise deep breathing and leg exercises
- The opportunity to discuss the operation, to anticipate what will happen in hospital and during the longer-term recovery at home, and to plan for any resulting change (for example, stoma formation or mastectomy).

In emergency situations where this is not feasible, physical and psychological recovery may be slower.

The factors outlined below influence the development of postoperative wound infection.

Age

People between the ages of 20 and 40 years have a lower infection rate, probably because their immune system is functioning optimally (Ayliffe *et al.*, 1977). This has major clinical implications as a high proportion of surgical patients fall into the older age group.

Gender

Gender also influenced the ability to withstand infection in the study undertaken by Ayliffe *et al.* (1977). After general surgical procedures (stripping varicose veins, hernia repairs and gut operations), males were more likely to develop infection, especially staphylococcal infection, than were females. Males carry staphylococci more often than females and disseminate them more easily, especially from the perineal area (Hare and Thomas, 1956).

Nutritional status

Cruse and Foord (1973) detected a significant association between postsurgical sepsis and obesity: for clean wounds overweight people had an infection rate of 13 per cent compared with 1.8 per cent for those of ideal body weight. Subcutaneous adipose tissue is poorly vascularised, and it may be difficult to secure haemostasis during closure. Secondary Gram-negative infection is probably also more common in this group. Moist skin folds may harbour sufficient bacteria to form a reservoir, the bacteria reaching the wound by contact spread.

Undernourishment is also important. The rate of post-surgical sepsis for people significantly below their ideal body weight was 16.6 per cent in the study by Cruse and Foord (1973). The inflammatory response, the immunological response and tissue repair all depend on adequate supplies of protein. A negative nitrogen balance impedes healing and increases the opportunity for infection to supervene.

Metabolic disorders

Metabolic disorders are believed to alter the ability of the tissues to withstand pathogenic invasion, but the mechanism is obscure and may vary between one type of patient and another. Diabetes mellitus is one of the most common metabolic disorders and therefore among the easiest to establish. The clean wound infection rate for diabetic patients was 10.7 per cent in the study by Cruse and Foord (1973). The physiological mechanism remains to be elucidated, but there are suggestions that neutrophil migration may occur more slowly than in people without diabetes.

Temperature

Maintaining the patient's normal body temperature around the time of surgery appears to decrease infection and promote healing (Kurz *et al.*, 1996).

Corticosteroids

The association between a depressed inflammatory response and corticosteroid therapy has been well established. Physical and psychological stress may, by increasing the release of corticosteroid hormones from the adrenal cortex, suppress healing, increase the rate of surgical wound infection and delay recovery (Boore, 1978).

Malignancy

Malignancy is often cited as a risk factor for post-surgical sepsis. In a study by Bucknall (1982), conducted on over a thousand patients undergoing laparotomy, malignancy and its associated problems of anaemia and malnutrition resulted in a significantly higher infection rate.

Aseptic dressing technique

The purpose of the aseptic (non-touch) dressing technique is to avoid contact between open tissue, the fingers and any other potentially contaminated item that could lead to cross-infection. Dressing procedures frequently take the form of time-consuming rituals that are not evidence based (Bree-Williams and Waterman, 1996). In the absence of supporting research, the following are offered as a means by which to save time, resources and patient discomfort:

■ Question the need to change the dressing at all. A larger, more absorbent dressing may be applied to deal with seeping exudate ('strike-through') in order to avoid discomfort, environmental contamination and cross-infection. Daily changes are usually unnecessary and may be painful. Transparent polyurethane dressings permit inspection without removal.

■ Cleanse the hands with an alcoholic handrub at the bedside immediately before handling the dressing. Time walking to a sink is saved, especially if the hands have to be decontaminated more than once during the procedure.

■ Avoid the application of solutions to wounds that are already clean. This increases the risk of contamination and cools the wound, slowing mitotic activity and the action of phagocytic cells (Thomas, 1989).

■ Research with occlusive and semi-permeable dressings such as hydrocolloids suggests that the surfaces of healthy granulating wounds may be colonised by, rather than infected with, saprophytic organisms, even though these are capable of pathogenic activity (Brennan *et al.*, 1985). A clean rather than a complicated aseptic procedure may be more appropriate for this type of wound. Micro-organisms can never be completely removed from the wound surface; they may even be beneficial. Strongly acidic or alkaline solutions (such as hydrogen peroxide and Eusol) are not recommended. They damage new tissue, destroy the delicately balanced microflora of the wound and soon lose their antiseptic properties (Leaper, 1996).

With chronic lesions, it is vital that the nurse responsible for providing treatment understands the aetiology of the wound, otherwise an inappropriate regimen may be selected and tissue repair will not be promoted. Occlusive, semi-permeable dressings are more appropriate than cheaper cotton wool or gauze. They provide a more effective physiological environment for healing, are less likely to traumatise the tissues and do not disseminate bacteria into the air when removed (Lawrence *et al.*, 1992). It is helpful to anticipate the way in which the wound is likely to respond to treatment. Occlusive, semi-permeable dressings promote auto-debridement so the wound may appear to become larger before the formation of granulation tissue, (Melhuish *et al.*, 1994) contraction eventually indicating that progress is occurring. The use of some hydrocolloids is associated with odour, which, although it may be unpleasant, is not an indication of infection or necrosis.

REVISION CHECKLIST: KEY AREAS

❏ Introduction to wounds and wound healing: Historical aspects of wound care, Classifying wounds

❏ Stages of wound healing: Proliferative phase, Phase of maturation, Surgical intervention and approaches to wound repair

❏ Wound infection: Auditing wound infection, Identifying wound infection, Factors associated with surgical wound infection

❏ Aseptic dressing technique

Activities – linking knowledge to clinical practice

1. **Are** the results of the studies undertaken by Cruse and Foord and the National Prevalence Survey of Infection in Hospital concerning surgical wound infection rates directly comparable? Explain your answer.

2. **Draw** up a table or flow chart to compare and contrast the ways in which surgical and chronic wounds heal.

SELF-ASSESSMENT

1. Which of the following wounds heal by first intention?
   (a) burns ☐
   (b) pressure sores ☐
   (c) a nick from scalpel blade ☐
   (d) a graze ☐

2. An abscess is defined as ....
   ....
   ....

3. Wounds heal best under moist conditions.
   True? ☐ False? ☐

4. Eusol (pH 8) is damaging to wounds.
   True? ☐ False? ☐

5. Contaminated wounds never heal.
   True? ☐ False? ☐

6. Cellulitis is caused by:
   (a) staphylococci ☐
   (b) streptococci ☐
   (c) *Bacteroides* ☐
   (d) *Salmonella* ☐

7. Angiogenesis begins at the surface of the wound. True? ☐ False? ☐

8. Preoperative shaving reduces the risk of surgical wound infection. True? ☐ False? ☐

References

Ayliffe GAJ, Brightwell KM, Babb BJ *et al*. (1977) 'Surveys of hospital infection in the Birmingham region'. *Journal of Hygiene* **79**: 299–313.

Babb JR, Lynam P and Ayliffe GAJ (1995) 'Risk of airborne transmission in an operating theatre, containing four ultra clean air units'. *Journal of Hospital Infection* **31**: 159–68.

Boore J (1978) *Prescription for Recovery*. RCN, London.

Borneside GH and Borneside BB (1979) 'Comparison between moist swab and tissue biopsy methods for quantitation of bacteria in experimental incision wounds'. *Journal of Trauma* **19**: 103–5.

Bree-Williams FJ and Waterman H (1996) 'An examination of nurses' practices when performing aseptic technique for wound dressings'. *Journal of Advanced Nursing* **23**: 48–54.

Brennan SS, Foster M and, Leaper DJ (1985) 'Antiseptic toxicity in wounds healing by secondary intention'. *Journal of Hospital Infection* **8**: 263–7.

Bucknall TE (1982) 'Burst abdomen and the incisional hernia – a prospective study of 1129 major laparotomies'. *British Medical Journal* **184**: 931–3.

Byrne DJ, Napier A and Cuschieri A (1990) 'Rationalising whole body disinfection'. *Journal of Hospital Infection* **15**: 183–7.

Coello R, Glenister H, Ferres J *et al*. (1993) 'The cost of infection in surgical patients: a case control study'. *Journal of Hospital Infection* **25**: 239–50.

Cruse PJE and Foord R (1973) 'A five year prospective study of 23,649 surgical wounds'. *Archives of Surgery* **107**: 206–10.

Cruse PJE and Foord R (1980) 'The epidemiology of wound infection: a 10 year prospective study of 62,939 wounds'. *Surgical Clinics of North America* **60**: 27–40.

Cutting KF and Harding KG (1994) 'Criteria for identifying wound infection'. *Journal of Wound Care* **3**: 198–201.

Easmon CSF (1984) 'Prevention is not always the best antibiotic cure'. *Hospital Doctor* **15**: 10–11.

Emmerson AM, Enstone JE, Griffin M *et al.* (1996) 'The Second National Prevalence Survey of Infection in Hospitals – overview of the results'. *Journal of Hospital Infection* **32**: 175–90.

Forrest RD (1982) 'Early history of wound treatment'. *Journal of the Royal Society of Medicine* **75**: 198–205.

Glenister H (1993) 'How do we collect data for surveillance of wound infection?' *Journal of Hospital Infection* **24**: 283–9.

Gristina AG, Price JL, Hobgood CD *et al.* (1985) 'Bacterial colonisation of percutaneous sutures'. *Surgery* **98**: 12–19.

Hallstrom R and Beck SL (1993) 'Implementation of the AORN skin standard'. *Association of Operating Room Nurses' Journal* **583**: 498–506.

Hare R and Thomas CGA (1956) 'The transmission of *Staphylococcus aureus*'. *British Medical Journal* **2**: 840–4.

Holmes J and Readman R (1994) 'A study of wound infections following inguinal hernia repair'. *Journal of Hospital Infection* **28**: 153–6.

Humphreys H and Emmerson AM (1993) 'Control of hospital-acquired infection: accurate data and more resources, not league tables'. *Journal of Hospital Infection* **25**: 75–8.

Hutchinson JJ and Lawrence JC (1991) 'Wound infection under occlusive dressings'. *Journal of Hospital Infection* **17**: 83–94.

Johnson A (1988) 'The cleansing ethic'. *Nursing Times* (Community Nursing Supplement) **84**(6): 9–10.

Jones PH, Willis AT and Ferguson IR (1978) 'Treatment of anaerobically infected pressure sores with topical metronidazole'. *Lancet* **28**: 214–15.

Kurz A, Sessler DI, Lenhardt R *et al.* (1996) 'Perioperative normothermia to reduce the incidence of surgical wound infection and shorten hospitalisation'. *New England Journal of Medicine* **312**: 1195–9.

Lawrence JC, Lilly HA and Kidson A (1992) 'Wound dressings and airborne dispersal of bacteria'. *Lancet* **339**: 807.

Leaper D (1995) 'Risk factors for surgical infection'. *Journal of Hospital Infection* (Supplement) **30**: 127–39.

Leaper D (1996) 'Antiseptics in wound healing'. *Nursing Times* **92**(39): 63–8.

Lynch W, Davey PG, Malek M *et al.* (1992) 'Cost-effectiveness of the use of chlorhexidine detergent in pre-operative whole-body disinfection in wound prophylaxis'. *Journal of Hospital Infection* **21**: 179–91.

Marks J, Harding LE and Hughes LE (1985) 'Pilonidal sinus excision: healing by open granulation'. *British Journal of Surgery* **72**: 637–40.

Melhuish JM, Plassman P and Harding KG (1994) 'Circumference, area and volume of the healing wound'. *Journal of Wound Care* **3**: 380–4.

Murray Y (1988) 'Tradition rather than cure?' *Nursing Times* **84**(38): 75–80.

National Research Council (1964) 'Post-operative wound infection'. *Annals of Surgery* (Supplement) **160**(2): 1–192.

Neal M (1994) 'Necrotising infections'. *Nursing Times* **90**(41): 53–9.

Nora PF (1972) 'Prophylactic abdominal drains'. *Archives of Surgery* **64**: 729–32.

Pollock AV and Evans M (1983) 'Microbiological prediction of abdominal surgical wound infection'. *Archives of Surgery* **122**: 33–7.

Pruitt BZ (1984) 'The diagnosis and treatment of infection in the burned patient'. *Burns* **11**: 79–81.

Ryan TJ (1985) *An Environment for Healing: The Role of Occlusion.* Royal Society of Medicine/Oxford University Press, Oxford.

Seropian R and Reynolds BM (1971) 'Wound infection after pre-operative depilatory versus razor preparation'. *American Journal of Surgery* **121**: 251–5.

Thomas ST (1989) 'Pain and wound management'. *Nursing Times* (Community Supplement) **85**(28): 11–15.

Thomlinson RH (1980) 'Kitchen remedy for malignant breast ulcers'. *Lancet* **2**: 707–8.

Wells FC (1983) 'Wound infection in cardiothoracic surgery'. *Lancet* **1**: 1209–10.

Westaby S (1985) *Wound Care.* Heinemann, London.

Whiteside MCR and Moorhead RJ (1994) 'Traumatic wound management. A guide to treatment of gunshot and bomb injuries'. *Journal of Wound Care* **3**: 183–6.

Wilson APR (1995) 'Surveillance of wound infection'. *Journal of Hospital Infection* **29**: 81–6.

Winter GD (1962) 'Formation of the scab and the rate of epithelialisation of superficial wounds in the skin of the young domestic pig'. *Nature* **193**: 293–4.

Wood RAB (1976) Disintegration of cellulose dressings in open granulating wounds. *British Medical Journal* **1**: 1444–5.

Further reading and information sources

Haley RW, Culver DH, Morgan WM, White JW, Emori TG and Hooton TM (1985) 'Identifying patients at high risk of surgical wound infection'. *American Journal of Epidemiology* **121**(2): 206–15.

Nicol M, Bavin C, Bedford-Turner S, Cronin P and Rawlings-Anderson K (2000) *Essential Nursing Skills.* Mosby, London.

Respiratory infections

CHAPTER OUTCOMES

After reading this chapter you should be able to:

■ State the prevalence of lower respiratory tract infection in hospital inpatients

■ List the organisms responsible for lower respiratory tract infection

■ Explain why postoperative and ventilated patients are at particular risk of developing lower respiratory tract infection and suggest strategies to help to reduce these risks

■ List the organisms responsible for upper respiratory tract infection and suggest preventative strategies in each case

Introduction – the importance of respiratory infections

Respiratory infections are commonly acquired in hospital; in fact nearly 23 per cent of nosocomial infections affect the respiratory tract, causing considerable morbidity and mortality. This type of respiratory infection generally affects those who are critically ill.

Lower respiratory tract infections

Lower respiratory tract infections involve the bronchi and alveoli (Figure 9.1). Bronchitis is usually a community-acquired infection. Pneumonia may be acquired in hospital or the community. Both are serious conditions.

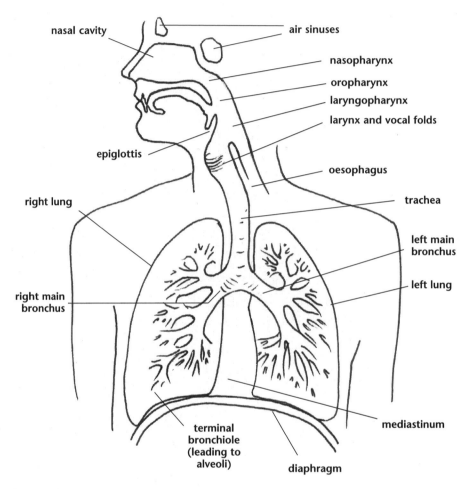

Figure 9.1   The respiratory tract

Bronchitis

Bronchitis (inflammation of the bronchi) is the label given to acute respiratory infections in which the dominant symptom is coughing without localised infection. It usually arises as a complication of upper respiratory tract infection caused by a virus, when bacterial infection supervenes. Some children seem prone to bronchitis. It appears to be related to poor living conditions (overcrowding, poor hygiene and poor nutrition) and is exacerbated by maternal smoking, especially during pregnancy. Individuals who have experienced childhood bronchitis are at risk of developing further symptoms during their teenage years if they then smoke.

Pneumonia

Pneumonia (inflammation of the lung) is a serious condition, responsible for most deaths caused by infection of the respiratory tract, especially in older adults and infants. The alveoli become filled with pus, air is excluded, and the lung is said to be 'consolidated'. In bronchopneumonia, consolidation is widely distributed; in lobar pneumonia, it is localised. Hospital admission is arranged to:

- **Administer antibiotics** – although many cases are viral, this may be difficult to determine, and time must not be lost in instituting treatment
- **Provide physiotherapy** – percussion, breathing exercises and postural drainage
- **Maintain the airway** – if necessary
- **Provide other supportive measures** – for example, maintaining fluid balance.

In the community, bacterial pneumonia is most frequently caused by *Streptococcus pneumoniae* and *Haemophilus influenzae,* which are often carried in the throats of healthy people. Infection is most common in people with pre-existing health problems, frequently developing as a complication of some other respiratory infection (for example, measles or influenza). Treatment is complicated because some strains of *Streptococcus pneumoniae* are now resistant to penicillin. Vaccination is recommended for people at risk of respiratory infection, following splenectomy and in older adults (Grist and Walker, 1991). Outbreaks occasionally develop in overcrowded, poorly ventilated environments (Hoge *et al.*, 1994).

Hospital-acquired pneumonia

In the second National Prevalence Survey of Infection in Hospitals, hospital-acquired pneumonia was the second most common infection, involving 22.9 per cent of patients, mainly postoperative patients and the critically ill (Emmerson *et al.*, 1996). Risk factors include obesity, impaired consciousness, a history of smoking and underlying respiratory disease. In hospital, pneumonia can be caused by bacteria, viruses or fungi, but most nosocomial pneumonia is caused by *Staphylococcus aureus* and Gram-negative opportunists (Inglis *et al.*, 1993).

Infection can arise from other people by cross-infection or from an environmental source (as, for example, with *Legionella*; see Chapter 14). Airborne transmission is not a major route in hospital except for *Legionella*. Instead, most cases of hospital-acquired pneumonia develop in patients who require mechanical ventilation (see Figure 9.2 below). These patients are at particular risk because they have lost the protective coughing and sneezing reflexes, their risk being increased further by antibiotic therapy and other invasive procedures. Ventilator-associated respiratory infection occurs when the bronchioles and alveoli become contaminated with pathogens. In health, they are kept free of micro-organisms by the mucociliary escalator: foreign particles become trapped in the mucus, are wafted upwards by ciliary action and are eventually swallowed. However, the upper respiratory passages harbour bacteria, including potential pathogens, and these may be transferred to the lower airways during invasive procedures.

Sources of pathogens for hospital-acquired infection

Aspiration of pathogens from the oropharynx

The aspiration of pathogens colonising the oropharynx is the most important source of bacterial pneumonia in hospital inpatients. Although many healthy people aspirate their secretions during sleep, these are dealt with by the body's immunological defences. In ventilated patients, the risk of aspiration is increased by the presence of endotracheal and tracheostomy tubes, and because the patients are sedated or have been anaesthetised.

Colonisation of the oropharynx

Colonisation of the oropharynx increases the risk of developing pneumonia and complicates its treatment. Gram-negative bacilli replace the normal flora if the patient receives antibiotics (Johanson et al., 1972).

Clinical Application

Reducing the Infection Risks Associated with Suctioning

Patients who require suctioning of their respiratory secretions have a high risk of developing nosocomial pneumonia. This risk is increased for patients with a tracheostomy and those being ventilated.

The main considerations are as follows:

- Select the smallest possible catheter to minimise the risk of trauma
- Wash or decontaminate the hands both before and after the procedure
- Wear gloves according to local hospital policy
- Use sterile solutions if a lubricant is required
- Withdraw the catheter if resistance is experienced
- Only suction as the catheter is being withdrawn
- Use a new catheter each time – never reintroduce a catheter into the airway
- Suction the mouth last (as it is considered to be clean rather than sterile)
- Change the suction container and tubing as per local protocol, for example between individual patients and daily where the equipment is being used for one patient only.

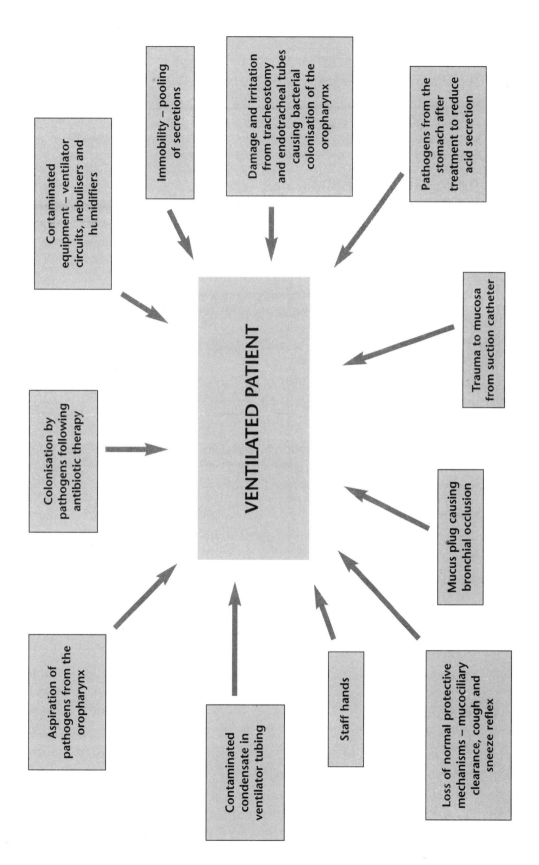

Figure 9.2 Infection risks in ventilated patients

Colonisation of the stomach

Colonisation of the stomach results if the patient receives drugs to neutralise or suppress the secretion of gastric acid (for example, antacids or cimetidine). These are commonly prescribed for the critically ill patient to reduce the risk of ulceration caused by stress (Craven *et al.*, 1986).

Endotracheal and tracheostomy tubes

Endotracheal and tracheostomy tubes irritate the respiratory mucosa and promote Gram-negative colonisation of the oropharynx. Contaminated secretions enter the trachea from the mouth and pharynx, secretions then seeping down through the space between the outer wall of the endotracheal tube and the tracheal wall. The endotracheal tube should provide an airtight seal sufficient to occlude this space, but leakage is possible during the periodic deflation of the cuff. Bacteria of the same strain have been isolated from the mouth and trachea of ventilated patients (Sanderson, 1983).

Contaminated ventilator circuits

Contaminated ventilator circuits may lead to cross-infection by delivering bacteria-laden air directly to the lower airways (Phillips, 1967).

Nebulisers

Nebulisers create aerosols of minute droplets that penetrate deeply into the narrowest airways and thus present a significant problem. This is especially so for small-volume medication nebulisers (Botman and de Krieger, 1987).

Humidification

Humidification of the circuit is essential to prevent dehydration of the airways. Humidifiers do not produce aerosols so if the water in the reservoir becomes contaminated, the bacteria are less likely to be inhaled. However, water vapour tends to condense in the tubing (Stucke and Thompson, 1980). The condensate may become heavily contaminated and can drain into the trachea, increasing the risk of infection (Craven *et al.*, 1984).

Tracheobronchial suction

Tracheobronchial suction, intended to reduce the risk of infection in pooled secretions, may contribute to its development if poor technique results in the transfer of bacteria (Fiorentini, 1992). Mucous membranes are more easily damaged by trauma than skin, and abrasions from the suction catheter further increase the risk of infection.

Bronchial occlusion with mucus plug

Postoperative respiratory infection arises when a bronchus becomes occluded with a plug of tenacious mucus. The patient may be frightened to move after an operation and reluctant to expectorate, especially if pain is poorly controlled. After some major surgery, immobility is complete because the patient is sedated and ventilated. Occlusion results in the pooling of secretions in the air passages distal to the obstruction, which then collapse when the air within the alveoli is absorbed but not replaced. Gaseous exchange in that area ceases. The tissue is still perfused, but the blood reaching it no longer receives oxygen and cannot be relieved of carbon dioxide. There is a change in the normal ventilation/perfusion ratio, which produces a right-to-left shunt. The bigger the mucus plug, the greater the problem because a larger airway is obstructed. An extensive area of the lung will thus be affected, leading to collapse (atelectasis). Conditions are now favourable for bacterial growth and multiplication.

Prevention of hospital-acquired pneumonia

The risk of developing nosocomial pneumonia can be reduced by early ambulation and physiotherapy to improve lung expansion in postoperative patients.

For the critically ill, nosocomial pneumonia remains difficult to prevent and expensive to treat (Kelleghan et al., 1993). Contaminated equipment has been incriminated in outbreaks (Gorman et al., 1993), but risks can be reduced by autoclaving any equipment used in respiratory therapy. This includes the ventilator and its circuits, nebulisers, humidifiers and non-disposable equipment used during endotracheal suction. If autoclaving is not possible, equipment can be decontami-

Clinical Application

Preventing Postoperative Chest Infection

Postoperative chest infections can be prevented by early ambulation and by teaching deep breathing exercises during the preoperative period, either individually or to groups of people (Lindeman and Van Aernan, 1971). As more operations are performed on a day-case basis with only a few hours before surgery, there will be an increasing need to organise presurgical appointments to provide instruction for the postoperative period. The importance of reducing smoking before surgery can be emphasised at the same time if necessary.

■ Anaesthetic equipment should be disinfected between patients, taking care to avoid recontamination during its assembly so that spread by contact is avoided

■ Postoperatively, physiotherapy is important to encourage coughing and expectoration. If infection occurs, the mucus plug may have to be removed by bronchoscopy and aspiration if physiotherapy is insufficient to dislodge it. Antibiotics are of secondary importance to mechanical clearing

■ Dehydration should be avoided as it increases the viscosity of respiratory secretions, which then become difficult to dislodge. Steam liquefies mucus so inhalations are helpful

■ Good pain control should be ensured in order to allow physiotherapy and ambulation.

Clinical Application

Suggested Protocol To Prevent Respiratory Infection in Ventilated Patients

Oral/nasopharyngeal/tracheostomy suctioning
(See also the Clinical Application box above, Reducing the Infection Risks Associated with Suctioning)

■ Decontaminate the hands both before and after the procedure
■ Employ aseptic technique to introduce the catheter with a gloved hand
■ Oxygenate the patient both before and after the procedure (to avoid hypoxaemia)
■ Clear secretions from the tubing.

General

■ Wash the hands after every contact with an intubated patient
■ Use clean gloves for all routine contact with respiratory equipment and wash the hands afterwards
■ Use HME filters if possible; otherwise, date and change the ventilator circuits every 48 hours (Craven *et al.*, 1982)
■ Date and change the connector tubing every 24 hours (Craven *et al.*, 1982)
■ Remove condensation from the ventilator tubing if humidification is being used: it may support the growth of Gram-negative bacteria, leading to colonisation and infection (Stucke and Thompson, 1980)
■ Change oxygen masks and tubing between patients
■ Provide oral care 2 hourly as the mouth can operate as a source of respiratory pathogens
■ Turn or reposition the patient every 2 hours to prevent the stagnation of respiratory secretions
■ Administer analgesia regularly in order to permit movement and physiotherapy
■ Store all equipment clean and dry.

nated in an automated washing machine or with chemical disinfectants followed by rinsing with tap water.

Ventilators

Ventilators need not be routinely decontaminated if filters are used to protect the inspiratory and expiratory circuits. The routine use of heat–moisture exchange (HME) filters and closed suction systems in ventilators has reduced the risk of hospital-acquired pneumonia. HME filters cut down the need to humidify the gases being administered to ventilated patients.

The routine disinfection of equipment is no longer necessary, the HME filter alone being changed every 24–48 hours. Where HME filters are not used, disinfection or disposal of the circuits themselves is recommended every 48 hours (Craven *et al.*, 1982). Condensate collecting in ventilator tubing should be regularly drained.

Humidifiers

Humidifiers should always be used during oxygen therapy to prevent dehydration of the respiratory mucosae. They should be filled with sterile water and decontaminated every 48 hours (Craven *et al.*, 1982).

Nebulisers

Nebulisers used to deliver medication easily become contaminated. They should be washed with detergent and dried every time they are used. Mouthpieces should be changed every 24 hours (Cobben *et al.*, 1996).

Upper respiratory tract infections

Upper respiratory tract infections involve the nasal passages, pharynx, tonsils and epiglottis (see Figure 9.1 above). Most are minor infections acquired in the community and are caused by viruses. Upper respiratory tract infections can, however, have serious consequences for the very young and older adults. They also account for a high proportion of days lost from work and school in the UK, so their impact on the health of individuals and their social and economic consequences should not be dismissed.

Coughs and colds

Coughs and colds are mainly caused by rhinoviruses, members of the picornavirus group. There are about 200 different types so somebody who has just recovered from one cold may succumb to another caused by a different rhinovirus. It was traditionally believed that transmission occurred by inhaling virus particles contained in airborne droplets, but there is evidence that it also takes place by contact, especially via the hands. In laboratory simulations, Gwaltney *et al.* (1978) showed that volunteers' hands became contaminated after shaking hands with infected subjects; they were more likely to develop colds than individuals exposed to viral aerosols released by sneezing. Rhinoviruses survive in the inanimate environment if they are protected by mucus. Objects that are handled frequently (doorknobs, light switches and crockery, for example) thus become contaminated, and the viruses are passed to a new host, reaching the eyes or nose when the face is touched. General hygiene and handwashing are especially important in schools to prevent infection by rhinoviruses. Self-inoculation is the most common form of transmission (Hendley *et al.*, 1973).

Colds are a nuisance and can cause problems in people with pre-existing respiratory difficulties, especially older adults (Nicholson *et al.*, 1996). There is no evidence that developing an upper respiratory infection is related to becoming wet or 'chilled'. Colds are common in the UK, which has been attributed to the damp climate, but they also develop in hot, dry countries. When older adults are admitted to hospital with hypothermia and lower respiratory tract problems after falling at home, the problem has arisen because secretions have pooled in the lower airways, setting in train a sequence of events similar to those arising after occlusion with a mucus plug. In babies and young children, upper respiratory tract infection is usually harmless, as it is in adulthood, but it can interfere with feeding and occasionally leads to acute otitis media or involvement of the lower airways. The community nurse's advice is helpful, reassuring parents and determining whether medical intervention is necessary (Taylor, 1988). Treatment is seldom necessary. The nasal discharge associated with colds contains virus particles, dead cells from the nasal mucosa and bacteria, but these are of the same type as are present in health. Bacterial invasion of the damaged epithelium is rare, and antibiotics are seldom required (see Chapters 1 and 4).

Other viruses responsible for 'colds' include:

- Parainfluenza virus
- Reoviruses
- Coxsackie viruses
- Adenoviruses
- Respiratory syncytial virus (RSV)
- Coronaviruses
- Echoviruses.

Clinical Application

Treating Upper Respiratory Tract Infections in Children

- **Antibiotics** – are not usually necessary as most infections are viral. They are of value only when there is evidence of bacterial infection (streptococcal throat infection or acute suppurative otitis media)
- **Antipyretics** – reduce an elevated temperature. Paracetamol dose calculated on body weight is safe and has valuable analgesic properties. Aspirin should not be given to children under 12 years old because it has been associated with the development of encephalopathy and hepatitis (Reye's syndrome) (Tarlow, 1986)
- **Decongestant drops** – are helpful before a feed to allow an infant to breathe as well as to swallow
- **Antihistamines** – may be useful in cases of allergy when the nasal mucosa is swollen, but they do not speed recovery. They cause drowsiness, which may be annoying in older children
- **Antitussives** – to suppress coughing, are of possible value if the household has been disturbed all night or the child is distressed.

Otitis media

Otitis media (inflammation of the middle ear) is a common childhood complaint. The middle ear is lined with respiratory mucosa and becomes inflamed during a cold. Pressure changes from obstruction of the pharyngotympanic (eustachian) tube give rise to discomfort in the ear.

Acute suppurative otitis media

Acute suppurative otitis media (an abscess in the ear) causes pain and fever, and should be suspected if a child awakes crying with a high temperature. Unless medical intervention is prompt, the tympanic membrane will rupture under pressure, bloodstained mucopurulent material escaping as a discharge. An antibiotic (penicillin or amoxycillin) is prescribed, along with an antipyretic and an analgesic. Recovery begins within 3 or 4 days. Most ruptured eardrums heal spontaneously without problems, but slight deafness may persist for a few days until mucus and debris lodged in the middle ear disperse.

Glue ear

Glue ear (secretory otitis media) is the term used to describe the accumulation of viscous secretion within the middle ear. It occurs when the child has had recurrent colds and associated otitis media. Surveys have shown that, in some areas, up to 40 per cent of school-age children have secretory otitis media, but it usually resolves without intervention within a few days or weeks (Taylor, 1988). Transient conductive deafness is common. Surgical intervention has become fashionable through fears that speech and language development will be impaired, leading to educational difficulties. The eardrum is incised, material from the cleft of the middle ear is removed by suction, and grommets (plastic aeration tubes) are inserted. The value of surgery is, however, now being questioned. Glue ear is usually self-limiting, but permanent scarring of the tympanum has been reported after surgery (Moran and Wilson, 1986). The relationship between upper respiratory tract infection, deafness and educational underachievement is difficult to disentangle because all these conditions are common in children from economically deprived backgrounds.

Croup

Croup (laryngeal spasm) is a feature of viral infection involving the larynx and trachea. The child initially develops a snuffly nose, inspiration then becoming noisy and sounding harsh (stridor). This is distressing for the patient and frightening for the parents. Treatment traditionally involved the use of steam kettles to liquefy secretions and relieve obstruction, the modern alternative being a steamy bathroom. Most children recover without treatment, but croup remains a worrying condition because:

- Children occasionally develop obstruction and exhaustion, and thus require emergency admission to ensure that the airway remains patent
- Rarely, acute epiglottitis supervenes, emergency treatment being essential. This is usually caused by bacteria such as *Haemophilus influenzae*
- Children occasionally experience repeated attacks of croup, suggesting allergy.

Respiratory syncytial virus

Respiratory syncytial virus (RSV) is an RNA virus responsible for acute respiratory infection in infants and young children, often severe in babies under the age of 6 months. Bronchopneumonia may result, and death is not uncommon. In older children, RSV infection is usually milder. By the age of 4 years, most children show serological evidence of previous infection, but this does not necessarily result in lasting immunity. Outbreaks of RSV have been documented in the community and may occur in hospital, especially among very sick children, contributing to morbidity and mortality. Virus particles are present in nasal secretions, nosocomial spread being via the hands. This is supported by the results of a study in which the incidence of RSV declined after a strict handwashing regimen was introduced among staff and parents (Isaacs *et al.*, 1991).

Pertussis

Pertussis (whooping cough) is caused by a small Gram-negative bacterium called *Bordetella pertussis*.

Following exposure to a source of infection, the bacteria become attached to ciliated cells lining the respiratory mucosa. Non-specific symptoms without the typical cough develop within 5–7 days. The child appears to have a cold but is highly infectious, releasing a large number of bacteria from the nasopharynx. Finally, the infection enters the paroxysmal phase, characterised by coughing that often ends in vomiting. Vaccination is an important public health measure in the control of this frightening and unpleasant infection, which can in severe cases be life-threatening. The bacteria are never carried in a healthy throat (Weiss and Hewlett, 1986).

Diphtheria

Diphtheria is caused by the Gram-positive bacillus *Corynebacterium diphtheriae*. It is a very rare infection in the UK, but travellers to Eastern Europe, countries of the former Soviet Union and areas in the developing world may be exposed to the organism. The disease results in an acute respiratory illness characterised by the formation of a tenacious 'membrane' (consisting of white blood cells, bacteria and respiratory epithelium) within the upper respiratory tract. This membrane can cause laryngeal obstruction, leading to death without emergency treatment, such as a tracheostomy, to maintain a patent airway. *Corynebacterium diphtheriae* also produces an exotoxin that circulates in the blood to cause complications such as myocarditis and peripheral neuropathy.

The management of patients and contacts with diphtheria includes:

- Informing the proper officer of the relevant public health authority as diphtheria is a notifiable disease
- Case isolation
- Protective clothing – gloves, aprons and masks – for staff and visitors
- Treating the patient with penicillin and diphtheria antitoxin
- Treating contacts with erythromycin and immunising them with diphtheria toxoid
- Meticulous attention to oral hygiene and pain relief
- Monitoring vital signs, especially respiration. Cardiac monitoring should be undertaken if myocardial involvement is suspected.

It is important to stress that active immunisation against diphtheria, administered during childhood, is very effective. Others who may need immunisation include contacts of a case of diphtheria, healthcare workers, laboratory staff and those who travel to countries where the disease is endemic.

Influenza

Influenza is caused by an RNA virus belonging to a group called the myxoviruses, which has an affinity for mucoproteins present on the surface of human and other mammalian cells. There are three types of influenza virus: A, B and C. The surface of each type is coated with a number of specific antigens (V, H and N) to which the host responds by secreting the corresponding antibody. Standard nomenclature is employed to classify the different strains according to their surface antigens.

Influenza is transmitted via infected nasopharyngeal secretions, resulting in an acute illness with fever, headache, myalgia and profound malaise, although (contrary to popular belief) relatively minor respiratory symptoms. Severe colds are sometimes erroneously labelled 'flu' by sufferers. In young people, influenza is an unpleasant, debilitating illness, disrupting work or school. The consequences can be grave for older adults or those in poor health (Nicholson, 1990). Pneumonia may supervene. This is usually attributed to colonisation of the traumatised respiratory epithelium by potential pathogens (*Staphylococcus aureus* and *Haemophilus influenzae*), but in some cases the virus itself may be responsible.

Influenza viruses are widespread throughout the world, producing epidemics every few years. Spread across the community is most common for type A, which is the most virulent (Grist, 1989), type C being least likely to cause epidemics. Worldwide pandemics have been recorded but are difficult to predict. In 1918, 20 million people – including young adults – died from influenza. More recently, the pandemic of Asian flu resulted in a high incidence of infection but a lower rate of mortality. Most major outbreaks represent the emergence of new variants of influenza virus with different surface antigens (antigenic drift). This is most marked with type A. The population has no immunity against the new antigens so infection becomes rife. The existence of the three different strains of the virus (A, B and C), the differences in the surface antigens displayed by members of the same strain and the phenomenon of antigenic drift contribute to the difficulties of controlling influenza. No single vaccine will give lasting immunity. Instead, vaccination is necessary as each new strain emerges. It is recommended for older adults in institutional care where rapid spread may occur and for those with chronic respiratory, cardiac or renal disease, with diabetes mellitus and those who are immunocompromised.

Clinical Application

Increasing the Uptake of Influenza Vaccination

The influenza vaccine, prepared from inactivated, highly purified viruses, is cheap and safe, with few side-effects (Govaert and Dinant, 1993, but only 40 per cent of those at risk receive it (Ogden, 1993). Most offers of immunisation are made within the primary care setting, and most people who accept request it the following year. Practice nurses are in a key position to run immunisation clinics, maintain registers of people at risk and liaise with practice managers so that reminders and repeat prescriptions are issued. The failure of susceptible people to accept vaccination leads to increased mortality, although many deaths will not be directly attributed to the influenza itself. Outbreaks are expensive because a large number of patients are admitted to hospital over a short period of time and normal services are disrupted (Grist, 1989).

Other respiratory infections and those arising from pathogens in the respiratory tract – pulmonary tuberculosis, Legionnaire's disease and meningococcal meningitis – are covered in Chapter 14.

REVISION CHECKLIST: KEY AREAS

❏ Introduction – the importance of respiratory infections

❏ Lower respiratory tract infections: Bronchitis, Pneumonia, Hospital-acquired pneumonia

❏ Upper respiratory tract infections: Coughs and colds, Otitis media, Croup, Respiratory syncytial virus, Pertussis, Diphtheria, Influenza

Activities – linking knowledge to clinical practice

1 **The viruses** responsible for colds and related upper respiratory tract infections are transmitted mainly by self-inoculation when contaminated fingers contact the nasal epithelium or conjunctivae (which is lined with the same type of epithelium). The next time you are in a public place, ideally sitting opposite other people, or if you teach, when you are in front of a group, observe how often the face, especially the nose and eyes, is touched. If possible, watch a few people for 10–15 minutes. Can you see why upper respiratory tract infections are so prevalent? On the basis of your findings, do you think that teaching the public about the importance of hand hygiene to prevent colds would be successful?

2 **Identify** the major problems associated with respiratory infection within your clinical area and suggest a strategy for its prevention.

SELF-ASSESSMENT

1. Which of the following never operate as respiratory pathogens?
   (a) staphylococci ☐
   (b) rhinoviruses ☐
   (c) *Bacteroides* spp. ☐
   (d) Gram-negative bacteria ☐

2. The prevalence of lower respiratory tract infection in hospital is .... per cent.

3. Pneumonia is a common hospital-acquired infection, especially after surgery.
   True? ☐ False? ☐

4. Antibiotics are of secondary importance to physiotherapy in the prevention and treatment of postoperative chest infection.
   True? ☐ False? ☐

5. Which of the following may operate as a possible source of lower respiratory tract infection in the ventilated patient?
   (a) the kidney ☐
   (b) the mouth ☐
   (c) the stomach ☐
   (d) the suction catheter ☐

6. The pathogen responsible for whooping cough is *Haemophilus influenzae.*   True? ☐ False? ☐

7. Influenza vaccination benefits which of the following?
   (a) patients in congestive cardiac failure ☐
   (b) those with chronic bronchitis ☐
   (c) children recovering from bronchitis ☐
   (d) anyone taking corticosteroids for more than a year ☐

8. A pyrexial child with a cough may benefit from which of the following?
   (a) paracetamol 2 tablets 4 hourly ☐
   (b) aspirin ☐
   (c) an antitussive ☐
   (d) paracetamol dose calculated on body weight ☐

References

Botman A and de Krieger RA (1987) 'Contamination of small volume medication nebulisers and its association with oropharyngeal colonisation'. *Journal of Hospital Infection* **10**: 204–8.

Cobben NAM, Drent M, Jonkers EFM *et al.* (1996) 'Outbreak of severe *Pseudomonas aeruginosa* respiratory infections due to contaminated nebulisers'. *Journal of Hospital Infection* **33**: 63–70.

Craven DE, Connolly M, Lichtenberg G *et al.* (1982) 'Contamination of mechanical ventilator tubing changes every 24 or 48 hours'. *New England Journal of Medicine* **306**: 1505–8.

Craven DE, Goularte TA and Make BJ (1984) 'Contaminated condensate in mechanical ventilator circuits: a risk factor for nosocomial pneumonia?' *American Review of Respiratory Diseases* **129**: 625–8.

Craven DE, Kunches LM, Kilinsky V *et al.* (1986) 'Risk factors for pneumonia and fatality for patients receiving continuous mechanical ventilation'. *American Review of Respiratory Diseases* **133**: 792–6.

Emmerson AM, Enstone JE, Griffin M *et al.* (1996) 'The Second National Prevalence Survey of Infection in Hospitals – overview of the results'. *Journal of Hospital Infection* **32**: 175–90.

Fiorentini A (1992) 'Potential hazards of tracheobronchial suctioning'. *Intensive Critical Care Nursing* **8**: 217–26.

Gorman LJ, Sanai L, Notman W *et al.* (1993) 'Cross-infection in an intensive care unit by *Klebsiella pneumoniae* from ventilator condensate'. *Journal of Hospital Infection* **23**: 17–26.

Govaert TME and Dinant GJ (1993) 'Adverse reactions to influenza vaccine in elderly people: randomised double blind placebo trial'. *British Medical Journal* **307**: 988–99.

Grist N (1989) 'Influenza update'. *Practitioner* **233**: 56–9.

Grist N and Walker E (1991) 'Pneumococcal immunisation'. *Practice Nurse* January: 454–6.

Gwaltney JM, Moskalski PB and Hendley JO (1978) 'Hand to hand transmission of rhinovirus colds'. *Annals of Internal Medicine* **88**: 463–7.

Hendley JO, Wenzel RP and Gwaltney JM (1973) 'Transmission of rhinovirus colds by self-inoculation'. *New England Journal of Medicine* **291**: 1361–4.

Hoge CW, Reichler ME and Dominguez EA (1994) 'An epidemic of pneumococcal disease in an overcrowded, inadequately ventilated jail'. *New England Journal of Medicine* **331**: 643–8.

Inglis TJJ, Sproat LJ, Hawkey PM *et al.* (1993) 'Staphylococcal pneumonia in ventilated patients: a twelve month review of cases in an intensive care unit'. *Journal of Hospital Infection* **25**: 207–10.

Isaacs D, Dickson H, O'Callaghan C *et al.* (1991) 'Handwashing and cohorting in prevention of hospital acquired respiratory syncitial virus'. *Archives of Disease in Childhood* **66**: 227–31.

Johanson WG, Pierce AK and Sandford JP (1972) 'Nosocomial respiratory tract infections with Gram-negative bacilli'. *Annals of Internal Medicine* **77**: 701–14.

Kelleghan SI, Salemi C, Padilla S *et al.* (1993) 'An effective continuous quality improvement approach to the prevention of ventilator-associated pneumonia'. *American Journal of Infection Control* **21**: 322–30.

Lindeman CA and Van Aernan B (1971) 'Effects of structured and unstructured pre-operative teaching'. *Nursing Research* **20**: 319–32.

Moran AGD and Wilson JA (1986) 'Glue ear and speech development'. *British Medical Journal* **293**: 713–14.

Nicholson KG (1990) 'Influenza vaccine and the elderly'. *British Medical Journal* **301**: 617–18.

Nicholson KG, Kent J, Hammersley V *et al.* (1996) 'Risk factors for lower respiratory complications of rhinovirus infections in elderly people living in the community'. *British Medical Journal* **313**: 119–23.

Ogden J (1993) 'A hard sell ('Flu immunisation)'. *Nursing Times* **89**(47): 54–5.

Phillips I (1967) '*Pseudomonas aeruginosa* respiratory tract infections in patients receiving mechanical ventilation'. *Journal of Hygiene* **65**: 229–35.

Sanderson PJ (1983) 'Colonisation of the trachea in ventilated patients: what is the bacterial pathway?' *Journal of Hospital Infection* **4**: 15–18.

Stucke VA and Thompson REM (1980) 'Infection transfer by respiratory condensate during positive pressure respiration'. *Nursing Times* (Infection Control Supplement) **76**(7): s3–s7.

Tarlow M (1986) 'Reye's syndrome and aspirin'. *British Medical Journal* **292**: 1543–4.

Taylor B (1988) 'Coughs and colds in children'. *Health Visitor* **612**: 313–15.

Weiss AA and Hewlett EL (1986) 'Virulence factors of *Bordetella pertussis*'. *Annual Review of Microbiology* **40**: 661–86.

Further reading and information sources

Begg NW and Balraj V (1996) 'Diphtheria: are we ready for it?' *Archives of Disease in Childhood* **74**: 568–71.

Demers RR (1982) 'Complications of endotracheal suctioning procedures'. *Respiratory Care* **27**: 453–7. (A practical guide useful for anyone performing this procedure)

Nicol M, Bavin C, Bedford-Turner S, Cronin T and Rawlings-Anderson K (2000) *Essential Nursing Skills*. Mosby, London.

10 Infections associated with intravascular devices

CHAPTER OUTCOMES

After reading this chapter you should be able to:

■ Draw a diagram to show the portals of entry and sources of infection associated with intravascular devices

■ Define the terms 'bacteraemia', 'phlebitis' and 'septicaemia'

■ List the factors that place patients at risk of developing sepsis related to the presence of an intravascular device

■ Explain how the risk of infection may be reduced for patients with intravascular devices

---

Introduction – infection risks and intravascular devices

Intravascular devices are used extensively in hospital and increasingly in domiciliary settings. Their insertion is an invasive procedure, breaching the skin, which is the body's primary defence against infection. Pathogenic invasion is possible from a number of sites and sources (Figure 10.1). Many infections result from microorganisms on the patient's skin gaining access extraluminally from the insertion point, or intraluminally following contamination of the hubs or stopcock (Elliott *et al.*, 1995).

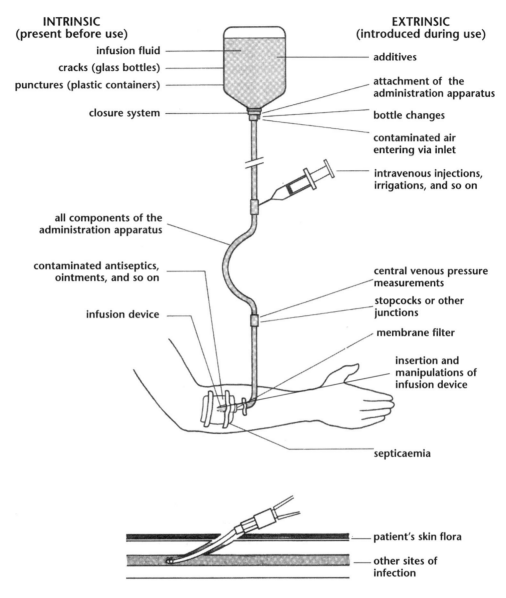

INTRINSIC
(present before use)

infusion fluid

cracks (glass bottles)

punctures (plastic containers)

closure system

all components of the
administration apparatus

contaminated antiseptics,
ointments, and so on

infusion device

EXTRINSIC
(introduced during use)

additives

attachment of the
administration apparatus

bottle changes

contaminated air
entering via inlet

intravenous injections,
irrigations, and so on

central venous pressure
measurements

stopcocks or other
junctions

membrane filter

insertion and
manipulations of
infusion device

septicaemia

patient's skin flora

other sites of
infection

Figure 10.1   Intravascular therapy – portals of entry

Morbidity and mortality from sepsis arising as a complication of intravascular therapy are increasing, findings reported from the Public Health Laboratory Service indicating an increase of 39 per cent between 1989 and 1991 (Elliott, 1993). Waghorn (1994), recording data collected in a district general hospital, listed 39 episodes of sepsis associated with intravascular devices over a 2-year period, including six fatalities.

Infections associated with intravascular devices

The risk of sepsis is increased when new techniques are introduced and the experience of staff is limited, particularly when infection control protocols are being developed. The introduction of intravascular volume control sets was initially associated with a poor level of maintenance, evidence being seen of leakage, dirty injection ports and breaches in asepsis during handling (Dumas *et al.*, 1971). Later studies recorded lower infection rates explained through the introduction of newer, less easily contaminated equipment and strict protocols for asepsis (Buxton *et al.*, 1979; Shinozaki *et al.*, 1983; Leroy *et al.*, 1989). Infection showed a definite association with breaches in asepsis in all of these studies, with clear links to poor hand hygiene. Protocols for managing intravascular devices differ between centres, contributing to the variation in infection rate that has been recorded (Nyström *et al.*, 1983). There are no national guidelines for the insertion and care of intravascular devices in the UK so auditing to identify problems is important (Elliot, 1993; Elliot *et al.*, 1995). Another factor contributing to the disparity in sepsis rate is the lack of consensus regarding the criteria accepted as evidence of infection. Authors employ different definitions so comparisons between findings are not meaningful (Table 10.1) (Johnson and Oppenheim, 1992). Clinically suspected intravascular catheter-related sepsis is defined as persistent pyrexia (of more than 38.5 ^{0}C) returning to normal when the device is removed (Haddock *et al.*, 1983). Most authorities believe that the device should only be considered responsible for the infection in the absence of any other explanation for the patient's symptoms.

Bacterial colonisation and infection of intravascular devices

The first step towards infection is colonisation of the catheter (Cercenado *et al.*, 1990). The organisms responsible are often those growing at the site of insertion. Bacteria and proteins adhere to the surface of the catheter, forming a biofilm (Chapter 7). As the biofilm develops, the organisms become incorporated into it and are protected. They multiply, eventually reaching a sufficient number to cause infection. The biofilm further protects the bacteria by offering mechanical protection from antibiotics so infection (once established) is more difficult to treat unless the device is removed.

Most colonisation and infection associated with intravascular devices is caused by bacteria forming part of the normal skin flora, especially *Staphylococcus epidermidis*. This originates from the patient's skin or from staff handling the device (Maki and Ringer, 1987). It colonises plastic more easily than other bacteria through its ability to adhere to plastic surfaces (Pascual *et al.*, 1993). However, a significant number of intravascular infections are also caused by Gram-negative opportunists (Vázquez *et al.*, 1994).

Table 10.1   Definitions of intravascular-associated infection

- Colonisation of the catheter (Maki and Ringer, 1987)
- Phlebitis (Tager *et al.*, 1983)
- Septicaemia (Ricard *et al.*, 1985)
- Culture of a newly withdrawn intravascular line (Maki *et al.*, 1977). Infection is considered to be present if 15 or more bacteria are isolated, allowing for accidental contamination during removal.

Presentation of infection associated with intravascular cannulation

Infection associated with intravascular cannulation may present in a variety of forms: localised cutaneous infection, phlebitis, bacteraemia or septicaemia.

Localised cutaneous infection

Localised cutaneous infection may develop at the point where the cannula enters the skin. It is characterised by the signs of inflammation, which include localised redness and heat.

Phlebitis

Phlebitis (inflammation of the vein), the most common complication associated with intravascular therapy, usually results from chemical or mechanical irritation. The main predisposing factors are the infusion of hypertonic solutions and the presence of particulate matter derived from incompletely reconstituted drugs, fragments of rubber or glass from vials and plastic from the cannula. Erythema develops proximal to the site of venepuncture, with pain. Bacteria are seldom responsible for phlebitis, but septicaemia is more common in patients who have developed it (Francombe, 1988).

Bacteraemia

Bacteraemia (the presence of bacteria in the blood) may be transient or may lead to septicaemia (Gray and Pedlar, 1994).

Septicaemia

Septicaemia (multiplication of bacteria in the blood) produces signs and symptoms of infection – fever and rigors. It is the most serious and life-threatening of all the above infectious conditions. Intravascular devices are not the only cause of bacteraemia and septicaemia, but in hospital they are the most common source.

Risk factors associated with intravascular infection

Patient's condition

The risk of infection is highest among immunocompromised patients, the group most likely to require intravascular therapy for parenteral nutrition and to administer drugs (such as antibiotics and cytotoxic therapy).

Length of time the catheter remains in situ

The longer the device remains in place, the greater the risk of biofilm formation, colonisation and infection (Clarke and Raffin, 1990).

Phlebitis

Phlebitis, whether from chemical or mechanical irritation of the blood vessel, predisposes to infection.

Clinical Application

Reducing the Incidence of Phlebitis

Staff education

- Increase staff awareness of infection control protocols in relation to intravascular devices and provide regular updates.
- Include education about intravascular devices in preregistration courses.

Duration of intravascular cannulation

- Keep a record of the date of cannula insertion in the nursing notes. Recent guidelines stress the importance of good record-keeping in protecting the welfare of patients (UKCC, 1998).
- Many studies and most specialists advocate the routine rotation of the cannula site every 48–72 hours, although an audit study by Stonehouse and Butcher (1996) found no correlation between length of time the cannula remained in situ and phlebitis.
- Cannulae should be replaced whenever signs of phlebitis are observed.

Recognising the problem

- Observe the site for signs of phlebitis at least once a day, and check the site prior to nursing interventions involving the cannula or intravenous infusion, for example intravenous injection.
- Grade signs of phlebitis using a recognised scale.
- Audit the incidence of phlebitis.

Clinical Application (cont'd)

Expert teams

- Where one exists, use the specialist cannulation team.
- Consult the infection control team.

Mechanical problems – trauma and irritation

- Use the smallest cannula appropriate for the situation.
- Secure the cannula properly to avoid movement.
- Select the insertion site carefully: some sites may cause discomfort or be inconvenient.
- Select cannulae made from material least likely to cause trauma.

Chemical problems

- Ensure that no hypertonic fluids are infused via a peripheral vein.
- Make sure that drugs for intravenous injection are prepared and administered correctly to avoid the possibility of problems caused by undissolved residues and changes in pH.

Filtration of particulate material

- Consider the use of filters to minimise the effects of particulate matter such as drug residues, rubber, plastic, glass and micro-organisms.

Problems of infection

- Use an aseptic technique during insertion of the cannula and any other dealings with the cannula or infusion.
- Clean the site prior to insertion of the cannula.
- Cover the insertion site with a well-secured dressing.
- Decontaminate or wash the hands before and after dealing with the cannula or infusion.
- Check the infusion fluid for signs of contamination, for example deterioration, colour change or damage to the container.
- Check the expiry date of the infusion fluid.
- Flush the cannula with heparin or sodium chloride (according to local protocols) to help to prevent blockage and subsequent bacterial colonisation of the device.

The material and type of device

The material used in the manufacture of the device influences the incidence of infection. Teflon and silastic catheters resist bacterial adherence and colonisation better than other plastics (Toltzis and Goldmann, 1990). Various different types of intravascular device carry different levels of risk (see below).

Types of intravascular device

The earliest peripheral intravascular devices, introduced in 1945, were made of plastic. They were superseded in 1950 by newer designs in which a plastic catheter covered a steel needle. In a modified form, these models are still used to establish short-term venous access (Brown, 1988), but single and multilumen catheters are now available. These have revolutionised the care of patients undergoing long-term nutritional and intravascular therapy, improving treatment prospects and quality of life by removing the need for difficult and repeated venepuncture. The most familiar examples include:

- **Broviac catheters** (Broviac *et al.*, 1973) – These consist of a narrow silicone rubber catheter 'tunnelled' subcutaneously between the point of insertion into the skin and entry into a central vein via a Dacron cuff. Tissue grows up into the cuff, securing the catheter into position. This helps to prevent bacterial invasion. The site heals within approximately 10 days of insertion. Dressings are no longer necessary.

- **Hickman catheters** (Figure 10.2) (Hickman *et al.*, 1979) – The catheter bore is wider as this model is intended for the administration of blood products and can be used for patients undergoing bone marrow transplantation.

Central venous and arterial catheters have been associated with a higher rate of sepsis than peripheral lines (Nyström *et al.*, 1983; Waghorn, 1994). However, complications appear to be less problematic when allowance is made for the extended time that they remain in situ compared with peripheral lines, and the high risk of infection seen in immunocompromised patients, who are most likely to use them (Decker and Edwards, 1988). There is no evidence that subcutaneously 'tunnelled' subclavian catheters reduce the incidence of sepsis arising through contamination of the skin–catheter junction, especially when highly trained staff are responsible for care (Garden and Sim, 1983; Keohane *et al.*, 1983).

Prevention of infection associated with intravascular devices

Infection control protocols should include guidelines for insertion and subsequent management.

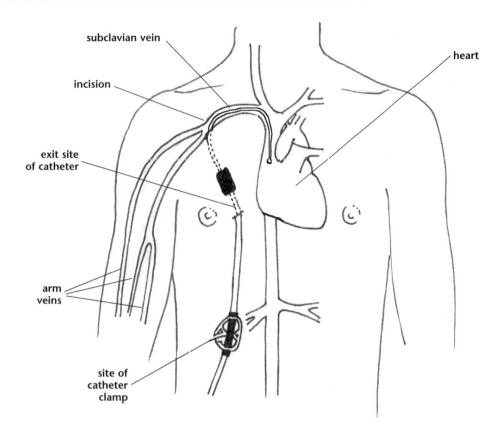

subclavian vein

heart

incision

exit site
of catheter

arm
veins

site of
catheter
clamp

Figure 10.2 A Hickman catheter – position and insertion

Insertion of the cannula

Aseptic technique

A strict aseptic technique is required to reduce the risk of transferring bacteria from the skin of the patient or health professional into the blood vessel. The hands should be decontaminated immediately before the catheter is introduced. Sterile gloves, gowns and drapes should be used during the insertion of central lines as this has been shown to reduce the infection rate (Raad *et al.*, 1993); this is easier to ensure if the insertion is performed in theatre. Once in situ, the catheter should be secured with sterile tape rather than sutured, in order to avoid traction. Traction could carry any bacteria present deeper into the wound or result in mechanical trauma, increasing the risk of non-bacterial phlebitis (Maki *et al.*, 1973).

Shaving the site

Shaving the site should if possible be avoided. It causes skin damage, increasing the number of micro-organisms present and therefore the risk of infection (Cruse and Foord, 1980).

Maintaining the intravascular system

Hand hygiene

Hand hygiene is essential to reduce cross-infection. The hands should be decontaminated before intravascular lines are accessed and connections should only be manipulated with gloved hands. Where possible, intravascular drugs should be given through latex membranes in order to avoid the use of stopcocks. Bacteria have been cultured from stopcocks and cannula hubs, but their significance has not been established. The incidence of infection has been reduced in some studies when colonised administration sets have been removed, but this may not always be practical. Cannulation at a new site may be difficult or impossible in a patient who urgently needs to continue treatment (Johnson and Oppenheim, 1992).

Skin preparation

Skin preparation and cleansing with 4 per cent chlorhexidine solution around the venepuncture site at each dressing change reduces infection more effectively than cleansing with povidone iodine or 70 per cent alcohol (Maki *et al.*, 1991). This is not surprising as the bacteria responsible for the infections associated with intravascular devices are often those normally present on the skin, especially *Staphylococcus epidermidis,* a Gram-positive coccus that chlorhexidine continues to destroy some time after its application.

Sterile dressings

Sterile dressings are used to protect the insertion site. There is a lack of consensus concerning the effect of the type of dressing on the incidence of infection. Transparent film dressings are often used because they permit inspection of the site without being removed so that early signs of phlebitis or infection are readily observed. Skin commensals may, however, build up underneath, and this may increase risks of infection. There is some evidence that films have no advantage over sterile gauze changed at regular intervals (Ricard *et al.*, 1985; Maki and Ringer, 1987). Dressings impregnated with antiseptics appear to be ineffective (Maki and Ringer, 1987).

Contamination of infusion fluids

The contamination of intravascular infusion fluids, although responsible for a number of outbreaks during the 1970s, is now a rare cause of sepsis because of the introduction of strict quality control during commercial preparation. Problems may still arise when fluids intended for parenteral administration are prepared on hospital premises without these high standards (Frean *et al.*, 1994). Before the bag is changed, the nurse should check that it has not reached the expiry date, that the bag is patent and that the fluid is clear. With contamination, the contents appear cloudy.

Filters

Filters positioned intraluminally between the cannula and fluid administration set reduce the risk of phlebitis and prevent bacteria gaining access to the vein (Francombe, 1988). They are particularly valuable when the administration set will be manipulated frequently but are not suitable for use with blood, blood products, lipid emulsions or with Swan-Ganz catheters (Quercia *et al.*, 1986).

Access to an intravascular therapy team

Access to the services of an intravascular therapy team is considered to be of key importance, especially in conjunction with centrally positioned catheters. Tomford *et al.* (1984) found that the rate of phlebitis fell from 32 per cent to 15 per cent after the involvement of a multidisciplinary team, while Keohane *et al.* (1983) reported a reduction from 25 per cent to 4 per cent when the team incorporated a nutrition nurse attending to patients undergoing parenteral therapy. The literature surrounding the insertion and care of intravascular lines is vast and frequently confusing. A regular review of new material by experts is needed to ensure that the latest research findings, for example concerning rotating the insertion site and changing the administration set, are incorporated into practice.

REVISION CHECKLIST: KEY AREAS

❑ Introduction – infection risks and intravascular devices

❑ Infections associated with intravascular devices: Bacterial colonisation and infection of intravascular devices, Presentation of infection associated with intravascular cannulation, Risk factors associated

with intravascular infection, Types of intravascular device

❑ Prevention of infection associated with intravascular devices: Insertion of the cannula, Maintaining the intravascular system

---

Activities – linking knowledge to clinical practice

1 **Find out** whether your ward or unit is currently auditing complications associated with intravascular devices.

(a) If a system of audit exists, comment on the criteria used, taking into consideration the types of patient catered for.

(b) If no system of audit currently exists, draw up a list of factors that should be considered, taking into account the types of patient catered for.

2 **Find out** what information is given to patients and/or relatives about caring for their central line (Hickman catheter) at home.

SELF-ASSESSMENT

1. Phlebitis is usually a complication of
   bacterial infection.   True? ☐ False? ☐

2. Bacteraemia is defined as ....

3. Septicaemia is defined as ....

4. According to research evidence, the sepsis
   rate is invariably higher when a
   centrally placed intravascular
   device is used.   True? ☐ False? ☐

References

Broviac JW, Cole JJ and Scribner BH (1973) 'A silicone rubber atrial catheter for prolonged parenteral alimentation'. *Surgery, Gynecology and Obstetrics* **136**: 602–6.

Brown J (1988) 'Peripherally inserted central catheters: use in home care'. *Journal of Intravascular Nursing* **13**: 144–7.

Buxton AE, Highsmith AK and Garner JA (1979) 'Contamination of intravascular infusion fluid: effects of changing administration sets'. *Annals of Internal Medicine* **90**: 764–8.

Cercenado E, Javier E and Rodriguez M (1990) 'A conservative procedure for the diagnosis of catheter-related infections'. *Archives of Internal Medicine* **150**: 1417–20.

Clarke DE and Raffin TA (1990) 'Infectious complications of indwelling long-term central venous catheters'. *Chest* **97**: 966–72.

Cruse PJE and Foord R (1980) 'The epidemiology of wound infection: a 10 year prospective study of 62,939 wounds'. *Surgical Clinics of North America* **60**: 27–40.

Decker MD and Edwards KM (1988) 'Central venous catheter infectious'. *Paediatric Nursing Clinics of North America* **14**: 503–9.

Dumas RJ, Warner JF and Dalton MP (1971) 'Septicaemia from intravascular infusions'. *New England Journal of Medicine* **284**: 257–60.

Elliott TSJ (1993) 'Line-associated bacteraemias'. *Public Health Laboratory Service CDR* **3** R: 91–6.

Elliott TSJ, Faroqui MH, Tebbs SE *et al.* (1995) 'An audit programme for central venous catheter-associated infections'. *Journal of Hospital Infection* **30**: 181–91.

Francombe P (1988) 'Intravascular filters and phlebitis'. *Nursing Times* **29**(84): 34–5.

Frean JA, Arntzen L, Rosekilly I *et al.* (1994) 'Investigation of parenteral nutrition fluids associated with an outbreak of *Serratia odorifera* septicaemia'. *Journal of Hospital Infection* **27**: 263–73.

Garden OJ and Sim AJW (1983) 'A comparison of tunnelled and non-tunnelled subclavian vein catheters: a prospective study of complications during parenteral feeding'. *Clinical Nutrition* **2**: 51–4.

Gray J and Pedlar SJ (1994) 'The changing face of bacteraemia'. *Journal of Hospital Infection* **27**: 317–18 (Letter to the Editor).

Haddock G, Barr J, Burns HJG *et al.* (1983) 'Reduction of central venous catheter complications'. *British Journal of Parenteral Therapy* **3**: 124–8.

Hickman RO, Bruckner CD, Clift RA *et al.* (1979) 'A modified right atrial catheter for access to the venous system on marrow transplant recipients'. *Surgery, Gynecology and Obstetrics* **148**: 871–5.

Johnson A and Oppenheim BA (1992) 'Vascular catheter-related sepsis: diagnosis and prevention'. *Journal of Hospital Infection* **20**: 67–78.

Keohane PP, Jones BJ, Attrill H *et al.* (1983) 'Effect of catheter tunnelling and a nutrition nurse on catheter sepsis during parenteral nutrition'. *Lancet* **2**: 1388–90.

Leroy O, Billiau V, Beussart C *et al.* (1989) 'Nosocomial infection associated with long-term arterial cannulation'. *Intensive Care Medicine* **15**: 241–5.

Maki DG and Ringer M (1987) 'Evaluation of dressing regimens for prevention of infection with peripheral intravenous catheters. Gauze, a transparent polyurethane dressing and an iodophor-transparent dressing'. *Journal of the American Medical Association*, **258**(17): 2396–403.

Maki DG, Goldman D and Rhame FS (1973) 'Infection control in intravascular therapy'. *Annals of Internal Medicine* **79**: 867–87.

Maki DG, Weise CE and Sarafin H (1977) 'A semi-quantative culture method for identifying intravascular catheter-related infection'. *New England Journal of Medicine* **296**: 1305–9.

Maki DG, Ringer M and Alvardo CJ (1991) 'Prospective randomised trial of povidone, iodine, alcohol and chlorhexidine for prevention of infection associated with central venous and arterial catheters'. *Lancet* **338**: 339–43.

Nyström B, Larson OS, Dankert J *et al.* (1983) 'Bacteraemia in surgical patients with intravascular devices: a European multicentre incidence study'. *Journal of Hospital Infection* **4**: 338–49.

Pascual A, Ramirez de Arellano E, Martinez-Martinez L *et al.* (1993) 'Effect of polyurethane catheters and bacterial biofilms on the *in vitro* activity of antimicrobials against *Staphylococcus epidermidis*'. *Journal of Hospital Infection* **24**: 211–18.

Quercia RA, Hill S, Klimek J *et al.* (1986) 'Bacteriologic contamination of intravascular infusion delivery systems in an intensive care unit'. *American Journal of Medicine* **80**: 364–8.

Raad II, Hohn DC and Gilbreath BJ (1993) 'Prevention of central catheter-related infections by using maximal sterile barrier precautions during insertion'. *Infection Control and Hospital Epidemiology* **15**: 231–8.

Ricard P, Martin R and Marcoux A (1985) 'Protection of indwelling vascular catheters; incidence of bacterial contamination and catheter-related sepsis'. *Critical Care Medicine* **13**: 542–3.

Shinozaki T, Deane PS, Mazuzan JE *et al.* (1983) Bacterial contamination of arterial lines. A prospective study. *Journal of the American Medical Association* **249**: 223–5.

Stonehouse J and Butcher J (1996) Phlebitis associated with peripheral cannulae. *Professional Nurse* **12**(1): 51–4.

Tager IB, Ginsberg M, Ellis S *et al.* (1983) An epidemiological study of the risks associated with peripheral intravascular catheters. *American Journal of Epidemiology* **118**: 839–51.

Toltzis P and Goldmann DA (1990) Current issues in central venous catheter infection. *Annual Review of Medicine* **41**: 169–76.

Tomford JW, Hershey CO, McLaren CE *et al.* (1984) 'Intravascular therapy team and peripheral venous catheter associated complications. A prospective controlled study'. *Archives of Internal Medicine* **144**: 1191–4.

United Kingdom Central Council for Nursing, Midwifery and Health Visiting (1998) *Guidelines for Records and Record Keeping*. London, UKCC.

Vázquez F, Mendoza MC, Villar MH *et al.* (1994) 'Survey of bacteraemia in a Spanish hospital over a decade'. *Journal of Hospital Infection* **26**: 111–21.

Waghorn DJ (1994) 'Intravascular device-associated systemic infections: a 2 year analysis of cases in a district general hospital'. *Journal of Hospital Infection* **28**: 91–102.

Further reading and information sources

Campbell L (1998) 'IV-related phlebitis, complications and length of hospital stay: 1'. *British Journal of Nursing* **7**(21): 1304–2.

Campbell L (1998) 'IV-related phlebitis, complications and length of hospital stay: 2'. *British Journal of Nursing* **7**(22): 1364–3.

Clark L (1994) 'Safety first'. *Nursing Times* **90**(5): 64–6.

Fuller A and Winn C (1998) 'The management of peripheral IV lines'. *Professional Nurse* **13**(10): 675–8.

Gabriel J (1994) 'An intravascular alternative'. *Nursing Times* **90**(31): 39–41.

Jackson A (1998) 'A battle in vein: infusion phlebitis'. *Nursing Times* (Infection Control Supplement) **94**(4): 68–71.

Wilson J (1994) 'Preventing infection during intravascular therapy'. *Professional Nurse* **9**(6): 388–92.

11 Enteric infection

CHAPTER OUTCOMES

After reading this chapter you should be able to:

■ Differentiate between foodborne infections and intoxications

■ List the main organisms responsible for foodborne infection

■ List the main organisms responsible for foodborne intoxication

■ Explain to a member of the public effective strategies for preventing foodborne illness at home

■ Explain why foodborne disease is a problem in hospital and identify the main steps taken to prevent and control it

---

Introduction to enteric infection

All food contains micro-organisms. Some cause spoilage by altering the appearance, taste or smell, but food that has 'gone bad' is unlikely to be consumed and therefore does not cause a threat to health. Items contaminated by enteric bacteria or their toxins, however, can give rise to unpleasant illness even though their appearance, smell and taste are unchanged. The illnesses caused by contaminated food can range from very mild to serious illness, which may lead to death in vulnerable people.

Incidence of enteric infection

Enteric infection is a major health problem. Official statistics collated by the Public Health Laboratory Service (PHLS) and published by the Office of Population Censuses and Surveys reveal an upward trend in the number of reported cases since the mid-1980s in the UK. This is, however, only the tip of the iceberg as isolated cases are not reported, large outbreaks occuring when several people have eaten the same food being more likely to be investigated (Tranter, 1990). The main contributory factors are:

- The advance preparation of food
- Inadequate cooking
- Inadequate cooling
- Improper storage
- Reheating.

Faults during food production, transport and storage before sale also contribute (North, 1989).

Risk factors

Risk factors are related to the immune status of the individual (intrinsic) and factors associated with modern lifestyle affecting food choice and preparation (extrinsic).

Intrinsic factors

The following are at particular risk:

- The very young – The immune system in the very young is not mature so susceptibility to infection is high. Traditionally, health visitors have played a major role in educating the public about the importance of hygiene, especially when infant feeds are prepared. The incidence of gastroenteritis is higher for bottle-fed babies, vomiting and diarrhoea developing either because feeds are too concentrated or because of infective gastroenteritis. Sick children are at greatest risk. The trend towards early discharge means that these infants are now likely to be cared for in the community. They often require special feeds administered enterally, and these feeds may become contaminated, especially if they are prepared by parents at home (Anderton *et al.*, 1993).

- Older adults – Fewer organisms are required to produce an infective dose, while diarrhoea and vomiting are more likely to result in dehydration and electrolyte imbalance.

- Patients with severe illnesses, especially those who are immunocompromised – This group includes cancer patients and those with AIDS.

Extrinsic factors

Those most at risk are:

- Frail people (including older adults) – Frail people may not be able to get out to buy fresh food.

- People with limited financial means – Individuals in this group cannot afford good-quality produce. Lacking transport, they may rely on local shops where turnover is slower and perishable items may remain longer on the shelves. They are also less likely to throw away suspect items because they cannot afford waste. Lack of refrigeration can be a problem, especially in bed and breakfast accommodation where families with young children are housed by the social services.

- People who frequently eat out or rely on a high proportion of preprepared food – Mass production and preprepared meals or snacks are associated with an increased risk.

- Travellers – Overseas travel has increased dramatically over the past 20 years, exposing people to lower standards of hygiene than at home (Cossar *et al.*, 1990).

- People living in institutions – This includes residents of schools, prisons, nursing homes and hospitals, where mass catering is inevitable.

Foodborne illness is usually mild, resolving spontaneously within a few days, but the consequences can occasionally be more serious. Dehydration can be severe, dangerous and expensive. It can also be difficult to treat in infants and older adults.

Food infection and intoxication

The term 'food poisoning' is used to describe vomiting or diarrhoea following the consumption of food contaminated with bacteria or their toxins. As it also encompasses illnesses resulting from the ingestion of natural poisons (berries or toadstools, for example), 'foodborne illness' is a more accurate term. There are two types of foodborne illness: invasive intestinal gastroenteritis and intoxication (Table 11.1).

Infection (invasive intestinal gastroenteritis) results when bacteria are ingested in contaminated food. They multiply within the gut, giving rise to a systemic, infectious illness characterised by malaise, pyrexia and cramping abdominal pain in addition to nausea, vomiting and diarrhoea. Symptoms generally develop and resolve more slowly than in cases of intoxication because there is an incubation period in which the bacteria establish themselves within the host and multiply before causing symptoms. The victim is infectious, and precautions must be taken when excreta and vomitus are handled. Heating the food to 60 ^{0}C kills most bacteria, but the temperature must be high enough and applied for long enough to destroy sufficient bacteria to result in a level below the infective dose. This may be impossible for some dishes likely to deteriorate with heat (such as custards or lightly boiled eggs) or when the food is heavily contaminated. It is not always possible to detect the presence of bacteria by odour.

Table 11.1   Food infections and intoxications

Infections	Intoxications
Salmonella	Bacillus cereus
Shigella	Staphylococcus aureus
Campylobacter	Clostridium perfringens*
Listeria	Clostridium botulinum

* Toxins are released after ingestion and not into the food

Intoxication develops when food containing bacterial toxins is consumed. Vomiting, sometimes with diarrhoea, develops within a few hours. The patient is not infectious. Toxins are heat stable so contaminated food is not rendered safe by normal cooking, pasteurisation and other heat treatments.

Invasive gastrointestinal infection

Salmonella

Salmonella is a Gram-negative, motile bacillus able to grow under aerobic and anaerobic conditions. The optimum temperature for growth is 37 ^{0}C, but it can multiply anywhere between 7 ^{0}C and 48 ^{0}C. It is readily destroyed by heat but can survive freezing and drying, especially if protected by protein in food. Bacteria have been isolated from the fingers even after the hands have been washed and dried (Pether and Gilbert, 1971). World wide, *Salmonella* is a major cause of foodborne illness. There has been a sharp increase in the number of reported cases in the UK in recent years, mainly owing to *Salmonella enteritidis* (Baird-Parker, 1990).

The increase in *Salmonella* infection is related to the overcrowding of livestock on farms, mass production and poor hygiene in premises where food is prepared, stored and sold. Contamination during transport has been documented (Hennessy *et al.*, 1996), and cross-contamination can occur to any food in contact with it (Johnston, 1990).

Salmonella is a zoonotic organism ubiquitous among domestic and wild warm-blooded animals, including poultry, although not usually giving rise to the clinical manifestations of infection in these hosts. Data from the PHLS reveal that

Clinical Application

Salmonella and Eggs

Salmonella can survive light cooking (Mitchell *et al.*, 1989), raw and undercooked eggs having been widely implicated as the cause of *Salmonella* foodborne illness in traditionally prepared and cook–chill dishes (Lacey and Buckingham, 1993). Several theories have been put forward to suggest the source of contamination:

■ **Faecal contamination** – via cracks in the shell. Bacteria lodged in the crack may reach the yolk when the egg is broken, or become sucked inside as it cools in the refrigerator. This is less likely with battery hens, for which there is a 'roll-away' system for newly laid eggs. Eggs produced in this way are, however, increasingly unacceptable to consumers.

■ **Vertical transmission** – via the oviduct of an infected bird. The bacteria are thought to gain access to the egg before the shell develops.

■ **Cross-contamination** – via the fingers or from other contaminated source to shelled eggs or their products during food preparation or storage.

Pasteurised eggs should be used to prepare lightly cooked and raw egg dishes (such as ice cream and mayonnaise) in all catering establishments and if possible at home (DoH, 1993), the Department of Health repeating this advice in 1998. The same document also advises vulnerable people to avoid foods prepared from raw or lightly cooked eggs. Other hygiene measures recommended include the following:

■ Wash the hands after handling eggs
■ Do not use eggs with damaged shells
■ Store the eggs in the refrigerator if possible, or in a cool, dry place
■ Store eggs separate from raw meat and other possible contaminants
■ Use the oldest eggs first
■ Clean kitchen surfaces and equipment after preparing egg dishes
■ Eat egg dishes soon after cooking or refrigerate them.

Salmonella enteritidis has been isolated from a high proportion of broiler chickens intended for retail sale and from the eggs of free-range and battery hens (Baird-Parker, 1990). This has prompted considerable media interest, some authorities concluding that the presence of *Salmonella enteritidis* has reached epidemic proportions.

Salmonella has an incubation period of 12–72 hours in the human host, symptoms appearing up to 7 days after ingestion. The illness lasts 2–5 days and is more severe in older adults and the very young. Although the acute stage of infection is usually over quickly, bacteria can be shed in the faeces of asymptomatic carriers for up to 3 months. Diagnosis is by stool culture; bacteria are not usually present in blood. Treatment is fluid replacement. Antibiotics prolong carriage, but if infection is severe with complications (for example, septicaemia or damage to the intestinal mucosa resulting in malabsorption and nutrient loss), ciprofloxacin is prescribed. This reduces the duration of diarrhoea and vomiting, and eliminates *Salmonella* from the stools (Ahmad *et al.*, 1991)

Nosocomial salmonellosis

Between 1992 and 1994, infectious intestinal disease accounted for 15 per cent of all reported outbreaks (189 out of 1275) in hospitals; of these, 125 were caused by salmonellae. Transmission was mainly by person-to-person spread rather than by the consumption of contaminated food. Hospital outbreaks lasted on average 16 days, with considerable disruption to hospital services. The cost of outbreaks was high as many staff and patients had to be screened, and infection was considered to have contributed to the deaths of five patients (Wall *et al.*, 1996).

Clinical Application

The Stanley Royd Incident

An outbreak of *Salmonella* infection at Stanley Royd Hospital in Wakefield, Yorkshire in 1984 involved over 400 patients and staff receiving food from the same kitchen, and the death of 19 elderly patients. This prompted a public enquiry with recommendations for the future investigation, control and prevention of outbreaks. Recommendations centred mainly on the improvement of kitchen facilities and practices. As a result, Crown Immunity was lifted from hospital kitchens in 1987. Hospital authorities and Trusts whose catering departments fail to comply with requirements are now liable to prosecution in the same way as are commercial premises (DoH, 1986).

More hospital outbreaks occur where there is a high incidence of faecal soiling (for example, paediatric, maternity and geriatric units), and many have been reported in patients with mental health problems (Joseph and Palmer, 1989). The opportunity for infection is increased by these patients' poor personal hygiene and by movement between different parts of the hospital (Cruikshank, 1984). Although person-to-person spread is the most important route, it cannot always be distinguished from transmission via contaminated clinical equipment (such as rectal thermometers, gastroscopes or faulty bedpan washers) because the bacteria can survive well in moist environments (Meara *et al.*, 1988). It is frequently impossible to trace the source of infection. Kitchen workers carrying *Salmonella* may cause infection in sick and healthy people (Dryden *et al.*, 1994).

Campylobacter jejuni

Campylobacter jejuni is a Gram-negative, highly motile bacterium. Infection was first reported to the PHLS in 1977. The number of reported cases has since increased every year, and it is now one of the most common causes of foodborne disease. Much of this apparent upsurge may be the result of improved diagnostic facilities (Cowden, 1992). Health professionals are more likely to see patients with *Campylobacter* infection than many other enteric infections because the symptoms of acute abdominal pain and bloodstained diarrhoea can be so severe and frightening that the victim will seek medical help. The incubation period is 2–10 days, and the illness lasts 10–14 days.

The bacteria are widespread within the environment and have been isolated from sewage, raw meat and unpasteurised milk. They do not multiply below 30 ^{0}C and are thus unlikely to grow on food at room temperature. Cross-contamination readily occurs between stored items, and foods as diverse as salads and cake icing have operated as vehicles for infection (Blaser *et al.*, 1982). Death is unusual but morbidity is considerable, and it has been suggested that *Campylobacter* infection may be linked with the later development of Guillain–Barré syndrome.

Campylobacter appears to be less infectious than many of the other bacteria causing foodborne illness. Person-to-person spread is rare, with only occasional reports among members of the same household (usually children during the acute diarrhoeal phase), and community outbreaks are uncommon. Infection has, however,

---

Clinical Application

Controlling an Outbreak of *Salmonella*

Galloway *et al.* (1987) report the following successful control measures in a hospital for long-term patients. The outbreak involved 11 patients and 12 members of staff over a period of 3 weeks:

- Screening stool specimens from all patients on wards where diarrhoea had been reported. Positive patients were isolated and looked after by staff not responsible for any of the other patients
- Screening staff from affected wards, catering staff and others with gastrointestinal symptoms. This helped to eliminate carriers
- Cleaning the central and ward kitchens
- Destroying soiled furniture
- Curtailing admissions until the outbreak was controlled.

Taking food histories from patients and testing food specimens did not help to identify the source of the infection.

resulted from handling family pets carrying the bacteria, and vertical transmission from mother to fetus has been documented. The illness is usually self-limiting but can if necessary be treated with erythromycin or aminoglycosides (Chapter 4).

Shigella sonnei

Shigella sonnei is a Gram-negative rod causing dysentery. Infection results in acute inflammation of the large bowel with the passage of loose stools containing blood, pus and mucus. Four species are responsible for clinical illness (Table 11.2). *Shigella sonnei* is the species encountered most often in the UK. It is disseminated by the faecal-oral route, outbreaks typically occuring in institutions among young children. Control is by improving standards of personal hygiene. Chronic carriage is rare, although those recovering from acute infection may continue to shed bacteria for a few weeks.

Table 11.2   *Shigella* species responsible for dysentery

Species	Distribution	Presentation
Shigella dysenteriae	Tropical and subtropical	Severe
Shigella flexneri	Tropical and subtropical	Moderate
Shigella boydii	Tropical and subtropical	Moderate
Shigella sonnei	Temperate	Mild

Escherichia coli

Escherichia coli is a commensal in the human bowel. Colonisation occurs within a few weeks of birth and is of benefit to the host because it reduces the risk of overgrowth by other potentially pathogenic bacteria. However, some serotypes of *E. coli* can cause foodborne infection. These fall into four groups, depending on factors contributing to their virulence and the way in which they interact with the intestinal mucosa (Gould, 1996).

Enteropathic E. coli

Enteropathic *E. coli* (EPEC) is a major cause of severe diarrhoea in infants in developing countries. Most outbreaks have been reported from hospitals or nurseries and in each case traced to a food-handler or to water contaminated with human sewage (Doyle, 1990). This serotype owes its pathogenicity to its ability to adhere strongly to the intestinal mucosa, destroying the microvilli and disrupting absorption.

Enterovasive E. coli

Enterovasive *E. coli* (EIEC) has been responsible for many outbreaks since its pathogenic activity was first described in the 1940s (Doyle, 1990). Food-handlers and contaminated water are the usual source, but person-to-person spread is also possible. EIEC causes invasive dysentery and bloodstained diarrhoea.

Enterotoxigenic E. coli

Enterotoxigenic *E. coli* (ETEC) is the principal agent implicated in travellers' diarrhoea reported by those visiting countries with poor standards of hygiene. Infection is uncommon in the UK except in those returning from overseas but it is a major cause of gastroenteritis among all age groups in developing countries. Outbreaks are generally traceable to a human source. The bacteria invade the intestinal mucosa but produce watery rather than bloodstained diarrhoea, and recovery is usually complete.

Enterohaemorrhagic E. coli

Enterohaemorrhagic *E. coli* (EHEC) causes a wide range of illnesses, from mild diarrhoea to severe abdominal pain with haemorrhagic colitis. Symptoms arise from the production of an enterotoxin called verocytotoxin, which is produced when the bacteria adhere to the intestinal wall. The organism is extremely virulent and relatively few bacteria will cause harm (Williams and Ellison, 1998).

The disease is usually self-limiting, and most people recover within about 8 days. However, approximately a third of those infected require hospital admission, and a small number (mainly children) develop haemolytic uraemic syndrome, a form of renal failure carrying a mortality rate of 17 per cent. Survivors may have residual renal problems.

The main serotype associated with EHEC is *E. coli* 0157. This is now recognised as an important pathogen and has caused outbreaks in the USA, Canada and the UK, in households, nurseries, residential homes and hospitals. Person-to-person spread is possible via the faecal-oral route, and asymptomatic carriage is possible. Outbreaks have been linked to the consumption of many types of meat, especially undercooked beef products, meat pies and hamburgers, unpasteurised milk and milk products, faecally contaminated water and vegetables washed in it. Dairy cattle may operate as a reservoir. EHEC is uncommon in the UK, but the number of cases reported annually to the PHLS is increasing.

Listeria monocytogenes

Listeria monocytogenes is a facultive Gram-positive, non-sporing bacillus present in soil and water as well as on vegetation. Although *Listeria* was identified as an animal pathogen early in the 20th century, it has only recently been recognised as a cause of human disease (Jones, 1990). Listeriosis can take the following forms (Levy, 1989):

- Intrauterine or perinatal infection
- Meningitis
- Septicaemia
- Cutaneous infection arising through contact with animals (rare).

Most people develop immunity through exposure to bacteria in the environment. Some are asymptomatic carriers, and only 10–15 per cent of infections occur in

Clinical Application

Outbreak of *E. coli* 0157 in Central Scotland during 1996

During 1996, a serious outbreak of *E. coli* 0157:H7 occurred in Lanarkshire, Central Scotland. There have been other outbreaks, both before and after, but this was the most serious to date, with 20 deaths, all of which occurred in people aged over 65 years.

The 1996 outbreak was eventually traced to a specific butcher's shop. Infected meat and meat products were supplied from this shop to various other business outlets, which increased the size of the outbreak (Williams and Ellison, 1998). The widespread distribution of infected foods also made tracing the source more difficult.

Various recommendations on food handling, training, minimising contamination, regulations and enforcement, and managing outbreaks have been published by the Pennington Group (see Further reading and Information sources), which was established by the government to investigate all aspects of the *E. coli* 0157:H7 outbreak in Central Scotland.

There are implications for nurses, midwives and health visitors in their role as health educators, and in the training and supervision of all staff, especially those who handle food. As with most aspects of infection control, the importance of proper handwashing protocols cannot be stressed enough.

healthy people (Levy, 1989). Infection follows the consumption of contaminated food (Schlech, 1991), the incubation period being 7–70 days.

Listeria causes severe infection in the immunocompromised host and in pregnant women. Cases are uncommon, even in these groups, but the mortality rate is high (Wilkinson, 1989). Pregnant women may remain asymptomatic after infection or develop flu-like symptoms. *Listeria* crosses the placenta and can cause spontaneous miscarriage, stillbirth or the delivery of an acutely ill baby. Neonatal listeriosis is classified as being of early (within 2–3 days of delivery) or late (5 days or more) onset. In early-onset cases, the infant develops septicaemia, the mortality rate being 40–50 per cent. With late-onset listeriosis, meningitis is the most common presentation. Mortality in the neonate is 25 per cent, but maternal recovery occurs spontaneously after delivery without treatment. Diagnosis is by blood or cerebrospinal fluid culture in adults. In cases of suspected neonatal infection, swabs are taken from the eyes, ears and placenta. Adults are treated with high doses of ampicillin. Infants are given gentamicin for at least 2 weeks, the dose being determined by weight.

Listeria infection has resulted from the consumption of unpasteurised milk (in Brie, Camembert and blue vein cheese), chilled cold meats, pâté, undercooked chicken, prepared salads such as coleslaw and cook–chill products. Hard cheeses (such as Cheddar) and processed and cottage cheese are safe, as are pasteurised milk and milk powder heated during production. There are moves to ban the sale of 'raw' (unpasteurised) milk in the UK at the time of writing.

Listeria grows at temperatures as low as 2 ^{0}C and multiplies in refrigerated food, although growth in temperatures up to 42 ^{0}C is possible. Outbreaks may be seasonal, occurring most often during the autumn, which is in contrast to most other agents responsible for foodborne disease. Food probably becomes contaminated from environmental sources during production, a situation exacerbated by modern methods of raising livestock since feed may be contaminated with *Listeria* (Fenlon, 1985).

Foodborne intoxication

Staphylococcus aureus

Staphylococcus aureus causes gastrointestinal symptoms by producing heat-stable enterotoxins. The amount necessary to cause symptoms is unknown but is thought to be as little as 1 μg/100 g of food. Symptoms usually appear within 2–6 hours of ingestion, depending on the amount consumed. The cause of vomiting and diarrhoea is poorly understood: presumably the toxin irritates receptors in the gut wall, relaying impulses to the vomiting centre in the medulla. Staphylococcal disease is not reportable in the UK so its incidence is not established. It is thought to vary between countries, depending on eating habits, and appears to be more common in the USA than in the UK (Tranter, 1990). Typical episodes last 2–3 days, and many people recover without seeking the advice of a health professional.

Staphylococcus aureus is a natural food contaminant, the source being always another person. Unwashed hands are usually to blame, especially if the food-handler has a septic lesion not covered by a waterproof dressing. The bacteria multiply in the warm, damp conditions so often provided by inadequately refrigerated display counters in shops, restaurants and fast-food outlets, releasing toxins. They survive in a saline environment and are particularly associated with salty foods such as ham, and sugary products. The salt or sugar discourages the growth of other bacteria, so a large number of staphylococci flourish unchecked. Other foods incriminated include fish, poultry, cakes with cream or custard fillings and salads. Cross-contamination between items stored close together is possible.

Clostridia

Clostridia are anaerobic, Gram-positive, spore-forming bacteria. They inhabit soil, playing an important role in the decomposition of dead organisms. Some species are commensals in the human gut but may also operate as human pathogens. The toxins are released after ingestion.

Clostridium perfringens

Clostridium perfringens is responsible for many outbreaks of foodborne illness, especially in institutions. The tough spores withstand cooking but germinate when the food, often meat, is inadequately reheated. The organism multiplies best between 37 ^{0}C and 41 ^{0}C. The source of the outbreak is usually difficult to establish because *Clostridium perfringens* is widespread within the environment and is often present within the human gut, especially among long-stay patients.

In a typical outbreak described by Pollock and Whitty (1991), the source was reheated mince. The outbreak involved 58 out of 647 elderly people, with two deaths. Cases were restricted to the four wards where the meals arrived earliest. Food destined for the other wards remained in the heated trolley for longer and reached a satisfactory temperature, halting the multiplication of bacteria. Contamination occurred in the hospital kitchen; samples from the remaining raw mince did not contain clostridia.

Clostridium difficile
See Chapter 4.

Clostridium botulinum
Botulism was first described during the early 19th century (Hutchinson, 1992). It is a paralytic illness resulting from the consumption of food contaminated with neurotoxins released by *Clostridium botulinum*. Symptoms develop within 2–6 hours. The muscles supplied by the cranial nerves are usually affected first, leading to visual disturbance, difficulty with speech and swallowing, and then paralysis. Symptoms are variable. This, coupled with the rarity of the disease, makes diagnosis difficult. It is not always possible to detect the toxin in the faeces, blood or gastric washings.

Most cases have been associated with preserved meat, fish or vegetables because the bacteria and their resistant spores can survive under anaerobic conditions that exclude competing bacteria. The toxin is destroyed by heating at 80 ^{0}C for 30 minutes; to eliminate spores, however, heat is necessary at 121 ^{0}C for 2.5 minutes. This is possible on a commercial scale but difficult to achieve domestically, with clear implications for those who preserve their own produce. The increased availability of frozen food, vacuum packing and the better distribution of fresh produce have reduced the incidence of botulism, which is a serious illness with a high mortality rate.

Bacillus cereus
Bacillus cereus is a Gram-positive rod contaminating rice. Its tough spores are not destroyed by boiling and germinate if the food is subsequently stored overnight without adequate refrigeration. The bacteria multiply and produce toxins. The bacteria are not destroyed during the gentle reheating used to produce 'special fried rice' the next day.

Clinical Application

Investigating Outbreaks of Enteric Infection in Hospital

■ The appearance and pattern of symptoms is an important indicator of the causative organism. A sudden outbreak involving several people is indicative of food intoxication (clostridial or staphylococcal). Cases of salmonellosis appear more sporadically from a common source because of the longer incubation period. Virus infections spread with no relationship to any food source.

■ Samples of food (raw and 'left-overs') are obtained if possible to identify a source. A recent meal involving mince or a meat pie suggests clostridial intoxication, the consumption of salty food implicating staphylococci. The food can be examined microscopically. If staphylococci or clostridia are the cause, they will be present in large numbers.

■ Stool specimens are obtained for microscopy and culture. Toxins may be revealed by enzyme-linked immunosorbent assay (ELISA) techniques. Infectious patients, and carriers, must be isolated. Staff with symptoms must remain away from work until they are well and have bacteriological clearance. Staff who are carriers must be identified and should not handle food until they are clear of the organism.

■ Practices will be examined in the central hospital and ward kitchens. Investigations should include the examination of trolleys used to transport meals.

■ Ward practices and facilities should be examined, especially in relation to handwashing. Person-to-person spread of gastrointestinal pathogens is possible, and clinical equipment may act as fomites.

Enteric infection caused by viruses

Outbreaks of diarrhoea and vomiting caused by viruses are common in hospitals and the community. Diagnosis is by electron microscopy but is not always made as many infections are mild and self-limiting. There are no published guidelines for the management of these infections in hospital, but Trusts are increasingly developing their own (Rao, 1995).

Viruses involved in enteric infections

Hepatitis A virus

Hepatitis A virus is an RNA virus. Small outbreaks have been reported from families and institutions, larger epidemics resulting from the consumption of contaminated water, milk and food. Symptoms include malaise, nausea, vomiting, abdominal pain and jaundice. Subclinical infection is common and gives lasting immunity in areas where sanitation is poor. The higher standard of living in the UK results in a reduced exposure and increases the risk of infection in adulthood, especially during foreign travel. A safe and reliable vaccine is available (Tilzey et al., 1992), but routinely immunising travellers is not cost-effective (Behrens and Roberts, 1994). There is no specific treatment.

Hepatitis E virus

Hepatitis E virus is a recently discovered hepatitis virus disseminated by the faecal-oral route. Carrier status has not been reported. The infection has been detected in travellers returning to the USA from Asia, Africa and Mexico.

Norwalk virus

The Norwalk virus is an RNA virus causing winter vomiting. Transmission is by the faecal-oral route and in droplets. Outbreaks have occurred in the community, schools, hotels and hospitals. The infection is usually mild and self-limiting, but early detection is vital for social and economic reasons (that is, to reduce the length of time away from work or school), because the Norwalk virus is highly infectious, up to 50 per cent of those exposed succumbing (Little and Jenkins, 1995). The Norwalk virus frequently contaminates water. As oysters, mussels and other bivalves feed by filtering particles from seawater, they tend to concentrate the virus and cause gastric illness if consumed.

Rotavirus

Rotavirus is an RNA virus responsible for outbreaks of winter vomiting. Cases sometimes show seasonal clustering, although they can occur at any time of the year. Most cases involve infants and young children. Rotavirus is responsible for significant infant mortality in developing countries, but in the UK the illness is not usually severe. For a long time, it was believed that rotavirus was spread by the droplet route, but, as with many other viruses, dissemination appears to depend more on direct contact between individuals, the hands playing a major role. Rotavirus particles have been isolated from the hands (Samandi et al., 1983), and the incidence of diarrhoea falls in nurseries when hygiene is improved, with emphasis on handwashing (Black et al., 1981).

Other causes of enteric infection

Giardia intestinalis

Giardia intestinalis (formerly *lamblia*) is an obligate protozoal parasite. It forms cysts, infection resulting when these are ingested. *Giardia* cannot multiply in food, but it contaminates water in parts of the world where hygiene is poor. Outbreaks have occasionally been reported in developed countries (Jephcott et al., 1986), and cases have occurred among children attending day nurseries (Galbraith et al., 1987). Transmission is by the faecal-oral route when the water is consumed or used to wash food served raw, food-handlers probably playing a part. The incubation period is 1–3 weeks, and unless treated, the infection persists for 4–6 weeks. The protozoa inhabit the small bowel, the main symptom being offensive diarrhoea with cramping abdominal pain, sometimes malabsorption, and weight loss. Asymptomatic carriage is common (Casemore, 1990). Cysts can withstand chlorination at concentrations used to disinfect water and may survive for more than 2 weeks in a damp, cool environment. They are destroyed by heat and prolonged freezing, but ice cubes in drinks have been associated with infection. The infectious dose is possibly no more than 10 cysts. Treatment is with metronidazole.

Cryptosporidium spp.

Cryptosporidium spp. are intestinal parasites not recognised as a human pathogen until 1976, although they were known to cause animal disease before this time. *Cryptosporidium* causes infection in the immunocompromised host but may also infect healthy people. The incubation period is 3–10 days. Symptoms include watery diarrhoea, abdominal pain and vomiting lasting up to 6 days in otherwise healthy people. Symptoms persist in patients with an impaired immune system (for example, those with HIV). Outbreaks have been reported, mainly from schools and nurseries, and water supplies are occasionally contaminated. No drug is currently effective against this infection, but it is usually self-limiting in otherwise healthy people.

Chronic cryptosporidiosis is an AIDS-defining condition.

Entamoeba histolytica

Entamoeba histolytica is an anaerobic amoeba causing infection when the cysts are ingested in food as a consequence of poor hygiene. The incubation period is usually 2–6 weeks but can be much longer – sometimes months (Casemore, 1990). Infection results in bloodstained, mucoid diarrhoea. *Entamoeba* is endemic in poor communities in tropical and temperate countries, but outbreaks in the UK are rare. Treatment is with metronidazole.

Preventing foodborne infection

Foodborne infection is largely preventable (Barrie, 1996). Good practices include:

- Complying with legal requirements for catering
- Protecting food from contamination at all stages from production to consumption
- Providing training in food and personal hygiene for all food-handlers
- Educating the public about food hygiene.

Legal requirements

The Food Safety Act 1990 and the Food Hygiene (General) Regulations 1970 are intended to ensure that premises where food is prepared are safe and properly maintained. According to the Regulations, food to be served hot should be at 63 ^{0}C or above, and cold food below 5 ^{0}C. All premises used to prepare, store or serve food must be registered with the local authority and may be inspected by their Environmental Health Officers. After an inspection, the officers can issue informal warnings, improvement notices specifying remedial action that should be taken within a given period, or prohibition notices, which result in immediate closure of the premises. Those responsible for breaches of the food hygiene laws are liable to prosecution.

Training for food-handlers

Providing training for food-handlers, including food-handlers in health and social care premises, is essential under the food hygiene legislation. Ward kitchens in hospital are subject to the Food Hygiene Regulations, and ward managers are responsible for ensuring they are adhered to:

- The kitchen should be clean
- Items in the refrigerator should be monitored. They should be labelled with the date and discarded if not used
- The temperature of the refrigerator should be monitored, and the refrigerator should be kept clean
- Staff should wash and dry their hands before food-handling
- Paper cloths should be used to dry kitchen equipment
- Staff with gastrointestinal symptoms should be aware that they must report to the occupational health department.

Food is frequently stored in hospital kitchens, but there is disturbing evidence of unsafe practice (Smith, 1991).

Educating the public

Understanding the circumstances likely to result in foodborne disease is the key to its prevention. Disease can only occur if the following events take place in sequence:

1. The item must be contaminated by micro-organisms able to operate as human pathogens
2. It must stand at a temperature favouring microbial growth and reproduction
3. Time is needed for microbial multiplication and invasion or toxin release.

Contamination may occur at source or at any stage during food production, transport or storage. Food manufacturers use different strategies to disrupt the chain culminating in foodborne disease. Eliminating contamination before storage is achieved by canning, freezing and the much older method of salting. Freezing holds the bacteria at temperatures too low for them to multiply and is acknowledged as one of the safest methods of preserving food. However, *Salmonella* already present can survive until it is thawed, then multiply. In theory, food can remain frozen safely for years provided the equipment is in good working order, but the colour and texture of some items may deteriorate. Vacuum packing is widely used to prevent botulism.

Safe practice in the home

Community nurses and health visitors have an important role in helping people to develop safe practices regarding food. A programme to educate the public should cover the buying, storing, preparing and cooking of food. A typical programme to promote awareness is shown below.

Buying food

- Avoid products that do not look fresh
- Avoid cans that are misshapen or pierced, and cracked eggs
- Avoid cartons with bulging lids
- Select raw and cooked items that have been displayed on separate cold counters.

Safe storage

- Discard suspect items. Sell-by dates are a suggestion only, whatever the date on the package
- Place the food in the refrigerator as soon as possible after purchase and not more than 1½ hours later
- Keep it refrigerated at 1–4 ^{0}C
- Cover all stored food
- Store raw and cooked items separately
- Place raw food such as meat in the bottom of the refrigerator where it will not drip onto items that will be consumed raw
- Store items intended for human and animal consumption apart.

Preparing food

- Wash and dry the hands before touching food and again after handling raw items
- Keep cuts and sores on the hands covered with a waterproof dressing
- Keep all kitchen surfaces scrupulously clean. Use separate chopping boards and utensils for cooked and raw food if possible, and wash them with detergent after use. Kitchen cloths should be kept clean and dry (Scott and Blomfield, 1990)

- Wash fruit and vegetables thoroughly in cold, running water
- Dismantle blenders and food processors after use, washing and drying all the parts thoroughly.

Cooking and reheating

- Thaw frozen food thoroughly before cooking
- Ensure that ovens reach the required temperature before the cooking time begins
- Stir liquids to avoid 'cold spots' around the sides of the saucepan
- Ensure that meat, poultry and fish are cooked thoroughly
- Cool food rapidly and place it in the refrigerator unless it is to be consumed immediately
- If food is to be kept hot before serving, hold it at 63 ^{0}C or above
- Never refreeze food that has thawed unless it has been cooked
- Take special care with microwave ovens. 'Cold spots' can develop where heat has failed to penetrate. Always follow the manufacturer's guidelines for the equipment and the food. Heating time should be adjusted if the machine is at a lower wattage, stirring halfway if there is no turntable.

Using new methods safely

New methods of preparation are sometimes blamed for cases of foodborne disease, but provided the system is monitored correctly, the risk is no greater than with conventionally prepared meals.

Cook–chill

Cook–chill is a method of precooking food in bulk, followed by its rapid cooling to 0–3 ^{0}C. The items are reheated immediately before serving, usually in a microwave oven (Armstrong, 1986). Cook–chill is used commercially to prepare convenience foods and has been introduced in many hospitals as well as in community-based meal provision for the housebound and disabled. Meals should not be stored for longer than 5 days and should be reheated at 70 ^{0}C (DoH, 1989). Cook–chill products are safe in hospital providing that production is operated in conjunction with a system of microbiological monitoring (Chudasama *et al.*, 1991; Shanaghy *et al.*, 1993). In a typical hospital system, food is prepared in a central kitchen, portioned, chilled, held under refrigeration for a maximum of 5 days, put onto cold plates and distributed to the wards in refrigerated trolleys before reheating. In a traditional system of bacteriological monitoring, audit occurs by taking samples at any stage in this process.

A more comprehensive method of quality control is offered by the Hazard Analysis Critical Control Point (HACCP) system. This is a system of control to assure food safety using a more standardised approach than traditional inspection and sampling. It has been used effectively within the food industry for over

20 years (Richards *et al.*, 1993). A flow chart is constructed to depict all stages in production from the arrival of raw articles to the meal reaching the consumer. A number of critical points are selected at which monitoring is considered vital, and sampling is performed with every batch. HACCP promotes the development and refinement of guidelines to ensure good practice and operates as a continual reminder to staff of the need for vigilance at every stage throughout food-handling. Its introduction has improved food quality in hospital (Shanaghy *et al.*, 1993).

REVISION CHECKLIST: KEY AREAS

❏ Introduction to enteric infection

❏ Incidence of enteric infection: Risk factors

❏ Food infection and intoxication: Invasive gastrointestinal infection, Foodborne intoxication

❏ Enteric infections caused by viruses: Viruses involved in enteric infections

❏ Other causes of enteric infection

❏ Preventing foodborne infection: Legal requirements, Training for food handlers, Educating the public

❏ Safe practice in the home

❏ Using new methods safely

Activities – linking knowledge to clinical practice

1 **Prepare** a checklist of good practice for food-handling in a health- or social care setting. This could be a ward or day centre, or a nursery where feeds are prepared. List possible real or potential risks and suggest a strategy for improvement.

2 **Prepare** a checklist of good practice for food-handling in commercial premises where staff prepare food to serve to the public (take-aways or delicatessen counters, for example). Visit a typical outlet and note the extent to which the key points on your checklist are being fulfilled.

SELF-ASSESSMENT

1. *Staphylococcus epidermidis* causes food intoxication.   True? ☐ False? ☐

2. *Campylobacter* causes infective invasive gastroenteritis.   True? ☐ False? ☐

3. *Salmonella* is spread:
   (a) via the faecal-oral route ☐
   (b) by person-to-person contact ☐
   (c) on contaminated fingers ☐
   (d) via fomites ☐

4. Rotavirus causes foodborne infection.   True? ☐ False? ☐

5. *Giardia* is:
   (a) protozoal ☐
   (b) not highly infectious ☐
   (c) able to survive disinfection of water ☐
   (d) a common hazard for the traveller ☐

6. Botulism is caused by:
   (a) *Clostridium perfringens* ☐
   (b) *Clostridium difficile* ☐
   (c) a Gram-positive sporing rod ☐
   (d) consuming improperly canned food ☐

7. *Escherichia coli* is:
   (a) a harmless commensal in the human gut ☐
   (b) a cause of travellers' diarrhoea ☐
   (c) spread by food-handlers ☐
   (d) able to produce enterotoxins causing severe foodborne illness ☐

8. The symptoms and signs of hepatitis A virus infection are:
   ....
   ....

9. 'Microwave ovens are a health hazard'. Comment.

References

Ahmad F, Bray G, Prescott RWG *et al.* (1991) 'Use of ciprofloxacin to control a *Salmonella* outbreak in a long-stay psychiatric hospital'. *Journal of Hospital Infection* **12**: 171–8.

Anderton A, Nwoguh CE, McCune I *et al.* (1993) 'A comparative study of the numbers of bacteria present in enteral feeds prepared and administered in hospital and at home'. *Journal of Hospital Infection* **23**: 43–9.

Armstrong GR (1986) 'Cook-chill catering'. *Environmental Health* **10**: 253–8.

Baird-Parker AC (1990) 'Foodborne salmonellosis'. *Lancet* **336**: 1231–5.

Barrie D (1996) 'The provision of food and catering services in hospital'. *Journal of Hospital Infection* **33**: 13–31.

Behrens RH and Roberts JA (1994) 'Is travel prophylaxis worth while? Economic appraisal of prophylaxis against malaria, hepatitis A and typhoid in travellers'. *British Medical Journal* **309**: 918–22.

Black RE, Dykes AD, Kern EA *et al.* (1981) 'Handwashing to prevent diarrhoea in day centers'. *American Journal of Epidemiology* **113**: 445–51.

Blaser MJ, Checko P, Bopp C *et al.* (1982) '*Campylobacter enteritis* associated with foodborne transmission'. *American Journal of Epidemiology* **116**: 886–94.

Casemore DP (1990) 'Foodborne protozoal infection'. *Lancet* **336**: 1427–32.

Chudasama Y, Hamilton-Miller JMT and Maple PAC (1991) 'Bacteriological safety of cook-chill food at the Royal Free Hospital, with particular reference to *Listeria*'. *Journal of Hospital Infection* **19**: 225–30.

Cossar JH, Ried D and Fallon R (1990) 'A cumulative view of studies on travellers – their experiences of illness and the implications of these findings'. *Journal of Infection* 21: 27–42.

Cowden J (1992) '*Campylobacter:* epidemiological paradoxes'. *British Medical Journal* 305: 132–3.

Cruikshank JG (1984) 'The investigation of *Salmonella* outbreaks in hospital'. *Journal of Hospital Infection* 5: 241–3.

Department of Health (1986) *Report of a Public Enquiry into the Outbreak of Salmonella Food Poisoning at Stanley Royd Hospital.* HMSO, London.

Department of Health (1989) *Chilled and Frozen: Guidelines on Cook-chill and Cook-freeze Catering Systems.* HMSO, London.

Department of Health, Advisory Committee on the Microbiological Safety of Food (1993). *Report on Salmonella in Eggs.* HMSO, London.

Department of Health (1998) *Expert Advice Repeated on Salmonella and Raw Eggs.* Press Release – 98/138. DoH, London. http://www.open.gov.uk/doh/dhhome

Doyle MP (1990) 'Pathogenic *Escherichia coli, Yersinia entercolitica* and *Vibrio parahaemolyticus*'. *Lancet* 336: 1111–15.

Dryden MS, Keyworth N, Gabb R *et al.* (1994) 'Asymptomatic foodhandlers as the source of nosocomial salmonellosis'. *Journal of Hospital Infection* 28: 195–207.

Fenlon DR (1985) 'Wild birds and silage as reservoirs of *Listeria* in the agricultural environment'. *Journal of Applied Bacteriology* 59: 537–43.

Galbraith NS, Barrat NJ and Sockett PN (1987) 'The changing pattern of foodborne disease in England and Wales'. *Public Health* 101: 319–28.

Galloway A, Roberts C and Hunt EJ (1987) 'An outbreak of *Salmonella typhimurium* gastroenteritis in a psychiatric hospital'. *Hospital Infection* 10: 248–54.

Gould DJ (1996) 'Hygienic practices (*E. coli* foodborne illness)'. *Nursing Times* 92(36): 77–80.

Hennessy TW, Hedberg C, Slutsker L *et al.* (1996) 'A national outbreak of *Salmonella enteritidis* infections from ice cream'. *New England Journal of Medicine* 334: 1282–6.

Hutchinson DN (1992) 'Foodborne botulism'. *British Medical Journal* 305: 264–5.

Jephcott AE, Begg NT and Baker IA (1986) 'Outbreak of *giardiasis* associated with mains water in the United Kingdom'. *Lancet* 1: 730–2.

Johnston AM (1990) 'Veterinary sources of foodborne illness'. *Lancet* 336: 856–8.

Jones D (1990) 'Foodborne listeriosis'. *Lancet* 336: 1171–4.

Joseph CA and Palmer SR (1989) 'Outbreaks of *Salmonella* infection in hospitals in England and Wales 1978–87'. *British Medical Journal* 298: 1161–4.

Lacey SL and Buckingham SE (1993) 'Isolation of *Salmonella enteritidis* from cook-chill food distributed to hospital patients'. *Journal of Hospital Infection* 25: 133–6.

Levy J (1989) '*Listeria* and food poisoning – a growing concern'. *Maternal and Child Health* 14: 380–3.

Little K and Jenkins M (1995) 'When winter makes you sick'. *Nursing Times* 91(46): 55–60.

Meara J, Mayon-White R and Johnston H (1988) 'Salmonellosis in a psychogeriatric ward: problems of infection control'. *Journal of Hospital Infection* 11: 86–90.

Mitchell E, O'Mahoney M, Lynch D *et al.* (1989) 'Large outbreak of food poisoning caused by *Salmonella typhimurium* definitive type 49 in mayonnaise'. *British Medical Journal* 298: 99–101.

North N (1989) 'Food scares: the role of the Department of Health' in Harrison A and Gretton J (eds*) Health Care UK – an Economic and Social Policy Audit.* Policy Journals, Newbury, pp. 65–77.

Pether JVS and Gilbert RJ (1971) 'The survival of *Salmonella* on the finger tips and the transfer of organisms to food'. *Journal of Hygiene* 69: 673–81.

Pollock AM and Whitty PM (1991) 'Outbreak of *Clostridium perfringens* food poisoning'. *Journal of Hospital Infection* 17: 179–86.

Rao GG (1995) 'Control of outbreaks of viral diarrhoea in hospitals – a practical approach'. *Journal of Hospital Infection* 30: 1–6.

Richards J, Parr E and Riseborough P (1993) 'Hospital food hygiene: the application of Hazard Analysis Critical Control Points to conventional hospital catering'. *Journal of Hospital Infection* 24: 273–82.

Samandi AR, Huq MI and Ahmed QS (1983) 'Detection of rotavirus in the handwashings of attendants of children with diarrhoea'. *British Medical Journal* 1: 188–9.

Schlech WF (1991) 'Listeriosis: epidemiology, virulence and the significance of contaminated foodstuffs'. *Journal of Hospital Infection* **19**: 211–24.

Scott E and Bloomfield S (1990) 'The survival and transfer of microbial contaminants via cloths, hands and utensils'. *Journal of Applied Bacteriology* **68**: 271–8.

Shanaghy N, Murphy F and Kennedy K (1993) 'Improvements in the microbiological quality of food samples from a hospital cook-chill system since the introduction of HACCP'. *Journal of Hospital Infection* **23**: 305–14.

Smith F (1991) 'Looking into the refrigerator'. *Nursing Times* **87**(38): 61–2.

Tilzey AJ, Palmer SJ, Barrow S *et al.* (1992) 'Clinical trial with inactivated hepatitis A vaccine and recommendations for its use'. *British Medical Journal* **304**: 1272–6.

Tranter HS (1990) 'Foodborne staphylococcal illness'. *Lancet* **336**: 1044–6.

Wall PG, Ryan MJ, Ward LR *et al.* (1996) 'Outbreaks of salmonellosis in hospitals in England and Wales 1992–1994'. *Journal of Hospital Infection* **33**: 181–90.

Wilkinson PJ (1989) 'Ignorance about *Listeria*'. *British Medical Journal* **299**: 276–7.

Williams P and Ellison J (1998) 'Food fears'. *Nursing Times* **94**(28): 72–5.

Further reading and information sources

Department of Health (1990) *Food Sense: A Guide from HM Government.* HMSO, London.

Hobbs BC (1993) *Food Poisoning and Food Hygiene.* Edward Arnold, London.

Lancet Review (1991) *Foodborne Illness.* Edward Arnold, London.

Mills I (1996) 'Not quite good enough to eat'. *Nursing Times* **92**(36): 72–6.

Pennington Group (1997) *Report on the Circumstances Leading to the 1996 Outbreak of Infection with E. coli 0157 in Central Scotland: the Implications for Food Safety and the Lessons To Be Learnt.* Stationery Office, Edinburgh.

Sharp JMC (1988) 'Salmonellosis and eggs'. *British Medical Journal* **297**: 1557–8.

12 Infection risks from blood and body fluids

CHAPTER OUTCOMES

After reading this chapter you should be able to:

■ Describe how HIV infection is transmitted and diagnosed

■ Describe how hepatitis B infection is transmitted and diagnosed, and outline its effect on the health of the individual

■ Name two other viruses causing hepatitis that are transmitted in the same manner as hepatitis B

■ List the precautions that should be taken when handling blood or body fluids and explain the rationale underpinning your recommendations

■ State community health measures taken to control the spread of HIV and hepatitis B

■ Debate the ethical dilemmas associated with the diagnosis of HIV or hepatitis B in:

   (a) health professionals
   (b) patients/clients
   (c) screening populations as part of epidemiological research

Introduction – the risk of infection and health professionals

Infection is an occupational health risk for health professionals. The most serious threat to health is exposure to blood and body fluids, leading to parenteral infection. In the UK, health professionals are most likely to have contact with patients carrying the hepatitis viruses and the human immunodeficiency virus (HIV).

Clinical Application

Nosocomial Infection as an Occupational Health Risk

Clinical work places nurses at risk of developing infections from parenterally transmitted viruses, chickenpox and tuberculosis (Moore and Kczmarek, 1990). The prevention of infection is a health and safety issue, falling within the remit of the Health and Safety at Work Act 1974. This applies throughout England, Wales and Scotland but not to Northern Ireland, where the Health and Safety of Work Order 1978 makes similar provisions. Section 2 of the Health and Safety at Work Act lays down the duties of employers to employees, stipulating that arrangements must be made for the safe use, storage and transport of all substances and equipment, and that staff should receive training to ensure that they adhere to agreed protocols. The Act applies to all employers, whether NHS Trusts, private hospitals and clinics or GPs employing a practice nurse. It also details the responsibilities of the employer to persons other than employees. On healthcare premises, these include patients and visitors. There is therefore a duty to protect staff and the public from the risks of cross-infection.

Human immunodeficiency virus

Human immunodeficiency virus (HIV) is an RNA virus containing an enzyme called reverse transcriptase. The virus has a long incubation period. Possessing antibodies to HIV demonstrates a previous exposure to the virus, but seroconversion can take months so a test yielding negative results should be repeated – it may have been performed too soon. Several serological tests have been developed. Core antigen p24 levels in the blood are used to indicate an increase in viral replication, progression of the disease and infectivity. Information about HIV tests can be obtained from GPs, genitourinary medicine clinics, helplines and, in the case of occupational exposure, the occupational health department. Testing is performed only after counselling and discussion to ensure that the individual understands the significance of a positive result and the need for repeat testing if it is negative.

Transmission of HIV

The transmission of HIV occurs sexually, perinatally and parenterally. Pratt (1994) outlines possible situations in which exposure is possible:

- **Transmission to haemophiliacs** – Since 1987, blood products in the UK have been heat treated to destroy the virus so this risk has been eliminated. However, over 1200 haemophiliacs (about 30 per cent of the total) in the UK are seropositive.

- **Drug misuse** through sharing contaminated injection equipment – The risk of transmission is probably enhanced through the recreational use of other substances, including alcohol: these alter behaviour and lower inhibition.

- **Sexual transmission** between adults – Men and women can become infected, the risk being especially high for homosexuals acting as the passive partner during anal intercourse. The rectal mucosa is much more delicate than the vaginal mucosa, the virus gaining access via tears and abrasions. Nevertheless, in some parts of the world an equal number of both sexes carry HIV. This is the situation in Africa, where the infection is believed to have originated.

- **Vertical transmission** from infected mothers to infants.

- **Iatrogenic transmission** to healthcare professionals – HIV is more easily destroyed than hepatitis B and is less common, but the consequences of infection are so grave that the risk of occupational exposure should never be overlooked.

Occupational health risks

The nature of the exposure is important. For surveillance purposes two types are considered:

- **Percutaneous exposure** – the skin is cut or penetrated by a sharp instrument
- **Mucocutaneous exposure** – the eyes, the inside of the nose or mouth, or non-intact skin is exposed.

The rate of infection following percutaneous injury, although higher than with mucocutaneous exposure, is still low, varying between 0.18 per cent and 0.56 per cent in large epidemiological studies (Henderson *et al.*, 1990; Leentvaar-Kuijpers *et al.*, 1990) and 2 per cent in studies where samples have been smaller (PHLS, 1993).

The risk of healthcare workers acquiring HIV or any other parenterally transmitted infection from patients also depends on:

- The prevalence of the virus in the hospital or community where they are employed.

■ Expertise – Junior staff sustain needlestick injuries more often than experienced staff (Jagger *et al.*, 1990). Thus, early clinical practice should be carefully supervised.

■ The types of procedure performed – Those who routinely handle blood and body fluids most often are at greatest risk.

■ The risk of transmission associated with each accidental exposure – The risk of seroconversion is about one in 300 (0.33 per cent) and varies depending on the injury, for example venepuncture or intramuscular injection (Heponstall *et al.*, 1993). HIV has been isolated from blood, semen, vaginal secretions, breast milk, saliva and tears. The level in saliva and tears is probably too low to result in transmission (Lifson, 1988).

■ The individual's immune status – Those less fit are likely to develop infection.

Treatment

See Chapter 13.

Community health measures

Community health measures include:

■ Promoting the use of barrier precautions (with the correct type of condom) and emphasising the need for 'safe sex'. Explicit advice can be obtained from organisations such as the Terence Higgins Trust.

■ Screening all donated blood and heat-treating blood products.

■ Discouraging members of the public likely to be carrying HIV from donating blood, semen or tissues. Organs cannot be used if the donor is known to be antibody positive.

■ Informing the public and health professionals of the risks associated with handling blood and body fluids, and of how to deal with these.

■ Alerting the public to the dangers of sharing potentially contaminated items (razors, toothbrushes, sewing needles and scissors).

■ Supplying needles and syringes to people who use intravenous drugs for recreational purposes. The use of 'needle exchange' is controversial.

NB. Immunisation is not available for HIV, but considerable research is occurring in this area.

Hepatitis

Hepatitis is a generic term for inflammation of the liver. It is caused by a number of viruses including rubella, cytomegalovirus, herpes simplex and the hepatitis viruses.

Hepatitis B

Hepatitis B is an inflammatory condition affecting the liver that is caused by a DNA virus (Figure 12.1).

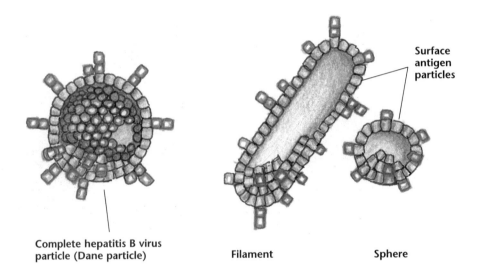

Complete hepatitis B virus particle (Dane particle)

Surface antigen particles

Filament

Sphere

Figure 12.1 The hepatitis B virus

Information concerning its structure has developed through studies of its surface antigens. The following terminology has been suggested by the World Health Organization (WHO):

- Dane particle – the entire virus particle
- HBV – hepatitis B virus
- HBsAg – hepatitis B surface antigen
- HBcAg – hepatitis B core antigen
- HBeAg – the e antigen associated with the core of the virus
- Anti-HBs – antibody to hepatitis B surface antigen
- Anti-HBc – antibody to hepatitis B core antigen
- Anti-HBe – antibody to the e antigen

The virus is detected by testing the blood for surface antigen. It may also cause a change in liver function tests, for example raised serum aminotransferase, bilirubin and alkaline phosphatase levels.

Infectious particles have been isolated from saliva and semen. Resolution of the infection is considered to have occurred when HBsAg and anti-HB are no longer detectable. Chronic carriers are those remaining HBsAg positive on at least two occasions 6 months apart. Infectivity is closely associated with the presence of the e antigen which indicates that active viral replication is occurring.

The incubation period ranges from 4 weeks to 6 months. Individuals are probably most highly infectious during the early, acute stages. Hepatitis B is usually self-limiting, but approximately 5 per cent of cases become chronically infected (Hart, 1990). The liver is inflamed and hepatocellular necrosis results.

The mortality rate of this condition is approximately 1 per cent. Only 30–40 per cent of those infected develop symptoms of acute infection, which tend to be non-specific, fever, malaise and anorexia being most commonly reported. Jaundice does not always develop, or it may be too mild to be noticeable. Between 50 and 60 per cent of patients develop a subclinical infection, remaining asymptomatic despite serological evidence of exposure.

These people are most likely to become chronic carriers, at greatest risk of developing cirrhosis and hepatocellular cancer, rare but grave complications for which treatment is not always successful (Main, 1991). Transmission occurs sexually (by vaginal or anal intercourse), through percutaneous sharps injury, by sharing infected needles and via contamination of the mucous membranes. The risk of infection after percutaneous exposure to the blood of a carrier for the e antigen is about 30 per cent (Shaw and Bell, 1993). The risk associated with mucocutaneous exposure does not appear to have been quantified. The hands, however, may carry minute abrasions so the contamination of apparently intact skin may present a significant risk. Many people who develop infection or become carriers cannot recall an injury (Denes *et al.*, 1978). As with HIV, the risk of seroconversion depends on the number of people carrying the virus within the local community and the individual's immunological status. Infants whose mothers developed acute hepatitis B infection during the third trimester of pregnancy or who are highly infectious carriers may also become infected.

Groups at high risk of infection

Despite the high rate of asymptomatic carriage, it is possible to identify a number of groups who are at high risk (Polakoff, 1986):

- Those who inject drugs intravenously
- Homosexual and bisexual men
- Prostitutes
- Healthcare professionals

- Immigrants from parts of the world where hepatitis B is endemic, for example Africa, South-east Asia and the Far East
- Those with learning difficulties, especially in institutional care where hygiene is difficult to control.

Community health measures: prevention of hepatitis B

Hepatitis B is a notifiable disease, the number of cases occurring being recorded by the Public Health Laboratory Service. Prevention involves:

- The development and implementation of guidelines to prevent spread from contaminated instruments
- Screening all blood for transfusion for HBsAg and excluding carriers from donation
- Using small pools (of not more than 10 donors) to prepare plasma products
- Offering vaccine to those at risk in hospital and the community.

Immunisation has been available for hepatitis B since the early 1980s (Szmuness *et al.*, 1982). Vaccine was originally produced from human plasma, but most is now obtained through a recombinant DNA technique that inserts HBsAg into yeast cells. Both types of vaccine are safe and approximately 90 per cent effective. The duration of immunity has been estimated at between 3 and 5 years. The vaccine should be routinely available to healthcare professionals, and nowadays most employers in the UK provide it (Trevelyan, 1991); uptake is, however, often poor (Spence and Dash, 1990) even though side-effects are minimal (Finch, 1987). Reasons for low uptake among health professionals include inconvenient appointment times in occupational health departments, pressures of work and misconceptions about the vaccine, especially overlooking the need for boosters (Briggs and Thomas, 1994).

It was initially estimated that only 1–4 per cent of those who had received the standard vaccination consisting of three injections failed to respond (Boxall, 1993), but it has since emerged that a higher proportion may be 'slow responders', requiring up to nine injections to seroconvert (Poole *et al.*, 1994). This suggests that it is not sufficient to evaluate the success of an immunisation campaign merely on uptake: serological testing to determine the effectiveness of the vaccine among the recipients is vital. Nevertheless, the number of health professionals becoming infected has declined in recent years. Good record-keeping in the occupational health department is essential to manage staff who have been exposed to blood-borne infections (Duthie *et al.*, 1994). Immunisation against hepatitis B also affords protection against hepatitis D, which depends upon the presence of HBV. The WHO recommends universal HBV immunisation in an attempt to reduce the number of deaths from hepatitis B and the number of people who carry HBV.

Risk to the public: hepatitis B and HIV

Although most cases of hepatitis B and HIV passed on within the clinical setting are transmitted from patient to health professional, there have been some instances of members of the public contracting the infection from a healthcare worker. Most have occurred when the individual has received treatment from a dentist or surgeon carrying the hepatitis e antigen or HIV. Nosocomial hepatitis B infections between patients have occurred during the use of medical devices (for example, endoscopes, autolets and vials) contaminated with blood and not properly disinfected (Drescher *et al.*, 1994). The first possible case of HIV transmission to six patients was reported in the USA in 1993 (CDC, 1993), and further cases have since been investigated (Chant *et al.*, 1993).

The United Kingdom Central Council for Nursing, Midwifery and Health Visiting (UKCC) stipulates confidentiality for members of the profession who are seropositive. It is, however, felt that the needs of the patient are paramount and that in those rare cases where a seropositive nurse, midwife or health visitor would present a risk to patients (for example, by performing invasive procedures), redeployment to another clinical setting should be arranged.

Clinical Application

Risk of Parenteral Infection Versus Confidentiality

Epidemiologists argue that, in order to trace changes in the pattern of disease within a community, it is necessary to have information about the number and type of people affected. However, members of the caring professions believe that individuals are entitled to confidentiality. At present, the UKCC rules that nurses involved in obtaining the blood of a known, named person for HIV testing without his or her consent should be open to disciplinary action. This does not, however, apply when the blood has been obtained for some other purpose, rendered anonymous and then tested as part of epidemiological monitoring. The UKCC is not in favour of routinely testing patients for HIV for ethical reasons, as well as because tests might fail to detect antibodies if performed before seroconversion, which can occur up to 3 months after exposure to the virus. The UKCC maintains that no nurse is justified in divulging a patient's antibody status to a third party except in the most exceptional circumstances, such as risk of transmission to an unsuspecting individual. In practice, 'exceptional circumstances' are likely to be difficult to define and to defend.

Hepatitis C

Once diagnostic tests had become available for hepatitis B, it became apparent that a number of post-viral cases of hepatitis must be associated with infection by another agent. This condition was initially called non-A, non-B hepatitis. It proved to be caused by an RNA virus subsequently named hepatitis C virus (Feinstone *et al.*, 1975). Hepatitis C virus is transmitted primarily via blood and body fluids, and appears to be most common among intravenous drug misusers and people who have had blood transfusions: it may now occur more frequently than HIV or hepatitis B infection in this population in some parts of the USA (Kelen *et al.*, 1992). Sexual transmission is thought to be possible, and asymptomatic carriage is common (Tedder *et al.*, 1991). Vertical transmission appears to be rare (Thaler *et al.*, 1991). Needlestick injury may lead to seroconversion in healthcare workers (Polish *et al.*, 1993) and has been estimated to give the individual a 3–10 per cent risk of infection (Mitsui *et al.*, 1992). Hepatitis C virus is more damaging than hepatitis B virus. So far, 50 per cent of those infected have become chronic carriers, of whom 20 per cent have developed hepatocellular cancer. Seroconversion may not occur until several months after exposure. Diagnostic tests are currently less sophisticated than those for hepatitis B virus: positive results cannot distinguish between active and old infections.

Hepatitis D

Hepatitis D virus (delta virus) is a defective RNA virus that can cause infection only in the presence of active hepatitis B virus infection. It is transmitted in the same way as hepatitis B, the same groups being at risk. The incubation period is 30–50 days. Mortality from acute hepatitis D virus infection is high: 2–20 per cent in these outbreaks so far reported. Infection is diagnosed by finding the antigen (HDAg) in the blood. Routine testing is not undertaken so the prevalence is not known, but it is more common in the countries of the former USSR, Middle East and Africa than in the UK. Vaccination against hepatitis B offers protection against both viruses (Murrell, 1993).

Hepatitis A

See Chapter 11.

Hepatitis E

See Chapter 11.

Other hepatitis viruses

An unidentified agent has recently been designated as hepatitis F; this is seen as a possible cause of fulminant hepatitis (Smales, 1998). A further virus has been identified – hepatitis G – which is transmitted via blood and blood products. Other modes of transmission, for example, via sexual intercourse, may occur.

Universal precautions

It is not possible to predict whether an individual is carrying a parenterally transmitted viral infection (Havlichek *et al.*, 1991), and as exposure to blood may occur before testing is possible in emergency situations (Gurevich, 1988), universal precautions must be taken whenever blood or body fluids are handled or if contact is possible (Wilson and Breedon, 1990). This means that risk assessment is of the procedure about to be undertaken rather than of the individual patient. Recent guidance from the Department of Health (1998) gives comprehensive information about protecting healthcare workers from infection with blood-borne viruses. The document stresses the practical advantages of having common infection control policies for these viruses.

Clinical Application

Should Known Carriers of Parenterally Transmitted Virus Infections be Treated Differently from Other Patients?

There is a powerful argument for treating all patients alike (Oakley, 1994): if the same precautions are taken for everybody, they will be regarded as routine and will be more acceptable. If patients or their families perceive that they are being treated differently, however, they may be resentful, suspicious and uncooperative. Genuine unhappiness has resulted because people have been needlessly incarcerated in single rooms or ostracised by rigid hospital policies. This is unnecessary and damaging to staff–patient relationships (King, 1990).

Protective clothing

Gloves

Gloves are worn to protect the patient during all invasive procedures and to protect the health professional whenever contact with blood or body fluids takes place or is anticipated. The following points need to be considered when policies for glove use are developed:

- Non-sterile, single-use gloves are adequate when universal precautions are taken. Sterile gloves are necessary for contact with parts of the body free of micro-organisms in health (Yanelli and Gurevich, 1988). They should conform to British Standard Institute Regulation (BSI) standards.

- Gloves should be changed between patients to prevent cross-infection. Washing is not recommended as it appears difficult to remove pathogens from the surface of latex and PVC (Dalgleish and Malkovsy, 1988), although this is now contested (Mulhall *et al.*, 1993). Further research is necessary in this area.

■ Gloves may have to be changed between different procedures involving the same patient to prevent endogenous infection (Goldmann, 1991).

■ The hands must be washed after gloves have been worn. Virus particles can leak through latex and PVC (Korniewicz, 1989), allergy may develop to the gloves or the lubricating powder they contain (Van Rijwisjk, 1992), and sweating is induced: bacteria are then leached out from beneath the nails and nail-beds, increasing the number available for cross-infection (Peireira *et al.*, 1990).

■ Gloves must be of sufficient gauge to avoid splitting and tearing, problems reported for numerous brands during tests that simulate clinical procedures (Korniewicz *et al.*, 1989). Double-gloving may be advisable with some brands of PVC glove. Trials have shown that they are more likely to leak than latex varieties, but this risk can be overcome when two pairs are used at once (Korniewicz *et al.*, 1994). Puncture is possible during clinical procedures: electronic testing indicates that, during elective surgical procedures, 24 per cent of gloves become perforated (Green and Grompertz, 1992). They should be removed at once if any defect is observed. Fingernails should be kept short to avoid puncture (Brookes, 1994).

■ Gloves must fit well and be available in a range of sizes so that manual dexterity is not compromised. Staff may otherwise be tempted to use expensive, sterile surgeons' gloves when they are unnecessary (Denton, 1991). Many Trusts now routinely monitor the use of gloves to check expense (Binney, 1994).

■ Some procedures are difficult to perform even with good-quality gloves. For example, needlestick injuries can result when venepuncture is performed clumsily, but this could be reduced by adopting a 'two-tier' system of glove use that would sanction experienced staff undertaking venepuncture without gloves (Jenner, 1990).

Aprons

Aprons must be worn if clothing is likely to be soiled. Plastic is a more effective barrier against liquid soiling than is cotton (Gill and Slater, 1991).

Eye protection

Eye protection conforming to BSI standards is required when splashing or aerosols are possible. This is unusual in ward situations but a risk in theatre or dentistry when high-speed drills are used. Eye protection (goggles or visors) may not be disposable and must be disinfected after use by washing in a liquid detergent solution, followed by thorough drying.

Other equipment

Equipment such as theatre shoes and phlebotomy cuffs may become splashed with blood and should be decontaminated or discarded (Forseter *et al.*, 1990, Thomas *et al.*, 1993). Hepatitis B virus can survive for at least a week in dry plasma (Bond *et al.*, 1983) and HIV survives for several days if protected by plasma (Hanson *et al.*, 1989).

Dealing with sharps

The handling of sharps should be performed with care to avoid injury. Ancillary as well as clinical staff may sustain injury (Dancocks and Hewitt, 1994). Health professionals should:

- Avoid resheathing needles. They should never be cut or bent as this is when most accidents occur (Wormser *et al.*, 1984)

- Never disconnect syringes from needles

- Consider themselves responsible for disposing of a sharp if they have used it: injuries may occur because the user has been careless of disposal (Weltman *et al.*, 1995). Protective devices are available to help to prevent needlestick injury. They are, however, expensive, and their effectiveness in the clinical situation still needs to be evaluated (Orenstein *et al.*, 1995).

Sharps disposal

Healthcare workers should adhere to the following examples of good practice:

- Sharps containers should comply with BSI regulations: they should be rigid and impermeable to leakage and puncture. No other containers should be used (Gwyther, 1989).

- Sharps should be placed in a designated container immediately after use. They should never be stored in open containers at the bedside, transported in pockets or carried in the hands.

- Sharps containers should be conveniently sited in all clinical areas. In critical care units, they should be placed at every bed space; in wards, they should be placed on the drugs trolley as well as in the treatment room.

- Sharps containers must be kept out of the reach of confused patients, those who may self-harm and children.

- No attempt must ever be made to retrieve items from a sharps container or to empty it.

- Sharps containers of the appropriate size must be available. Accidents are more likely when large objects are forced into small containers.

■ Where appropriate, patients should be educated about safe disposal. For example, diabetic patients responsible for administering their own insulin should be supplied with sharps containers at home, which are then collected by authorised handlers of clinical waste (see Chapter 5).

■ Sharps containers should be discarded when no more than three-quarters full, sealed and stored in a secure, dry place ready for collection. They must be incinerated.

Dealing with sharps injuries

■ Encourage the wound to bleed and then wash it thoroughly under running water before drying it.

■ Apply a waterproof dressing.

■ Complete the necessary documentation. In hospital, this will involve filling in an accident form. In clinics, an accident book should be available for reporting incidents.

■ Report the injury. In hospitals, reports are usually made to the occupational health department, or to the accident and emergency department when the former is closed. The need to report all incidents should be emphasised, as underreporting is common (Harmory, 1983).

■ Hepatitis B vaccine is effective prophylactically (Dienstag *et al.*, 1984). If the victim has not been immunised, a course of vaccination will be suggested. For those who have already completed the course, a booster will be offered. Staff

---

Clinical Application

Alternatives to Sharps

In the wards, sharps injuries could be reduced by using needleless devices. An analysis of all reported sharps injuries over a 2-year period in a major university hospital indicated that 82 per cent of the incidents resulted through needlestick injury, usually when intravenous lines were manipulated. The number of injuries declined when steel needles were replaced with plastic ones (Yassi and McGill, 1991). The introduction of a needleless heparin lock system has also been associated with a reduction in the number of injuries (Adams *et al.*, 1993).

In theatre, it is possible to replace scalpels with diathermy, ultrasonic dissectors and laser knives. Staples can replace sutures for the formation of gastrointestinal anastomoses and skin closure, and forceps may replace fingers during dissection and suturing. Retractors can be used to hold tissues away from the operative field instead of hands. Keyhole surgery is associated with more sharps injuries than conventional procedures because the hands are not visible.

exposed to HIV may be offered postexposure prophylaxis with zidovudine. This should if possible be given within an hour of exposure, and certainly no more than 4 hours later. Its effectiveness, however, remains to be evaluated. Few people have been exposed to percutaneous injury likely to place them at risk of HIV infection, and it has not been possible to test the efficacy of the drug in prophylaxis. Side-effects – headaches, nausea, myalgia, insomnia and bone marrow suppression – can be severe.

Dealing with blood contamination of the conjunctivae and mucous membranes

The following precautions are recommended:

■ Irrigation of the area with water
■ Recording and reporting the incident.

Spillage of blood and body fluids

Any spillage of blood and body fluids must be dealt with immediately by covering with sodium dichloroisocyanurate (NaDDC) powder, granules or hypochlorite solution. A plastic apron and gloves should be worn.

Using NaDDC:

■ Leave the powder or granules in contact with the fluid for 2 minutes
■ Scoop up the debris with disposable wipes
■ Discard everything in a yellow bag for incineration
■ Clean the area with water and detergent
■ Ensure that ventilation is optimal during this procedure; NaDDC may release chlorine, which is toxic.

Using hypochlorite solution:

■ Cover the spillage with paper towels to absorb the excess fluid
■ Pour the hypochlorite solution over the towels. Use a 1 per cent solution containing 10 000 ppm of available chlorine
■ Leave this for at least 2 minutes
■ Scoop all the debris into a yellow plastic bag for incineration
■ Clean the area with water and detergent
■ In domiciliary settings, employ the same procedure, using a solution consisting of one part household bleach to 10 parts water.

Emergencies are unavoidable, and it is inevitable that accidental exposure to blood or body fluids will occasionally occur. Routine good practice enables staff to cope in these situations.

Clinical Application

Should some Clinical Settings be Designated 'High-risk' Areas for Occupational Exposure to Blood and Body Fluids?

All are at risk of occupational exposure to blood through contamination or sharps injury and should be protected by hepatitis B vaccination (Goodlad, 1991). The risk is, however, higher for some people than others. Yassi and McGill (1991) discovered an association between the type of nursing procedure undertaken and the incidence of sharps injury, while Jagger *et al.* (1990) found that most accidents involving nurses occurred in clinics or theatre, where, next to the surgeon, the scrub nurse is the person most likely to have contact with blood (Closs and Tierney, 1990). Studies of this kind are valuable because they represent a first step towards the development of policies towards prevention; acknowledging the existence of high-risk situations does not detract from the right of all nurses to be protected against the hazards of parenterally transmitted infection.

REVISION CHECKLIST: KEY AREAS

- ☐ Introduction – the risk of infection and health professionals

- ☐ Human immunodeficiency virus: Transmission of HIV, Occupational health risks, Treatment

- ☐ Hepatitis: Hepatitis B, Hepatitis C, Hepatitis D, Hepatitis A, Hepatitis E, Other hepatitis viruses

- ☐ Universal precautions: Protective clothing, Other equipment, Dealing with sharps, Dealing with sharps injuries, Dealing with blood contamination of the conjunctivae and mucous membranes, Spillage of blood and body fluids

Activities – linking knowledge to clinical practice

1 'The right of the health professional to confidentiality is always paramount.' Debate this statement in relation to:

(a) A midwife newly diagnosed with HIV infection who routinely performs invasive procedures (such as episiotomy and suturing)
(b) A health visitor found to be a chronic hepatitis B virus carrier.

2 Develop a health and safety policy for dealing with blood and/or body fluid exposure in:

(a) A primary school (children aged 4–11)
(b) A community hostel for adults with learning disabilities.

SELF-ASSESSMENT

1. Which of the following are classified as body fluids for the purpose of universal precautions?
   - (a) semen ☐
   - (b) packed cell transfusions ☐
   - (c) unfixed tissues ☐
   - (d) synovial fluid ☐

2. Which of the following are transmitted parenterally?
   - (a) hepatitis B ☐
   - (b) hepatitis C ☐
   - (c) delta virus ☐
   - (d) hepatitis E ☐

3. All subjects infected with hepatitis B virus become chronic carriers.
   True? ☐ False? ☐

4. All chronic carriers of hepatitis B virus develop hepatocellular cancer.
   True? ☐ False? ☐

5. The most infectious part of the hepatitis B virus is:
   - (a) HBsAg ☐
   - (b) Anti-HBe ☐
   - (c) HBeAg ☐
   - (d) HBcAg ☐

6. Effective immunisation is available for:
   - (a) hepatitis B virus ☐
   - (b) HIV ☐
   - (c) hepatitis C virus ☐
   - (d) hepatitis D virus ☐

7. The hepatitis B virus is more virulent than the HIV virus. True? ☐ False? ☐

8. Providing that no cuts or abrasions are visible on the hands, it is safe to assume that contact with blood carries no health risk.
   True? ☐ False? ☐

References

Adams KS, Zehrer CL and Thomas W (1993) 'Comparison of a needleless system with conventional heparin locks'. *American Journal of Infection Control* **21**: 263–9.

Binney A (1994) 'Barrier method'. *Nursing Times* **90**(38): 68–70.

Bond WW, Favero MF, Peterson MJ *et al.* (1983) 'Inactivation of hepatitis B virus in intermediate to high level disinfectant chemicals'. *Journal of Clinical Microbiology* **18**: 535–8.

Boxall EH (1993) 'Risks to surgeons and patients from HIV and hepatitis'. *British Medical Journal* **306**: 652–3.

Briggs M and Thomas J (1994) 'Obstacles to hepatitis B vaccine uptake by health care staff'. *Public Health* **108**: 137–48.

Brookes A (1994) 'Surgical glove perforation'. *Nursing Times* **90**(21): 60–2.

Centers for Disease Control (1993) 'Update: investigations of persons treated by HIV-infected health care workers'. *Journal of the American Medical Association* **269**: 2622–3.

Chant K, Lowe D, Rubin G *et al.* (1993) 'Patient-to-patient transmission of HIV in private surgical consulting rooms'. *Lancet* **342**: 1548–9.

Closs SJ and Tierney A (1990) 'Theatre gowns: a survey of the extent of user protection'. *Journal of Hospital Infection* **15**: 375–8.

Dalgleish AG and Malkovsy M (1988) 'Surgical gloves as a mechanical barrier against human immunodeficiency viruses'. *British Journal of Surgery* **75**: 171–2.

Dancocks A and Hewitt S (1994) 'Hepatitis B immunisation status of A&E healthcare workers'. *Occupational Health* **46**(1): 20–3.

Denes AE, Smith JL, Maynard JE *et al.* (1978) 'Hepatitis B infection in physicians. Results of a nationwide seroepidemiological study'. *Journal of the American Medical Association* **239**: 210–11.

Denton I (1991) 'Taking stock'. *Nursing Times* **87**(96): 32–3

Department of Health (1998) *UK Health Departments Guidance for Clinical Health Care Workers: Protection Against Infection with Blood-borne Viruses.* DoH, London.

Dienstag JL, Werner BG and Polk BF (1984) 'Hepatitis B vaccine in health care personnel: safety, immunogenicity and indicators of efficacy'. *Annals of Internal Medicine* **101**: 34–40.

Drescher J, Wagner A, Haverich A *et al.* (1994) 'Nosocomial hepatitis B infections in cardiac transplant recipients transmitted during transvenous endomyocardial biopsy'. *Journal of Hospital Infection* **26**: 81–2.

Duthie R, Morgan-Capner P, Wilson M *et al.* (1994) 'Problems in management of health care workers exposed to HBeAg positive body fluids'. *Journal of Hospital Infection* **26**: 129–32.

Feinstone SM, Kapitan AZ and Purcell RH (1975) 'Transmission-associated hepatitis not associated to viral hepatitis A or B'. *New England Journal of Medicine* **292**: 767–70.

Finch RG (1987) 'Time for action on hepatitis B vaccination'. *British Medical Journal* **294**: 197–8.

Forseter G, Joline C and Wormser GP (1990) 'Blood contamination of tourniquets used in routine phlebotomy'. *American Journal of Infection Control* **18**: 386–90.

Gill J and Slater J (1991) 'Building barriers against infection'. *Nursing Times* **87**(50): 53–4.

Goldmann DA (1991) 'The role of barrier precautions in infection control'. *Journal of Hospital Infection* **18** (Supplement A): 515–23.

Goodlad J (1991) 'Work place risks'. *Nursing Times* **87**(9): 54–5.

Green SE and Grompertz RKH (1992) 'Glove perforation during surgery'. *Annals of the Royal College of Surgery* **74**: 306–8.

Gurevich I (1988) 'Complications of ICU hospitalisation. Transmissable infections in critical care'. *Heart and Lung* **17**: 331–4.

Gwyther J (1989) 'Sharps disposal containers and their use'. *Journal of Hospital Infection* **15**: 287–94.

Hanson PJ, Gor D and Jeffries DJ (1989) 'Chemical inactivation of HIV on surfaces'. *British Medical Journal* **298**: 862–4.

Harmory BH (1983) 'Under-reporting of needlestick injuries in a university hospital'. *American Journal of Infection Control* **11**: 174–7.

Hart S (1990) 'Hepatitis B: guidelines for infection control'. *Nursing Standard* **4**(45): 24–7.

Havlichek DH, Greenman E and Plaisier K (1991) 'High prevalence of historical risk factors for blood-borne infections among in-patients in a community hospital'. *American Journal of Infection Control* **19**: 67–72.

Henderson D, Fahey B and Willy M *et al.* (1990) 'Risk for occupational transmission of human immunodeficiency virus type 1 (HIV-1) associated with clinical exposures'. *Annals of Internal Medicine* **113**: 740–6.

Heponstall J, Porter K and Gill ON (1993) 'Occupational transmission of HIV: summary of published reports'. *PHLS Internal Report* September.

Jagger J, Hunt EH and Pearson RD (1990) 'Sharp object injuries in hospital: causes and strategies for prevention'. *Americal Journal of Hospital Infection* **18**(4): 227–31.

Jenner E (1990) 'Preaching safe practice'. *Nursing Times* **86**(28): 68–9.

Kelen GD, Green GB and Purcell RH (1992) 'Hepatitis B and hepatitis C in emergency department patients'. *New England Journal of Medicine* **326**: 1399–1404.

King R (1990) 'Hepatitis B: more care less scare'. *Nursing Times* **86**(5): 54–5.

Korniewicz DM, Laughon BE, Butz A *et al.* (1989) 'Integrity of vinyl and latex procedure gloves. *Nursing Research* **38**: 144–6.

Korniewicz DM, Kirwin M, Cresci K *et al.* (1994) 'Barrier protection with examination gloves: double versus single'. *American Journal of Infection Control* **22**: 12–15.

Leentvaar-Kuijpers G, Dekker MM, Cuutinho RA *et al.* (1990) Needlestick injuries, surgeons and HIV risks'. *Lancet* **335**: 546–7.

Lifson AR (1988) 'Do alternative modes for transmission of human immunodeficiency exist? A review'. *Journal of the American Medical Association* **259**: 1352–6.

Main J (1991) 'Therapy of chronic viral hepatitis'. *Journal of Hospital Infection* **18** (Supplement A): 177–83.

Mitsui T, Iwano K and Masuka K (1992) 'Hepatitis C virus infection in medical personnel after needlestick accident'. *Hepatology* **16**: 1109–14.

Moore RM and Kaczmarek RM (1990) 'Occupational hazards to health care workers: diverse, ill-defined, and not fully appreciated'. *Journal of the American Medical Association* **18**: 316–27.

Mulhall AB, King S and Wiggington E (1993) 'Maintenance of urinary drainage systems: are practitioners more aware of the dangers?' *Journal of Clinical Nursing* **2**: 135–40.

Murrell A (1993) 'Unlocking the virus'. *Professional Nurse* **8**(12): 780–3.

Oakley K (1994) 'Making sense of universal precautions'. *Nursing Times* **90**(27): 35–6.

Orenstein R, Reynolds L, Karabaic M *et al.* (1995) 'Do protective devices prevent needlestick injuries among health care workers?' *American Journal of Infection Control* **23**: 344–51.

Peireira LJ, Lee GM and Wade FJ (1990) 'The effect of surgical handwashing routines on the microbial counts of operating room nurses'. *American Journal of Infection* **18**: 354–64.

Polakoff S (1986) 'Acute viral hepatitis B: laboratory reports 1980–1984'. *British Medical Journal* **293**: 37–8.

Polish LB, Toing MJ and Co RL (1993) 'Risk factors for hepatitis C virus infection among health care personnel in a community hospital'. *American Journal of Infection Control* **21**: 196–200.

Poole CJM, Miller S and Fillingham G (1994) 'Immunity to hepatitis B among health care workers performing exposure prone procedures'. *British Medical Journal* **309**: 94–5.

Pratt R (1994) 'Safe practice'. *Nursing Times* **90**(21): 64–7.

Public Health Laboratory Service (1993) 'Health care workers and HIV: surveillance of occupationally acquired infection in the United Kingdom'. *Communicable Diseases Report* **3**(11): 147–53.

Shaw DJ and Bell DM (1993) 'Risk of occupational infection with blood-borne pathogens in operating and delivery room settings'. *American Journal of Infection Control* **21**: 343–51.

Smales C (1998) 'Hepatitis: symptoms, treatment and prevention'. *Nursing Times* **94**(44): 58–60.

Spence MR and Dash GP (1990) 'Hepatitis B: perceptions, knowledge, and vaccine acceptance among registered nurses in high risk occupations in a university hospital'. *Infection Control and Hospital Epidemiology* **11**: 129–33.

Szmuness W, Stevens CE, Harley EJ *et al.* (1982) 'Hepatitis B vaccine in medical staff of haemodialysis units: efficacy and subtype cross-protection'. *New England Journal of Medicine* **307**: 1481–6.

Tedder RS, Gibson RJC andd Briggs M (1991) 'Hepatitis C virus: evidence for sexual transmission'. *British Medical Journal* **302**: 1299–302.

Thaler MM, Park CK, Landers D *et al.* (1991) 'Vertical transmission of hepatitis C virus'. *Lancet* **338**: 17–18.

Thomas JA, Fligelstone LJ, Jerwood TE *et al.* (1993) 'Theatre footwear: a health hazard?' *British Journal of Theatre Nursing* **3**(7): 5–9.

Trevelyan J (1991) 'Hepatitis B and the law'. *Nursing Times* **87**(9): 52–3.

Van Rijwisjk L (1992) 'Gloves and other rubber-based devices: benefits, problems and guidelines'. *Wounds: A Compendium of Research and Practice* **4**: 65–73.

Weltman AC, Short LJ, Mendelson MH *et al.* (1995) 'Risk of disposal-related sharps injuries'. *Infection Control and Hospital Epidemiology* **16**(5): 268–74.

Wilson J and Breedon P (1990) 'Universal precautions'. *Nursing Times* **86**(37): 67–9.

Wormser GP, Joline C and Duncanson F (1984) 'Needlestick injuries during the care of patients with AIDS'. *New England Journal of Medicine* **310**: 1461–2.

Yanelli B and Gurevich I (1998) 'Infection control in critical care'. *Heart and Lung* **17**: 596–9.

Yassi A and McGill M (1991) 'Determinants of blood and body fluid exposure in a large teaching hospital: the hazards of intermittent exposure'. *American Journal of Infection Control* **19**: 129–35.

Further reading and information sources

Advisory Committee on Dangerous Pathogens (1995) *Protection against Blood Borne Infections in the Workplace. HIV, Hepatitis.* HMSO, London.

Royal College of Nursing (1997) *Hepatitis Guidelines.* RCN, London.

National Aids Helpline 0800 567 123.

Terence Higgins Trust, 52–54 Grays Inn Road, London WC1X 8JU. Tel: 0207 242 1010.

13 Sexually transmitted infections

CHAPTER OUTCOMES

After reading this chapter you should be able to:

- Explain why sexually transmitted infections are a significant health problem in the UK

- Define the term 'sexual health'

- List the functions of genitourinary medicine clinics

- List the common infections transmitted by the sexual route, name the organisms responsible and outline the methods used in diagnosis, prevention and treatment

Introduction to sexually transmitted infections

In the UK, the diagnosis and treatment of sexually transmitted infections (STIs) is available in genitourinary medicine (GUM) clinics, from GPs, from some family planning clinics and privately. STIs represent a significant health problem within the UK as many of the infections can lead to permanent problems such as infertility and can, in pregnant women, damage the fetus.

Incidence of STI in the UK

There is a well-established system of recording the number of cases of STI. Every GUM clinic is required to submit quarterly returns to the Department of Health.

These figures are vital for planning control measures, including health promotion campaigns, but the data underestimate the real incidence of infection: some infections are undiagnosed, and cases seen outside GUM clinics are excluded.

The latest figures show that the incidence of gonorrhoea and syphilis is declining but all other STIs are becoming more common. Most cases occur in young people in their teens to early 30s (DoH, 1995). In the early 1990s, the incidence of gonorrhoea and syphilis declined, probably with the increase in the use of barrier precautions and 'safe sex' in response to the public health campaign against HIV disease (Evans, 1994). As mentioned above, there has, however, been an upsurge in the incidence of all other conditions.

Possible reasons for the upsurge in some STIs

These may include:

- Today's more liberal approach towards sexual behaviours
- Improved public awareness and a greater willingness to seek help
- Improved contact tracing
- Increased travel, both within the UK and around the world
- An increasing tendency for young people to move away from home to work or study. This creates loneliness and insecurity, which helps to fuel sexual experimentation.

The control of gonorrhoea and syphilis (historically, two of the diseases defined as 'venereal' by law) has traditionally featured prominently in community health programmes. Both diseases are highly contagious and can be difficult to detect, with severe effects on the health of the individual if untreated. Recently concern has focused on limiting the spread of HIV. This has involved a considerable expenditure of public money through publicity campaigns. However, the public also needs to be aware that other conditions, such as *Chlamydia trachomatis,* human papilloma virus (HPV) and herpes simplex virus (HSV) infection, also have long-term effects.

Sexual health and the role of GUM departments

The control of sexually transmitted infection has been considered an important area of public health endeavour since the early part of the 20th century. The Venereal Disease Regulations (1916) required all local authorities to provide clinics where diagnosis and free treatment were available in strict confidence. Contact tracing became an essential feature of the service, contributing to its success. A second advance was made in 1924 with the establishment of the Venereal Disease Reference Laboratory: for the first time, it was possible to standardise methods of diagnosis and treatment and to collate statistics.

Nowadays, a broad view of sexual health is taken – it is seen as the integration of all aspects of sexual being including its physical, emotional, intellectual and social components. Sexual health is therefore an integral part of overall health and involves much more than helping people to avoid infection (Jones, 1994). Nurses working in this clinical setting provide information and advice, perform tests to diagnose infection and give treatment. GUM clinics play a central role in meeting the previous government's Health of the Nation targets (DoH, 1992) through efforts to reduce the incidence of HIV and other sexually transmitted infections. Community health issues addressed include:

- The availability of a confidential self-referral service without a waiting list for anyone wishing to discuss sexual health matters
- Examination and testing for genital infections
- Health education and counselling
- Partner notification
- Free prescriptions.

Clinical Application

Securing Adherence to Treatment at the GUM Clinic

Patient adherence to treatment is increased through GUM clinics because it is possible to process many specimens immediately. Diagnosis is swift and accurate, and treatment can begin at the same visit. The patient's reception in the clinic and the attitude of staff also play an important role in securing willingness to return for follow-up tests.

Sexually transmitted infections

Syphilis

Syphilis is caused by the spirochaete *Treponema pallidum*, which is exclusively a human pathogen.

Syphilis is a past example of a 'new' disease. It appeared suddenly in Europe in the late 15th century, engendering the same fear and speculation as HIV does today (Evans, 1994). There are two theories to explain its origins:

- **The Colomban theory** – syphilis endemic in the West Indies was brought to Europe by sailors returning with Columbus.

- **The unitarian theory** – syphilis is a form of yaws, a tropical treponemal infection caused by a spirochaete indistinguishable from *T. pallidum*. Yaws is a skin condition spread by direct skin contact. It was prevalent in the West Indies throughout the 15th century, reaching Europe as a result of slave-trading. It has been suggested that in a colder climate where more of the body is clothed, transmission gradually became dependent on the sexual route (Wasley, 1988). Infection results in a wide range of symptoms; in the past, syphilis was called the 'great imitator' (Roberts, 1982). Today, infection, although still considered serious, appears less virulent than when the first cases appeared in the 15th century.

Stages of syphilis

In adults, syphilis is transmitted mainly by sexual intercourse. The incubation period is 9–90 days. It progresses in four stages:

- **Primary syphilis** – A chancre (ulcer) appears at the site of infection on the genitalia, rectum, mouth or rarely finger. The early signs of infection are easily overlooked as chancres are painless and often difficult to see. Spirochaetes spread rapidly to other parts of the body, probably within a few hours.

- **Secondary syphilis** – About 2 months after infection, the victim may experience a vague, flu-like illness with malaise, fever and aching joints. Symptoms may be mild and dismissed because they are so non-specific. Some sufferers develop a rash. Patients are highly infectious because the surfaces of the lesions team with treponemes. The other manifestations of secondary syphilis include elongated ulcerated lesions ('snail-track' ulcers) and flattened warty growths (condylomata lata). Again, these are easily overlooked, or their significance may not be appreciated.

- **The latent stage** – The stage that follows may persist for years. The individual appears well but shows serological evidence of infection if tested.

- **Tertiary syphilis** – This arises years later. It is characterised by the development of chronic ulcers called gummata, which can develop anywhere on the skin or in the tissues. Gummata cause particular damage if they involve bone, cardiovascular or nervous tissue. A gumma developing on the wall of the aorta leads to weakening and the formation of an aneurysm. This is a grave complication of late syphilis. Involvement of the nervous system leads to tabes dorsalis (locomotor ataxia – a lack of co-ordination with disturbed sensation in the legs) and dementia (general paralysis of the insane). Many authorities classify the late complications affecting the cardiovascular and nervous systems as quaternary syphilis. The mechanism by which *T. pallidum* evokes damage remains obscure: it does not produce toxins, and it evokes only a weak immune response.

Congenital syphilis

Congenital (prenatal) syphilis occurs vertically from mother to fetus via the placenta. It causes spontaneous miscarriage, stillbirth or the delivery of a child with the signs and symptoms of syphilis (Table 13.1). The earlier the maternal infection occurs during pregnancy, the more grave the prognosis for the infant. Congenital syphilis is extremely rare in the UK, having been eliminated by routinely testing all pregnant women as part of their antenatal screening programme.

Table 13.1   The hallmarks of congenital syphilis

Early – appearing within 2 weeks of delivery

■ **Skin lesions** – a weeping, crusted rash ('syphilitic pemphigus') principally affecting the peripheries, followed by a papular rash and condylomata lata reminiscent of adult secondary syphilis. Scarring may result in areas subject to friction, such as the mouth

■ **Mucous membranes** – discharging lesions develop in the nose, mouth, throat, larynx and pharynx, interfering with feeding

■ **Viscera** – enlargement of the spleen and liver, with altered plasma protein levels

■ **Neurological** – meningitis

■ **Bone lesions** – syphilis involving the long bones results in pain, immobility and decalcification

Late – the stigmata of congenital syphilis result from maldevelopment of the tissues through the damage caused by treponemes at or soon after birth. They include:

■ A perforated nasal septum

■ Maldeveloped, notched, peg-shaped teeth (Hutchinson's incisors)

■ Scarring (rhagades) from the early rashes around the nose and mouth

■ Keratitis

■ Effusion of the joints (Clutton's joints)

■ Bony deformities, especially of the maxilla and long bones

■ Eighth cranial nerve deafness

Any of the conditions arising during the adult form of tertiary syphilis may also develop

Diagnosis

Diagnosis at the primary stage involves scraping exudate from the surface of the chancre for microscopy. Treponemes are too small and too difficult to visualise even under the high power of the light microscope so a special technique called dark ground microscopy is used. Most people with syphilis are, however, detected because they have been alerted to the risk through contact tracing or during routine testing for other STIs. The diagnosis is then made by serological testing (Table 13.2).

Table 13.2   Serological tests for syphilis

Venereal disease research laboratory test (VDRL) – a rapid precipitation test quantifying the number of treponemal antibodies in the blood, used routinely in screening to confirm the diagnosis and to monitor the course of infection once treatment has started

Fluorescent treponemal antibody test (FTA) – sometimes used in early diagnosis as it yields a result at an earlier stage in the course of disease than most other tests. Too expensive for routine screening

Treponema pallidum **haemagglutination assay (TPHA)** – a highly specific agglutination test for treponemal antigens that can be used in routine screening

NB: **Wasserman reaction (WR)** – a complement fixation test now superseded by modern tests that are more accurate

Treatment

Treatment involves the intramuscular administration of high doses of penicillin given for 10–14 days, the exact regimens varying between clinics. There have been no recorded cases of treponemal resistance to penicillin. Patients allergic to penicillin are usually given tetracyclines (Nettina, 1990). The injections are painful, and daily attendance can disrupt usual activities. Thus, as well as giving medication, the nurse has an important role in maintaining compliance, especially with clients who feel well or for whom the diagnosis was unexpected. Patients are asked to refrain from sexual activity until the course of treatment has finished and must return to the clinic to ensure that it has been successful. They may need to undergo neurological investigations. They must also be warned about the possibility of experiencing the Jarisch–Herxheimer reaction: fever, headache, nausea, chills, myalgia, tachycardia and dizziness (caused by hypotension) within 6–12 hours of receiving antibiotics. The cause of the reaction is unknown, but it is thought to be due to the release of endotoxins from the treponemes as they are destroyed. The Jarisch–Herxheimer reaction is usually short lived and is not harmful. Patients are advised to rest in bed and take fluids and antipyretics. Once the course of treatment has been completed, the infection is eradicated, but previous exposure does not produce immunity: it is thus possible to develop syphilis more than once.

Gonorrhoea

Gonorrhoea has been known since antiquity. Some biblical references to contagious disease probably refer to gonorrhoea and it was certainly known to the Greeks and Romans. There has been considerable confusion between this disease and syphilis. John Hunter's *Treatise of Venereal Disease* published in 1818, for example, describes experiments in which he infected a healthy subject with syphilis by puncturing his penis with a lancet dipped in pus. This pus must, however, have contained the organisms responsible for both syphilis and gonorrhoea. Further work performed towards the end of the 19th century indicated the existence of two separate infections, the agent responsible for gonorrhoea eventually being identified by Albert Neisser in 1879.

Gonorrhoea is caused by a Gram-negative diplococcus, *Neisseria gonorrhoeae* (also known as the Gonococcus or GC). It attaches to the urethral and cervical mucosae by pili, laboratory strains without pili being non-pathogenic. The bacteria survive in neutrophils (Figure 13.1). The adult vaginal wall is not invaded, probably because its tough squamous epithelium is inhospitable to the delicate bacteria. *Neisseria gonorrhoeae* rapidly succumbs to cold and drying. It is unable to survive long outside the host, explaining why transmission is primarily via the sexual route. The eyes of infants become infected during passage down the birth canal in the presence of cervical secretions containing gonococci (causing 'sticky eyes' or ophthalmia neonatorum).

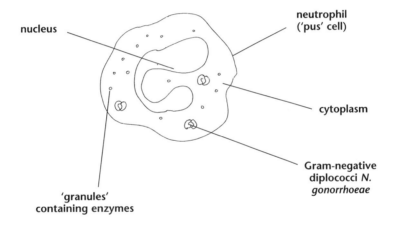

Figure 13.1   Neutrophil containing *Neisseria gonorrhoeae*

In both sexes, acute infection presents as urethritis, with discharge and pain on micturition. The incubation period is between 2 and 10 days. Approximately a third of infected women remain asymptomatic. The consequences are serious both from the perspective of the individual and in community health terms. Gonococci migrate from the cervix to the uterus and uterine tubes, where they cause severe scarring that may result in occlusion, thus impairing fertility. Escape from the fimbriated ends of the uterine tubes may lead to peritonitis, but this is less common. More often, female carriers experience symptoms of vague, debilitating chronic ill-health and are highly infectious. Gonococcal vulvovaginitis in young girls may be a sign of sexual abuse. In men, untreated infection causes scarring, urethral stricture, epididymitis and prostatitis.

The involvement of the joints, with the development of gonococcal arthritis, is another late occasional complication of infection in either sex.

Diagnosis

Diagnosis is by the examination of wet films of material collected using swabs. The survival of *N. gonorrhoeae* outside the host is so poor that microscopy must be performed in the clinic as soon as the swabs have been obtained.

Treatment

Treatment is usually successful using oral ampicillin with probenecid to delay its renal clearance. Penicillin-resistant strains were first reported in the 1970s. These release beta-lactamase enzymes, which destroy the beta-lactam part of the penicillin molecule (see Chapter 4), rendering it ineffective. Patients carrying resistant strains must be given another antibiotic, often spectinomycin. Infection does not result in immunity so it is possible to develop gonorrhoea more than once.

Chlamydia

Chlamydia trachomatis causes genital infection in both men and women. Its incidence is difficult to determine because, until recently, only the larger GUM clinics had the equipment necessary to perform the diagnostic tests. *Chlamydia* cannot be cultured outside living cells so infection is difficult to detect. A sensitive urine test has recently become available (Lee *et al.*, 1995).

Chlamydia infects the urethra and in men is responsible for most cases of non-specific urethritis (nongonococcal urethritis). Complications include prostatitis and epididymitis. In women, its behaviour is similar to that of *N. gonorrhoeae* and it may be carried asymptomatically. The cervix is a common site of infection. It ascends the genital tract, causing salpingitis and impaired fertility (Pearce, 1990). Infection with *Chlamydia* is serious and highly damaging, meriting early detection and treatment (Abel and von Unwerth, 1988). Contact tracing is not routinely performed in the UK as it is in the USA and Sweden. However, clinic staff introducing trial protocols to follow up the contacts of patients presenting with chlamydial infection have found them highly receptive to health promotion (White, 1992) and have been able to provide treatment to a high proportion of men and women who would not otherwise have received it (Cameron and Blately, 1993). Contact tracing is being increasingly used within the UK.

Treatment

Treatment involves tetracyclines, sulphonamides being prescribed when scarring involves the deeper tissues.

Genital warts

Genital warts are caused by the human papilloma virus (HPV). They are the most common sexually transmitted virus infections, accounting for up to 25 per cent of all attendance at GUM clinics (Barton, 1994), and are a source of anxiety for patients

(Chandler, 1996). The incubation period is 2 or 3 months, but the virus can remain latent for years so contact tracing is not practical. The mode of transmission is poorly understood. Entry is thought to occur via minor abrasions in the mucous membranes developing through trauma during sexual intercourse. Warts are unsightly, catch on clothing and contribute to the development of malignancy. HPV types 16 and 18 appear to have the greatest oncogenic potential and are important causative agents of cervical cancer both in women who have warts and in those whose partners are affected. Annual cervical smears are recommended for those at risk, and some authorities now recommend tests for HPV to complement cytology

Treatment

Treatment involves the topical application of a cytotoxic agent, podophyllin used as a 0.5 per cent solution being the most popular. This contains a number of plant extracts. Podophyllotoxin is therapeutically the most active treatment and is included in a number of proprietary preparations (for example, Warticon, Fem and Pharma). In the past people, were obliged to attend clinics for all their treatment, but providing the lesions are sited in an area where they may be visualised (with a mirror if necessary), self-treatment is now possible, although it should still occur under the supervision of a health professional. A typical regimen involves twice-daily application for 3 days and then a 4-day break, lasting for 3 or 4 weeks, with follow-up attendance at intervals to ensure that treatment is progressing. Resolution should begin during the first week of treatment but can take longer. Podophyllin necroses tissues by arresting nuclear division. It causes painful ulceration if applied to healthy tissues. Podophyllum resin products should not be used during pregnancy. Where genital warts are severe, treatment may involve cryotherapy.

Herpes simplex

HSV is a DNA virus responsible for cold sores (involving the oral mucosae) and genital ulceration. By the age of 5 years, over 60 per cent of the population have become infected. There are two types, distinguished on the basis of biochemical and antigenic properties:

- HSV-1, primarily isolated from oral lesions
- HSV-2, primarily isolated from genital lesions, and less common.

There is an increasing tendency for HSV-1 to be isolated from genital lesions. People already infected with HVS-1 can become infected with HVS-2 and vice versa.

Primary oral herpes infection

Primary oral herpes infection usually occurs early from contact with an asymptomatic salivary carrier or someone who has an actively discharging lesion. Characteristic vesicles appear around the mouth or eyes, sometimes associated with febrile illness. Encephalitis is a rare complication that may be fatal. Infection, however, is more often mild and overlooked.

Recurrent oral herpes infection

Recurrent oral herpes infection occurs throughout adult life. After primary infection, the virus migrates up the sensory nerves to their associated ganglia where it lies dormant, occasionally becoming active through some challenge to the immune system (a cold, influenza or sometimes even exposure to sunshine or during menstruation). Virus particles travel back down the nerves, and as these supply a localised area on the face, crops of vesicles develop at the same site, usually around the nostrils or lips.

Primary genital herpes

Primary genital herpes infection is acquired sexually, probably through small breaks in the mucosae. The main viral reservoirs are the cervix and the male genital tract. Painful ulceration develops on the glans and shaft of the penis or the vulva, where it may interfere with micturition. Individuals feel most unwell during the prodrome before the lesions have fully developed. Treatment of first-episode HSV is with oral antiviral agents, for example acyclovir or famiciclovir (Chard, 1998). Antiviral drugs should not be used during pregnancy.

Recurrent genital herpes

Recurrent genital herpes infection occurs throughout life, causing considerable guilt and anxiety (Williams, 1994). There is no treatment. Symptoms are controlled with idoxuridine (5-iodo-2-deoxyuridine), which interferes with DNA replication so that the virus cannot multiply. Some of those affected may, however, prefer to use complementary therapies, for example tea tree oil. Herpes virus plays a role in the development of cervical cancer so annual smears are recommended for female carriers. Delivery during primary infection may result in the baby developing fatal encephalitis unless elective caesarean section is performed.

Candidiasis

Candida is a yeast-like, spore-forming fungus. It causes a white, highly irritant vaginal discharge, often most troublesome just before menstruation. There are numerous species, the most common being *Candida albicans*. Spores are visible when wet films are Gram stained and examined under the microscope. Hyphae are difficult to visualise.

Candida occasionally causes balanitis in men. It is not always sexually transmitted but is most common in sexually active women, especially during the childbearing years. Infection is said to be more common in women taking oral contraceptives, but there is little supporting evidence for this (Odds, 1988). Some women suffer from repeated attacks which may be the result of reinfection. Boiling or disinfecting clothing is, however, not effective as a treatment, even though it is recommended in 'self-help' material for patients (Rashid *et al.*, 1991). The incidence is higher among diabetics than members of the general population and may be a sign

Clinical Application

General Advice and Support for People with Genital Herpes

Nurses, midwives and health visitors are well placed to offer general advice and support to people with genital herpes. A diagnosis of genital herpes will affect all aspects of the person's life and health – there will be psychological and social implications and not just the physical effects of the infection. Individuals may feel unclean, that their sex life is at an end and stigmatised by misinformed opinion on the nature of herpes. It is easy to see why those affected may become depressed, especially when one considers the recurring nature of herpes, which has no cure.

Several general pointers should be followed:

- Provide information about all aspects of genital herpes – treatments, recurrence, risk to sexual partners and pregnancy.
- Provide teaching that allows people to recognise when they have genital herpes.
- Provide teaching that allows people to recognise the 'early warning' signs of a recurrent episode of herpes.
- Provide written back-up information about genital herpes, including treatment, complementary therapies and self-help groups.
- Provide a relaxed and non-judgemental environment in which people have the opportunity to talk through their feelings about having genital herpes with a well-informed health professional.
- Advise patients to take simple symptomatic remedies, for example paracetamol, for the systemic illness that occurs with the primary infection, to rest and to take extra fluids.
- Give information about keeping the lesions clean and dry.
- Advise patients about when to stop having sexual intercourse; during the primary infection, for example, this would be until the lesions have healed and all other symptoms of genital herpes have passed.
- Stress the importance of women telling health professionals about a pregnancy or a plan to conceive in the future.
- Encourage patients to return for follow-up consultations and make sure that tests for other STIs are completed.
- If necessary, encourage sexual partners to visit the clinic.
- Ensure that the individual is involved in decisions about his or her management.

of undetected diabetes mellitus. It has been suggested that an elevated blood glucose level alters vaginal pH by interfering with lactic acid production. The situation may be similar in pregnancy, when *Candida* infection is also common. Increased oestrogen levels stimulate the formation of glycogen from glucose, again resulting in the excess production of lactic acid.

The personal, social and economic consequences of *Candida* infection tend to be overlooked. Many women suffer recurrent inconvenience, embarrassment and discomfort. The irritation is often most intense at night, interfering with sleep and the following day's activities. Micturition becomes painful. Time is lost from school or work, and underperformance may result (Odds, 1988). Contact tracing is not routinely performed, many cases being self-treated as topical fungicide creams are available without prescription. *Candida* has been responsible for nosocomial outbreaks, mainly among the critically ill (Lee *et al.*, 1991). Infection often develops in the mouth or large bowel in response to antibiotic therapy and can be transmitted via the hands of health professionals (Findik *et al.*, 1996). It is a common complication of immunosuppression, including HIV disease.

Treatment

Treatment is possible locally with nystatin or clotrimazole pessaries and cream to control itching. If this is unsuccessful, women may be given fluconazole orally. Contraception is vital during treatment as it is teratogenic.

Trichomoniasis

Trichomonas vaginalis is a highly motile, flagellated protozoon that may be carried asymptomatically or may cause an offensive, frothy, yellow-green vaginal discharge. Speculum examination reveals an inflamed cervix and vaginal walls. In severe cases, the vulva, perineum and insides of the thighs may become sore. The distress and inconvenience experienced by patients are frequently overlooked. The organisms are easily visualised in wet microscope preparations made from vaginal swabs and examined under low power, but they are difficult to isolate from men even though they may be present in prostatic fluid or cause mild urethral discharge. *Trichomonas vaginalis* forms cysts under adverse environmental conditions.

Sexual transmission is thought to be the most usual mechanism of dispersal because partners often show evidence of infection if examined thoroughly and it is sometimes possible to identify chains of infection when there have been multiple partners (Krieger *et al.*, 1993). Non-sexual transfer has been suggested but never demonstrated.

Treatment

Both partners should be treated with metronidazole. This may be difficult to organise because routine contact tracing is not performed.

Bacterial vaginosis

Bacterial vaginosis is not always sexually transmitted, although it is often diagnosed in conjunction with other STIs. It is a distressing condition most commonly diagnosed among women during the fertile years, especially if they have had several partners or a recent change of partner (Temple, 1994). It is beginning to attract more attention as it has recently been established that affected women are more likely to experience late miscarriage or preterm delivery (Hay *et al.*, 1994).

The most commonly reported symptom is an unpleasant, fishy odour from the genital area, not linked to poor hygiene. Some women also complain of a frothy, non-irritant grey discharge. Bacteriological examination of the vagina reveals an abnormally high number of anaerobic bacteria coupled with a reduction in the *Lactobacillus* count, suggesting a disturbance in the usual ecology of the vaginal flora and perhaps general ill-health. *Gardnerella vaginalis* is one of the bacteria most frequently isolated. An association was initially made between this organism and the presence of vaginal irritation in 1955 (Gardner and Dukes, 1955). However, it may also be present in healthy women. Diagnosis involves placing a piece of pH indicator paper inside the vagina to test the pH. A value greater than 4.5 indicates infection but is not specific. Swabs from the vaginal wall and cervix are cultured to demonstrate the presence of anaerobes and a reduction in lactobacilli.

Treatment

Treatment is with metronidazole or by applying 2 per cent clindamycin cream for 7 days.

HIV

HIV is an RNA retrovirus. The virus multiplies aggressively, damaging the host by progressively destroying the immune system, especially the CD4 (T helper) lymphocytes (see Chapter 2). These play a key role in activating the immune response, especially cell-mediated immunity. New CD4 lymphoctes are produced to replace those lost, but the immune system cannot sustain this effect indefinitely (Cooper and Mergigan, 1996). The result is profound immunosuppression, with the appearance of characteristic opportunistic infections (Table 13.3) and tumours (Kaposi's sarcoma and lymphomas). Many of the opportunistic infections and tumours are considered to be AIDS-defining by the Centers for Disease Control (Atlanta) and the World Health Organization.

Reverse transcriptase, an enzyme released by HIV, manufactures DNA blueprints of viral RNA. This reversal of the usual mechanism of nucleic acid synthesis permits HIV to take control of normal cellular function. Several new copies of the virus are made but lie dormant until some event or environmental insult triggers their release, the host cell being destroyed in the process. The total number of CD4 lymphocytes can be taken as a reflection of the extent of HIV infection. As the number of CD4 lymphocytes falls the risk of opportunistic infection increases dramatically.

A discussion of HIV as a parenterally transmitted infection can be found in Chapter 12.

Table 13.3   Opportunistic infections associated with HIV disease

Micro-organism	Presentation
Bacteria	
Mycobacterium *(M. tuberculosis, M. avium intracellulare, M. kansasii)*	Pulmonary or disseminated infection
Shigella	Diarrhoea
Salmonella	Diarrhoea
Viruses	
Herpes simplex	Mucocutaneous lesions of the gastrointestinal tract
Herpes zoster	Shingles
Cytomegalovirus	CNS, gastrointestinal and pulmonary lesions
Fungi	
Candida	Oesophageal and pulmonary lesions
Cryptococcus	Pulmonary, CNS and disseminated infection
Aspergillus	CNS and disseminated infection
*Coccidioides immitis**	Disseminated infection
*Histoplasma capsulatum**	Disseminated infection
Protozoa	
Pneumocystis	Pneumonia
Cryptosporidium	Diarrhoea
Toxoplasma	Pneumonia and disseminated infection
*Leishmania**	Lesions in the spleen, liver and bone marrow. Anaemia

* When patients have travelled to areas where the micro-organism is endemic

Transmission of HIV

Transmission occurs sexually, through exposure to infected blood and body fluids, and perinatally. Situations in which exposure is possible (Pratt, 1994) include:

- Iatrogenic transmission to healthcare professionals, or to haemophiliacs who have received blood products that have not undergone heat treatment (Chapter 12)
- Drug misuse (see Chapter 12)
- Sexual transmission
- Vertical transmission from infected mothers to infants.

Historical aspects of HIV infection

HIV was first reported in the USA in 1979. As the number of affected individuals increased, it became apparent that the characteristic opportunistic infections and Kaposi's sarcoma occurred in young, previously healthy homosexual men. In the UK, the first cases were reported in homosexual men who had had sexual contact with people from the USA. By 1983, a syndrome had been recognised. Towards the end of that year, HIV was identified as the causative agent, an antibody test being developed in 1984. This is a test for antibodies produced in response to HIV. HIV infection is now an established health problem world wide. The number of new HIV infections in Western Europe and North America is static (Unaids/WHO, 1998). HIV infection is, however, on the increase in sub-Saharan Africa, Asia, Latin America and Eastern Europe. A prevalence study of HIV infection undertaken in 1998 indicates that numbers of individuals living with HIV in the UK have grown considerably during the last 3 years, the estimated figure is 30,000 (DoH, 1999).

Manifestations of HIV infection

In adults, HIV infection is possible via the sexual route in both sexes. The risk of this is especially high for homosexual men acting as the passive partner during anal intercourse. The rectal mucosa is much more delicate than the vaginal mucosa, and the virus probably gains access via tears and abrasions. Sexual transmission between lesbians is extremely rare (Raiteri et al., 1994).

Antibodies appear about 3 months after exposure. In the earliest phase of the disease when they are being produced, the individual may experience a transient, non-specific illness: myalgia, pharyngitis, malaise, lymphadenopathy and a rash. It is possible to divide symptoms into three phases (Pinching, 1986):

- **Persistent generalised lymphadenopathy (PGL)** – during which patients display few symptoms and are mostly well
- **AIDS-related complex (ARC)** – when the first signs and symptoms of opportunistic infection appear
- **Acquired immune deficiency syndrome (AIDS)** – the full manifestation of the disease, with weight loss, fever and diarrhoea. Kaposi's sarcoma does not develop in all cases but it can affect the skin, mucous membranes or internal organs.

Other problems associated with AIDS

- Gastrointestinal involvement becomes increasingly common as the disease progresses because the gut is host to many potentially pathogenic agents able to cause opportunistic infection as the immune system fails. Lymphoid tissue in the gastrointestinal mucosa may be invaded by the virus and operate as a reservoir (Winson, 1994). Over 80 per cent of those with progressive HIV infection eventually develop diarrhoea, vomiting, malnutrition and wasting, which contribute to mortality. Quality of life is severely affected by *Candida* infections in the mouth and oesophagus, leading to anorexia and dysphagia, and by ulceration through cytomegalovirus and other opportunistic infections.

■ Cerebral involvement occurs late, indicated by memory loss, poor concentration and dementia. In rare cases, encephalopathy develops before the appearance of opportunistic infection.

■ Nosocomial infection is a major risk for hospital patients with HIV disease, staphylococcal infection being a particular problem (Goetz *et al.*, 1994).

Treatment of HIV infection and AIDS

Treatment should begin as early and as intensively as possible and should be targeted against the virus itself (Gallo, 1996). Before 1995, antiviral drugs were given to slow down viral replication. This prolonged the period before the immune system collapsed and delayed the development of opportunistic infections but did not effect a cure. A number of new drugs have, however, now become available, the aim of therapeutic intervention being to prevent the replication of HIV. If these drugs are successful, it may be possible to halt the disease itself.

Zidovudine (Azidothymidine or AZT) was the first nucleoside shown to improve survival and decrease the incidence of symptoms arising from opportunistic infection (Abouker and Swart, 1993). Zidovudine inhibits the action of reverse transcriptase so that the virus cannot reproduce. Used alone, however, it is only of short-term benefit as HIV rapidly develops resistance to it. Fortunately, other nucleosides became available in 1994, and there is a new group of drugs called protease inhibitors that are able to disrupt other metabolic reactions vital for the multiplication and survival of HIV. Triple therapy with two nucleosides and an HIV protease inhibitor seems to be the most effective treatment currently available (Collier *et al.*, 1996). This is because a combination of agents can be used to destroy HIV at different stages in its life cycle, and the use of more than one antiviral drug reduces the risk of resistance (Lipsky, 1996). Concurrent therapy with appropriate antimicrobial agents is used to reduce the incidence of opportunistic infection.

Community health measures

See Chapter 12.

Women and HIV infection

More than 3 million women are infected world wide, mainly in Africa (Quintanilla, 1996), about 90 per cent being of childbearing age. This is significant in public health terms as it increases the risk of vertical transmission. Vertical transmission is possible (Francis, 1994) during:

■ Pregnancy – HIV crosses the placenta
■ Delivery – HIV present in cervical secretions or blood contaminates the infant. This appears to be the most frequent mechanism as most infection occurs at or near delivery
■ Breastfeeding, via the milk

It is difficult to determine the most important route of transmission because all infants born to infected mothers have maternal antibodies at birth (passive immunity), which do not clear until the child is 18 months old. The transfer of the virus across the placenta is thought to be the most significant route. The need for further research is imperative as it will permit the development of evidence-based policies for delivery and infant feeding.

Clinical Application

Management of HIV-positive Mothers and Infants

Method of delivery – This risk of vertical transmission appears to be reduced when a caesarean section is performed (Newell *et al.*, 1994).

Breastfeeding – The advice given depends on circumstances. It is recommended by the World Health Organization in countries where safe water supplies cannot be guaranteed because the risk of gastroenteritis outweighs the risk of transmitting HIV via breast milk (Cutting, 1992).

HIV during childhood

Childhood HIV has received comparatively little publicity but the problem is considerable, an estimated 500 000 individuals being infected (WHO, 1993). The first case was reported to the Centers for Disease Control in Atlanta in 1982, but the number has since escalated. HIV infection progresses more rapidly in children because their immune system is immature. Most succumb to bacterial infections through depleted B lymphocyte activity, and a high proportion develop AIDS within their first year (Newell, 1994). In some centres, there is a policy to prescribe co-trimoxazole routinely to all children of HIV-positive women as protection against opportunistic infection, especially *Pneumocystis carinii*, which is that most commonly encountered.

REVISION CHECKLIST: KEY AREAS

- ❏ Introduction to sexually transmitted infections
- ❏ Incidence of STI in the UK: Possible reasons for the upsurge in some STIs
- ❏ Sexual health and the role of GUM departments
- ❏ Sexually transmitted infections: Syphilis, Gonorrhoea, Chlamydia, Genital warts, Herpes simplex, Candidiasis, Trichomoniasis, Bacterial vaginosis, HIV

Activities – linking knowledge to clinical practice

1 **The eradication** of congenital syphilis can be regarded as one of the greatest triumphs of community health medicine. Every pregnant woman in the UK is routinely tested during the course of antenatal care.

(a) Do you think that this is still justified?

(b) Is it ethical?

(c) Do you think that a similar approach could be used to identify women who might transmit HIV infection to their infants?

2 'HIV is a problem only to members of the gay community.' Debate this statement in relation to:

(a) the UK and Western Europe

(b) Africa.

SELF-ASSESSMENT

1. Sexual health is primarily concerned with avoiding infection.   True? ☐ False? ☐

2. The primary lesions of syphilis are:
   (a) gummata ☐
   (b) chancres ☐
   (c) condylomata lata ☐
   (d) snail-track ulcers ☐

3. A patient residing in the UK with syphilis will have to pay for primary prescriptions.
   True? ☐ False? ☐

4. Gonorrhoea is caused by:
   (a) *Neisseria gonorrhoeae* ☐
   (b) *Neisseria meningitidis* ☐
   (c) *Neisseria perfringens* ☐
   (d) *Treponema pallidum* ☐

5. Chlamydia may be carried asymptomatically.
   True? ☐ False? ☐

6. The lesions caused by human papilloma virus are treated with:
   (a) penicillin ☐
   (b) idoxuridine ☐
   (c) trimethoprim ☐
   (d) podophyllin ☐

7. Herpes simplex virus type 2 is isolated only from oral lesions   True? ☐ False? ☐

8. The organism responsible for trichomoniasis is:
   (a) fungal ☐
   (b) protozoal ☐
   (c) helminthic ☐
   (d) viral ☐

9. HIV infection is diagnosed according to plasma antigen levels.
   True? ☐ False? ☐

References

Abel E and von Unwerth L (1988) 'Asymptomatic chlamydia during pregnancy'. *Research in Nursing and Health* **11**: 359–65.

Abouker JP and Swart AM (1993) 'Preliminary analysis of the Concorde Trial'. *Lancet* **341**: 889–90.

Barton S (1994) 'New therapies for the treatment of genital warts'. *Nursing Times* **90**(20): 38–40.

Cameron S and Blately A (1993) 'Clinical genitourinary medicine, a protocol for the detection of chlamydia'. *Nursing Standard* **8**(5): 25–7.

Chandler MG (1996) 'Genital warts: a study of patient anxiety and information needs'. *British Journal of Nursing* **5**(3): 174–9.

Chard S (1998) 'Diagnosing and treating genital herpes'. *Nursing Times* **94**(46): 58–62.

Collier A, Coombes R, Schoenfield D *et al.* (1996) 'Treatment of human immunodeficiency virus infection with saquinavir, zidovudine and zalcitabine'. AIDS Clinical Trials Group. *New England Journal of Medicine* **334**: 1011–17.

Cooper DA and Mergigan TC (1996) 'Clinical treatment'. *AIDS* **10** (Supplement A): S133–4.

Cutting W (1992) 'Breastfeeding and HIV infection: advice depends on the circumstances'. *British Medical Journal* **305**: 788–9.

Department of Health (1992) *The Health of the Nation.* HMSO, London.

Department of Health (1995) *Statistical Bulletin: Sexually Transmitted Diseases, England 1994.* HMSO, London.

Department of Health (1999) *Unlinked Anonymous Prevalence Monitoring Programme in the United Kingdom.* DoH, London.

Evans G (1994) 'A history of sexually transmitted diseases'. *Nursing Times* **90**(18): 29–31.

Findik D, Ural O and Baysal B (1996) 'Bacterial colonisation and yeast carriage on the hands of nurses'. *Journal of Hospital Infection* **34**: 234–5.

Francis B (1994) 'The incidence of HIV/AIDS in children and their care needs'. *Nursing Times* **90**(26): 47–9.

Gallo RC (1996) 'AIDS as a clinically curable disease: the growing optimism'. *AIDS, Patient Care and STD's* **10**(1): 7–9.

Gardner JL and Dukes CD (1955) '*Haemophilus vaginalis* vaginitis. A newly defined specific infection previously classified "non-specific vaginitis"'. *American Journal of Obstetrics and Gynecology* **69**: 962–76.

Goetz AM, Squier C, Wagener MM *et al.* (1994) 'Nosocomial infections in the human immunodeficiency virus-infected patient: a two year survey'. *American Journal of Infection Control* **23**: 334–9.

Hay PE, Taylor-Robinson D, Lamont RF *et al.* (1994) 'Abnormal bacterial colonisation of the genital tract and subsequent pre-term delivery and late miscarriage'. *British Medical Journal* **308**: 295–8.

Jones M (1994) 'Genitourinary medicine'. *Nursing Times* **90**(18): 31–3.

Krieger JN, Verdon M, Siegal N *et al.* (1993) 'Natural history of urogenital trichomoniasis'. *Journal of Urology* **149**: 1455–8.

Lee H, Cernesky MA and Schachter J (1995) 'Diagnosis of *Chlamydia trachomatis* genitourinary infection in women by ligase chain reaction assay of urine'. *Lancet* **345**: 213–16.

Lee W, Burnie UP, Matthews RC *et al.* (1991) 'Hospital outbreaks with yeasts'. *Journal of Hospital Infection* **18** (Supplement A): 237–40.

Lipsky JJ (1996) 'Antiretroviral drugs for AIDS'. *Lancet* **348**: 800–3.

Nettina SL (1990) 'Syphilis: a new look at an old killer'. *American Journal of Nursing* **90**(4): 68–70.

Newell ML (1994) 'Mother to child transmission of HIV-1. The AIDS letter'. *Royal Society of Medicine Services* No 41. Royal Society of Medicine.

Newell ML, Dunn DT, and Peckham CS (1994) 'Caesarean section and risk of vertical transmission of HIV-1 infection'. *Lancet* **343**: 1464–7.

Odds FC (1988) *Candida and Candidosis.* Baillière Tindall, London.

Pearce MJ (1990) 'Pelvic inflammatory disease'. *British Medical Journal* **300**: 1090–1.

Pinching A (1986) 'AIDS and Africa: lessons for us all'. *Journal of the Royal Society of Medicine* **79**: 501–2.

Pratt RJ (1994) 'Safe practice'. *Nursing Times* **90**(21): 64–8.

Quintanilla K (1996) 'Can HIV be transmitted through breastmilk?' *Nursing Times* **92**(31): 35–7.

Raiteri R, Fora R and Sinicco A (1994) 'No HIV-1 transmission through lesbian sex'. *Lancet* **344**: 270–1.

Rashid S, Collins M and Kennedy RJ (1991) 'A study of candidosis: the role of fomites'. *Genitourinary Medicine* **67**: 137–42.

Roberts A (1982) 'The pox and the people'. *Nursing Times* **78**(28): 1177–85.

Temple CA (1994) 'Diagnosis and treatment of bacterial vaginosis'. *Nursing Times* **14**(90): 43–4.

Unaids/WHO (1998) AIDS Epidemic Update. December 1998 at www.unaids.org.

Wasley G (1988) 'No ordinary microbe'. *Nursing Times* **84**(38): 50–1.

White K (1992) 'Sterile conditions'. *Nursing Standard* **88**(44): 34–6.

Williams K (1994) 'Sexually transmitted diseases: fact from fiction'. *Nursing Times* **90**(3): 38–40.

Winson G (1994) 'Gastrointestinal problems in patients with AIDS'. *Nursing Times* **90**(25): 36–9.

World Health Organization (1993) *Thirteen Million HIV-positive Women by 2,000*. WHO, Geneva.

Further reading and information sources

Alder MW (1995) *ABC of Sexually Transmitted Diseases*, 3rd edn. British Medical Association, London.

Csonka GW (1990) *Sexually Transmitted Diseases: A Textbook of Genitourinary Medicine*. Baillière Tindall, London.

Pratt RJ (1995) *HIV and AIDS. A Strategy for Nursing Care*. Edward Arnold, London.

Sonnex C (1996) *A General Practitioner's Guide to Genitourinary Medicine and Sexual Health*. Cambridge University Press, Cambridge.

14 Epidemiology: changing trends of infectious disease

CHAPTER OUTCOMES

After reading this chapter you should be able to:

- Define the epidemiological terms 'prevalence', 'incidence', 'epidemic', 'endemic' and 'pandemic'

- Interpret the classic epidemiological curve and its derivations

- Recognise the points to look for when critically interpreting epidemiological data

- Name the organism(s) responsible for malaria, meningococcal meningitis, toxoplasmosis, BSE, Legionnaires' disease, tuberculosis, typhoid, cholera, the viral haemorrhagic fevers and rabies

Introduction to epidemiology

Epidemiology is the study of diseases and the ways in which they are distributed within the population. This traditionally meant contagious disease, but today the scope of epidemiology has expanded to include all diseases whether transmissible or not. Contagious diseases may occur in epidemics or pandemics, or they may be endemic within a community.

- **Epidemics** – In hospital, epidemics are recognised when two or more patients are infected by the same organism. In the community, a sudden increase in the number of infections of the same kind in a specific area (for example, a school or hotel) is defined as an epidemic.

- **Pandemics** – A pandemic is the simultaneous occurrence of a large number of the same infection. The Black Death (bubonic plague) sweeping across Europe in the 14th century is an example of a pandemic.

- **Endemic disease** – This is disease always present in a population. The number of cases varies depending on factors allowing the organisms to multiply and the susceptibility of potential hosts. Malaria is endemic in several regions of the world, including parts of Africa.

Epidemiological patterns – the distribution of contagious disease

Classical epidemiological curve

The classical epidemiological curve is drawn when the number of new cases of an infection is plotted against time (Figure 14.1). On the left-hand side of the graph, the number of people infected rises gradually, reaching a peak at the midpoint. On the right-hand side, recovery proceeds faster than the emergence of new infections until the epidemic wanes.

Much of our knowledge about the behaviour of contagious disease has come from studying the pattern of infection in geographically isolated regions. Spitzbergen, an island on the edge of the Arctic Circle, was once used to study the distribution of respiratory infections. Until the 1930s, it received no visitors throughout the winter. In spring, respiratory disease was absent from the population, the first colds appearing with the arrival of the earliest trade ship, being brought by the crew. The epidemic curve rose to its peak as an increasing number of the islanders caught colds from one another. As the year progressed, the number of new cases declined.

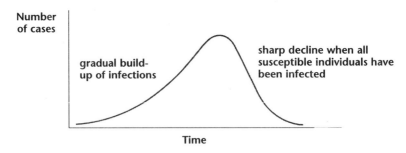

Figure 14.1　Classical epidemiological curve

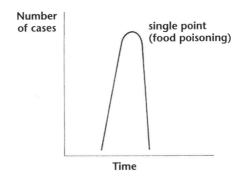

Figure 14.2   Single-point epidemiological curve

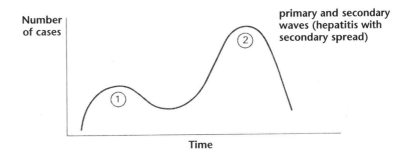

Figure 14.3   Epidemiological curve illustrating secondary spread

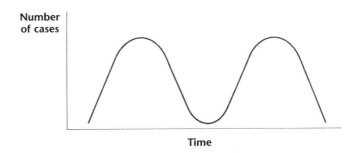

Figure 14.4   Epidemiological curve with cyclical infection

Single-point epidemiological curve

Other epidemiological curves include the single-point curve. In an outbreak of food-borne disease (see Chapter 11) with a short incubation period, many people will be affected simultaneously if the food is eaten at the same time. Their simultaneous recovery results in a single-point curve (Figure 14.2).

Secondary spread and longer incubation period

When the incubation period is longer (weeks or months), with the possibility of secondary spread, the curve develops a second peak (Figure 14.3). This is typical of an outbreak of *Salmonella* in a household where person-to-person transmission has occurred.

Cyclical epidemiological curve

Many infectious diseases appear cyclically every few years (Figure 14.4). Before the availability of vaccine, measles and whooping cough followed this pattern. Outbreaks resulted when a cohort of children lacking immunity had developed and waned once all were infected. Between outbreaks, cases occurred sporadically.

Factors affecting the incidence of infectious disease

Infectious agents depend on a supply of new victims. Thus, transmission is more likely when a large number of susceptible people are gathered together. Poor standards of hygiene, overcrowding and poverty increase the risk of spread. Early man probably escaped relatively unscathed because the total population was small and mobile, moving from one locality to another in search of food. Then, with better health resulting through improved hygiene, nutrition, living conditions and the introduction of public health measures such as vaccination, contagious diseases again caused less morbidity and mortality. The discovery of antibiotics led to an expectation that they would be eliminated altogether. This has not, however, been possible because of the emergence of antibiotic-resistant strains of bacteria. Moreover, many people still live in poor conditions, and this has contributed to the resurgence of infectious diseases. Several outbreaks have occurred in recent years, notably the Stanley Royd incident in which 19 frail patients died as a result of *Salmonella* food poisoning (DoH, 1986a) and an outbreak of Legionnaires' disease in Stafford (DoH, 1986b). These provided stimulus for the Acheson Report (DoH, 1988), proposing better strategies for the control of communicable disease. An outbreak of *Escherichia coli* in Central Scotland in 1996, which caused 20 deaths, led to further recommendations being made (Pennington, 1997).

It is clear that infections remain a major health problem. In developing countries, millions of people die from tuberculosis and malaria every year. The speed of air travel means that many apparently well people incubating these conditions develop symptoms after their arrival in other countries, importing infectious disease to the Western world. There are, however, other problems of infection in

Western countries. Recent years have witnessed the emergence of 'new' diseases caused by transmissible agents made possible by advances in technology and more accurate methods of surveillance. Both the acquired immune deficiency syndrome (AIDS) and bovine spongiform encephalopathy (BSE) are caused by transmissible agents, and some cancers have been linked to infection. For example, there is an established association between the papilloma wart virus and cervical cancer (Barton, 1994) and between the Epstein–Barr virus and Burkitt's lymphoma.

Interpreting epidemiological data

Epidemiological studies provide information about the ways in which micro-organisms are spread and the types of people most likely to be infected, and suggest risk factors. They also reveal genuine changes in the pattern of infection occurring over time, for example as a result of the emergence of antibiotic resistance.

Clinical Application

Epidemiological Data

To evaluate the results of epidemiological investigations, it is essential to have key knowledge about the way in which the information was collected. The results of different studies are often compared, but this is not meaningful unless the data were collected from similar groups of patients in the same type of clinical setting. Data collected prospectively, when the event occurred, are more likely to be more accurate than data collected retrospectively (after the event) (Kreger et al., 1989). Now that surveillance data are routinely stored on computer, prospective studies are easier to conduct and more accurate (Gransden, 1991). Data may be collected as part of a prevalence or incidence study, the proposed use affecting the interpretation of findings.

The **prevalence** is the number of the existing cases of a condition in a population at a particular point in time (Farmer et al., 1996). Prevalence studies give little explanation of risk factors so they are not useful as a means of suggesting control measures. The extent of a problem may be under-estimated because each case is counted only once. Infected patients who have successfully completed their antibiotic treatment or have died at the time of data collection are excluded. Prevalence studies may, however, reveal problems that merit more detailed investigations.

Incidence studies report the number of new cases of a condition arising within a population over a period of time. They are more expensive and more time-consuming but suggest possible risk factors contributing to the development of infection. From this approach, it has become apparent that critically ill patients are most susceptible to nosocomial infection (Evans et al., 1992). In the most sophisticated experimental incidence studies, different treatment regimens are tested. Patients are assigned to an experimental group to receive treatment (antibiotics or immunisation, for example), and the number of infections developing is compared with that seen in a control group that has not received treatment. Donowitz (1986) used this approach to show that the incidence of infection declined in a group of critically ill children when hand hygiene was scrupulously performed, cotton gowns making no difference.

International recommendations

The World Health Organization (WHO) holds overall responsibility for the administration of international health programmes to control disease, including infectious conditions. An example of successful collaboration between member nations is shown by the eradication of smallpox in 1970. Other areas dealt with under the WHO regulations include:

- Control of the spread of serious infectious conditions such as cholera, yellow fever and plague
- The disinfection of aircraft
- The control of vermin in ships.

The WHO provides advice about controlling infection by:

- Assisting individual nations to collect and analyse data, which it then disseminates to other countries.

- Acting as a resource for health workers by collecting, consolidating and publishing epidemiological data from different countries.

- Providing technical advice and training to encourage countries to standardise the methods they use to collect and present epidemiological data so that comparison is possible between them all. This is necessary because of the enormous difference between methods used to notify, investigate, diagnose and report diseases. Interpretation is straightforward if a universal method is employed.

- Offering blueprints for the role of public health laboratories in the surveillance and control of infectious disease so that information concerning new technology is shared.

Control of communicable disease in the UK

The Public Health Laboratory Service (PHLS) plays a key role in the control of infectious conditions. It comprises a network of laboratories in England and Wales as well as the Central Public Health Laboratory and the Communicable Disease Surveillance Centre (CDSC), both in Colindale, London. The PHLS was established in 1946 to protect the public from infection. This initially involved considering communicable disease in the community as nosocomial infection was still an emerging problem. However, since the 1950s when the PHLS helped to control staphylococcal wound infection, it has played an important role in the control of hospital infection.

Today, the PHLS provides infection control services to hospitals, public health microbiology such as testing water, food and milk, and epidemiological surveillance at national, regional and local levels. It also contributes to the control of communicable disease by investigating outbreaks and formulating policies for its control. A sudden increase in the number of infections caused by a specific organism in England or Wales is reported to the consultant in communicable disease control (CCDC) who will monitor the outbreak.

The role of the CDSC is to assemble, analyse and disseminate data relating to all communicable diseases. The early recognition of a problem and prompt action by the CDSC can contain an emerging outbreak. For example, an outbreak of botulism in 1989 was rapidly curtailed by an investigation that traced 27 cases to a particular brand of hazelnut yoghurt. Botulism is an uncommon but extremely serious infection, and without the prompt action of the CDSC there would have been a much higher mortality rate (only one death being recorded). It is also possible to predict possible epidemics and avert them. The 1995–96 rubella immunisation campaign in schools is an example of successful control. In Scotland, the Communicable Disease Surveillance Unit fulfils the same functions as the CDSC does for England and Wales.

Notifiable infections

Notifiable infectious conditions are reported to the CDSC to help to trace contacts who may have been exposed to infection so that they can be monitored and treated as necessary. In Scotland, notifiable diseases are reported to the Director of Public Health. In the case of food or waterborne infection, it is important to determine and eliminate the source. The data generated at local and national level help to monitor fluctuations in the incidence of infection and identify potential outbreaks, allowing preventative action or the recognition of a particular need for health promotion. Responsibility for notification falls to local authorities, which have a statutory responsibility to control infectious conditions within their boundaries. They can add to the statutory list of notifiable infectious conditions shown in Table 14.1. For example, HIV disease is not notifiable, but there is a confidential voluntary referral scheme at the CDSC. Similarly, sexually transmitted infections do not appear in Table 14.1 because they are reported anonymously to the Department of Health.

Changing trends of infectious disease

Malaria

Malaria is a disease of great antiquity (Najera-Morrondo, 1991) caused by protozoal parasites belonging to the genus *Plasmodium* (Table 14.2). The vector is the female *Anopheles* mosquito. Infection causes intermittent fever with haemolytic anaemia.

Table 14.1   Notifiable diseases in England and Wales

Public Health Control of Diseases Act 1984

Cholera	Plague	Smallpox
Food poisoning	Relapsing fever	Typhus

Public Health (Infectious Diseases) Regulations 1988

Acute encephalitis	Ophthalmia neonatorum
Acute poliomyelitis	Paratyphoid fever
Anthrax	Rabies
Diphtheria	Rubella
Dysentery	Scarlet fever
Leprosy	Tetanus
Leptospirosis	Tuberculosis
Malaria	Typhoid
Measles	Viral haemorrhagic fever
Meningitis	Viral hepatitis
Meningococcal septicaemia	Whooping cough
Mumps	Yellow fever

Table 14.2   Malarial parasites

Genus	Distribution	Severity	Fever
Plasmodium falciparum (malignant malaria)	Tropics	+++	Every 2 days
Plasmodium vivax	Temperate zones	++	Every 2 days
Plasmodium malariae	Subtropics	++	Every 3 days
Plasmodium ovale	Variable and patchy	++	Every 2 days

The life cycle of *Plasmodium* is complex (Figure 14.5). The protozoa are injected into the human host by the mosquito, then passing through a stage of division called the exoerythrocytic stage. Some plasmodia enter the red blood cells, the erythrocytes (erythrocytic stage), where they undergo asexual division. Their increasing number causes the cell to rupture, the escaping plasmodia being free to enter and destroy more erythrocytes in turn, thus giving rise to the haemolytic anaemia. Bouts of fever recur when the plasmodia enter the bloodstream. Their frequency depends on the length of time taken to complete the asexual stages of reproduction and to escape. Malaria kills more people world wide than any other specific pathogen and is responsible for enormous suffering. This is especially true of *P. falciparum,* which causes the most severe form of the disease.

Most cases of malaria occurring in the UK are contracted abroad, although travellers incubating the disease may not exhibit symptoms until after their arrival. There have been a number of cases of 'airport malaria' caused when mosquitoes have been transported to the UK in aircraft and then escaped (Conlon, 1990).

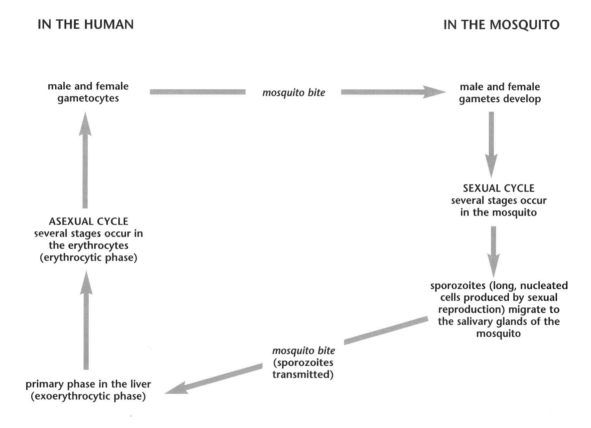

Figure 14.5 Simplified description of the life cycle of *Plasmodium*

Transmission

Person-to-person infection does not occur, and isolation is unnecessary unless a patient arriving from overseas with pyrexia and a presumptive diagnosis of malaria is considered to be at risk of harbouring another tropical fever.

Prevention

Malaria is controlled by draining the stagnant water used by *Anopheles* as a breeding ground. Small areas (puddles, ponds, wells and water butts) may be covered by a thin film of oil, and the introduction of fish preying on the larvae is a helpful measure. Insecticide sprays to kill adult *Anopheles*, repellents, mosquito-proof clothing and screens are recommended inside the home. A new insect repellent called Peripel 55 has recently become available. This represents a significant advance over other insecticides as it can be added to rinsing water after washing clothes. Numerous drugs are used in malarial prophylaxis, but resistance is widely reported so travellers should be advised to seek the latest information from travel centres. It may be necessary to take several drugs in combination to reduce the possibility of the plasmodia developing resistance. The interiors of aircraft should be treated with insecticide to reduce the risk of importing malaria. It has been suggested that public awareness of the dangers of malaria in relation to travel should be increased, especially as prophylaxis is highly cost-effective (Behrens and Roberts, 1994). A campaign by the WHO to eradicate malaria failed because of the problem of drug resistance and a lack of co-operation on the part of some member states. Prevention would be more of a reality if an effective vaccine could be developed.

Diagnosis

Diagnosis is confirmed by the microscopic examination of stained blood films, which reveal the malarial parasites.

Treatment

Chloroquine has traditionally been the mainstay of treatment and prophylaxis, but plasmodia are increasingly developing resistance to it (Moreland, 1991). A number of other drugs are available, including mefloquine, proguanil and primaquine.

Meningitis

Meningitis is an inflammation of the meninges caused by a range of bacteria and viruses (Table 14.3). Its symptoms and signs are listed in Table 14.4.

Table 14.3   Organisms causing meningitis

Viral meningitis	Bacterial meningitis
Echovirus	*Streptococcus pneumoniae*
Coxsackie virus	*Haemophilus influenzae type B*
Mumps virus	*Neisseria meningitidis*
	Escherichia coli
	Group B streptococci
	Listeria monocytogenes
	Mycobacterium tuberculosis

Viral meningitis is milder than bacterial infections, and most patients recover spontaneously (Davies, 1996). Bacterial meningitis has a mortality rate of 3–6 per cent, tends to be severe and can have an extremely rapid rate of onset (Kornelisse *et al.*, 1995). An individual with meningococcal disease can deteriorate and die within hours of feeling unwell. It is thus hardly surprising that considerable fear and anxiety surrounds meningitis.

Table 14.4   Signs and symptoms of meningitis

Fever	Drowsiness	Early on – vague flu-like symptoms
Neck stiffness	Kernig's sign	Painful joints
Photophobia	Headache	Fits
Cloudy cerebro-spinal fluid	Nausea and vomiting	

In infants, the signs of infection may be non-specific, for example irritability and poor feeding

NB. A characteristic rash will be present in meningococcal septicaemia – a dark red/purple petechial rash that does not disappear with pressure

Until recently, *Haemophilus influenzae* caused 40 per cent of all cases of meningitis in early infancy and early childhood, but since the introduction of vaccination in 1992 the incidence of this organism has declined sharply. Most cases of meningitis are now caused by *Neisseria meningitidis,* the incidence of which is rising (Davies, 1996).

Meningococcal meningitis is caused by *N. meningitidis*, a Gram-negative, aerobic coccus that affects primarily children and young adults, although people of any age can become infected. There are three serological groups: A, B and C. In 1994, serotype B caused 70 per cent of all cases of mengingococcal meningitis in the UK. The path resulting in clinical infection occurs in three stages:

1. Growth of the organism in the nasopharynx. This causes local inflammation but in most cases does not progress, and the individual becomes a carrier.
2. Invasion of the bacteria into the blood, with the appearance of a petechial rash and life-threatening mengingococcal septicaemia.
3. Invasion of the meninges and infection of the cerebrospinal fluid (CSF). Acute symptoms and fatality can develop within 12 hours.

Transmission

Neisseria meningitidis is carried asymptomatically in the nasopharynx of 5–10 per cent of healthy people, transmission being via droplets. The rate of carriage rises dramatically with overcrowding, which in the past has been associated with a higher incidence of infection. Spread also occurs by contact: saliva and nasal secretions easily contaminate bedding, and when they are shaken the bacteria are liberated into the surrounding air, settling as dust that is inhaled. *Neisseria meningitidis* dies rapidly in the environment.

Prevention of spread

Prevention is as follows:

- Isolating the patient for the first 24–48 hours of antibiotic therapy may be recommended. (A single room is usually appreciated for longer because the symptoms of meningism include intolerance of light and noise).

- Chemoprophylaxis for close contacts and staff who have performed mouth-to-mouth resuscitation. Susceptible carriers identified by throat swabbing are given rifampicin or ciprofloxacin.

- The vaccination of named people at risk. The effects of vaccination are short lived, and it is protective only against serotypes A and C. During 1999, a long-acting vaccine against group C meningococcal infection was introduced in the UK (see Chapter 2). Further research continues in the development of a vaccine effective against serotype B.

Diagnosis

Diagnosis is made by clinical examination and is confirmed by culturing CSF obtained by lumbar puncture.

Treatment

Treatment is with benzylpenicillin, patients allergic to penicillin being given chloramphenicol or a cephalosporin. The prompt administration of parenteral benzylpenicillin to suspected cases increases the chances of survival (Cartwright *et al.*, 1992).

Toxoplasmosis

Toxoplasmosis is caused by the protozoan *Toxoplasma gondii*, which is carried asymptomatically by many wild and domestic animals. Its life cycle is complex (Figure 14.6).

Transmission

Human infection occurs when infected meat is consumed or during contact with infected pets or livestock (Griffiths, 1990). Cats frequently harbour *Toxoplasma gondii*, having consumed infected prey. Human infection is possible through handling cat faeces (for example, litter trays or gardening in earth soiled by cats). It is usually asymptomatic, or the symptoms of malaise, myalgia and fatigue are mild so that diagnosis is never established. For some people however, toxoplasmosis is serious:

- The immunocompromised – especially people with HIV disease. Reactivation of latent infection occurs, giving rise to severe disseminated toxoplasmosis or encephalitis.

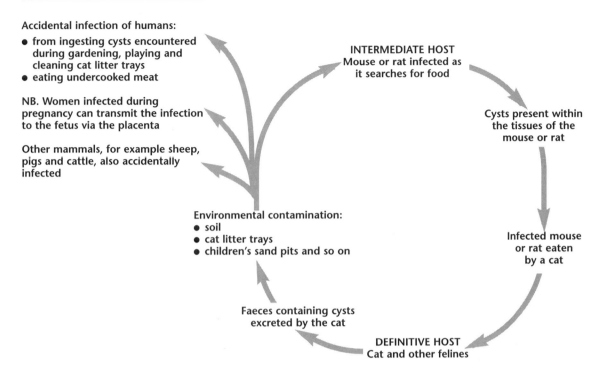

Figure 14.6 Simplified illustration of the transmission of *Toxoplasma gondii*

■ Organ transplant recipients – infection acquired from the donated organ becomes active with immunosuppressive therapy.

■ Pregnant women – vertical transmission occurs via the placenta from mother to fetus when primary infection occurs during pregnancy. Approximately 50 per cent of mothers developing primary infection will have an affected child or a stillbirth unless treated (Desmonts and Couvreur, 1974). Damage involves the central nervous system. The infant may also have jaundice, liver damage, rashes and haemolytic defects including anaemia. Surviving children may develop later-onset cirrhosis, encephalitis and eye damage, becoming blind after a latent period lasting many years.

The nature of toxoplasmosis makes it difficult to assess. In the UK an enzyme-linked immunosorbent assay test for detecting specific antitoxoplasma IgM has been used to demonstrate that the overall rate of primary infection is about two cases per thousand, suggesting that there may be 1200 maternal toxoplasma infections every year (Joynson and Payne, 1988). The cost of introducing a screening programme for pregnant women was investigated in 1984 but was dismissed as not being cost-effective.

Diagnosis

A rapid, safe, accurate screening test that became available in 1994 may lead to a more comprehensive screening programme in the UK (Hohlfeld et al., 1994). The test was developed in France, where the awareness of the risk associated with maternal toxoplasmosis is much higher than in the UK because there is a much higher incidence of infection, associated with eating rare meat. In France, screening during pregnancy is mandatory.

Treatment

Primary toxoplasma infection can be treated with spiromycin or sulphonamides.

Slow virus infections

Slow virus infections cause a range of diseases called the transmissible spongiform encephalopathies, characterised by slow progression and an incubation period of more than 10 years. The brain develops minute perforations, eventually assuming a spongy appearance. Slow virus infections include bovine spongiform encephalopathy (BSE or 'mad cow disease'), scrapie, which infects sheep, and Creutzfeldt–Jakob disease (CJD), which affects the human host. All have a long incubation period but eventually progress rapidly and are inevitably fatal.

BSE

BSE was first reported in 1985. Further cases became apparent the following year and the number has increased steadily since (Matthews, 1991) so that by 1996 150 000 cases had been reported (Institute of Food Science and Technology, 1996). Infection is caused by an unconventional viral agent called a prion (Holmes, 1996). Prions are self-replicating proteins that do not contain nucleic acid.

Transmission

Transmission appears to occur between cattle in affected herds, but the mechanism of this is not clear. There is less evidence to suggest vertical transmission between the cow and her affected calf (Institute of Food Science and Technology, 1996). BSE can be transmitted between members of different species, but whether this takes place under natural conditions remains a matter for conjecture. Epidemiological investigations suggest that the outbreak reported in the late 1980s stemmed from giving cattle high-protein feed containing the remains of sheep infected with scrapie: in the 1970s, feed was processed at a low temperature insufficient to destroy prions. There have been fears that infected milk and meat could enter the food chain and that BSE could be transmitted to humans.

Prevention

BSE is extremely resistant to heat and chemicals, and is therefore difficult to destroy. There has, however, been a dramatic reduction in the incidence of BSE since bone-meal and other animal products have been excluded from cattle feed as a result of the Bovine Offal (Prohibition) Regulations (Amended) 1989. Other control measures include the destruction of infected cattle and carcasses, tighter slaughterhouse controls and preventing BSE entering the human food chain by banning the use of bovine brain, spinal cord and thymus. Milk from infected cattle is destroyed.

A set of stringent restrictions was initially implemented, including a worldwide ban on the export of British beef and beef products, and a ban on the sale of certain cuts of beef in the domestic market. At the time of writing, the European Union had lifted various export restrictions, but some European governments and consumers still felt anxiety regarding the safety of British beef. The restriction concerning certain cuts of beef within the UK was lifted late in 1999.

Creutzfeldt-Jakob disease

CJD (a form of presenile dementia) is a rare, degenerative neurological condition causing demyelination of the brain and producing lesions similar to those seen in BSE. Prions have been isolated from brain tissue at postmortem. In the past, most cases of CJD affected people between 40 and 60 years of age, but cases are now seen in teenagers, possibly representing a new strain (new variant CJD). There is concern that if BSE were transmitted to humans, it would cause a condition similar to CJD.

Transmission

Transmission has occurred from cataract transplants, pituitary extracts used as a source of human growth hormone, and fertility drugs. Infection appears to occur only when defective prions are present. There is currently no confirmed evidence that BSE can be transmitted from cattle to humans. CJD appears world wide, and its incidence is not at present associated with the incidence of BSE.

Diagnosis

Diagnosis is on clinical grounds. CJD is differentiated from other forms of pre-senile dementia by its rapid onset and progression. Death usually occurs within a year of diagnosis. The typical spongiform changes in the cerebral cortex are seen at postmortem.

No treatment is currently available.

Enteric fevers

Enteric fevers are caused by *Salmonella typhi* and *Salmonella paratyphi* (causing typhoid and paratyphoid fevers respectively). The incubation period is approximately 14 days. Infection is usually severe, producing malaise, aching prostration, vomiting and abdominal pain. Pyrexia may continue for weeks, and septicaemia develops about 10 days after the onset of infection, with bacteria appearing in the blood, urine and stools. Bacteria may be carried for months, sometimes years. The usual seat of infection is the gallbladder, but other organs, including the liver, may be involved.

Transmission

Transmission is by the faecal-oral route. Both bacteria are virulent, only a low infective dose being needed to cause disease.

Diagnosis

A diagnosis is made by stool or blood culture and an agglutination test for antibodies (the Widal reaction).

Prevention

Prevention is achieved by eliminating the source of infection, including carriers, and public health measures focusing on the provision of safe water supplies, food preparation and the pasteurisation of milk. Travellers to regions where typhoid is endemic may receive active immunisation, but this is not highly effective (Grist and Reid, 1991).

Treatment

Treatment is with chloramphenicol in addition to the appropriate supportive measures, such as the correction of dehydration.

Cholera

Cholera is caused by *Vibrio cholerae*, an aerobic, Gram-negative bacterium. It is exclusively a human pathogen, endemic throughout Asia, occasional cases being reported when travellers return to Europe (Dawood, 1987). Cholera is no longer endemic in the British Isles, but in the 19th century Britain was seriously affected by four cholera pandemics, 14 000 people dying of it in 1866. During the 1854 epidemic, Dr John Snow carried out a piece of epidemiological research plotting the cases of cholera on a map of London. He identified a concentration of cases in Soho around the public water pump in Broad Street. At Snow's instigation, the pump handle was removed, and the epidemic, which was already in decline, soon ceased (BMA, 1989).

The incubation period for cholera ranges from a few hours to 5 days. The bacteria release an enterotoxin that alters the metabolism of the cells in the gastrointestinal mucosa so that they secrete a large quantity of fluid faster than it can be reabsorbed, resulting in copious diarrhoea and vomiting. Adults can lose up to a litre of fluid in 1 hour. Stools and vomitus are watery and specked with small white flocculi (fragments of the intestinal epithelium; 'rice water stools'). This is followed by massive dehydration, circulatory collapse and renal failure unless treated. Mortality, without proper medical intervention, is high.

Transmission

Transmission is by the faecal-oral route. The infective dose is high, many vibrios being required to cause symptoms. Thus, person-to-person transmission is rare. Chronic carriage is unusual, although the contacts of acutely infected patients may carry vibrios asymptomatically for a few days.

Prevention

Prevention depends on good-quality water supplies without contamination from human sewage. Active immunity is provided by killed vaccine, but protection is short (3 months) and only partial.

Diagnosis

Diagnosis is made by microscopy confirmed by faecal culture.

Treatment

Tetracycline reduces diarrhoea and the duration of vibrio excretion, but the mainstay of treatment is oral or intravenous rehydration. Vibrios are developing resistance to tetracycline so doxycycline or trimethoprim may be given instead.

Clinical Application

Water and Health

Today, water collection, distribution and purification systems in the UK are designed to ensure that every household receives a safe supply of drinking water. Its quality is monitored continuously through the collaborative efforts of Environmental Health Officers, the CCDC, the Environment Agency and staff from the regional water companies. Although access to clean water has been accepted as fundamental to human health for over 100 years in developed countries, poor sanitation continues to represent a major health threat throughout many parts of the world. Ironically, it is in the UK, where the original epidemiological studies relating to sanitation were undertaken, that the cost of domestic water supplies is now rising so that health may once again be threatened. Costs increased sharply in many areas in 1989 following privatisation, problems being acute in areas where metering has been introduced. The heaviest consumers and therefore those most severely affected are families with young children, people who are incontinent, and individuals with skin conditions requiring medicated baths. Health visitors have become concerned at the steep rise in the number of households where supplies have been disconnected through a failure to meet bills and the plight of clients struggling to reduce water consumption. More recent government measures have, however, curtailed the ability of the water companies to cut off supply to consumers unable or unwilling to pay.

Helicobacter infection

Helicobacter pylori is a Gram-negative bacterium causing inflammation of the gastric mucosa. Infection is linked to the development of gastritis, gastric and duodenal ulcers (peptic ulceration) and possibly stomach cancer.

Transmission

Transmission is via the oral-oral and oral-faecal routes. Asymptomatic carriage is possible, and 20–50 per cent of the population has been exposed to the bacteria. Nosocomial transfer via secretions contaminating endoscopes has been documented.

Prevention

Prevention is through attention to infection control protocols and by the thorough decontamination of clinical equipment.

Treatment

Treatment consists of bismuth with a combination of drugs – metronidazole, amoxycillin or tetracycline with an H_2-receptor antagonist. The addition of omeprazole (a proton pump inhibitor) speeds healing.

Legionnaires' disease

Legionnaires' disease is caused by *Legionella pneumophila*, a tiny, motile, Gram-negative bacillus found in soil and water that grows between 20 ^{0}C and 40 ^{0}C. Legionnaires' disease is not uncommon, but patients are slow to seroconvert, and the bacteria are difficult to detect and isolate. This may explain why the infection was unknown until recently. The first recorded outbreak occurred in 1976 among delegates attending a convention of the American Legion in Philadelphia (Fraser *et al.*, 1977). Epidemics have since occurred in several countries, mainly in hotels and hospitals. The largest outbreak in the UK occurred in Stafford District General Hospital in 1985. The design of the ventilation system was faulty, leading to contamination of the water supply (DoH, 1986b); there were 28 deaths.

Transmission

Epidemiological links between *Legionella* infection and contaminated hospital water are now well documented, with air conditioning, ventilation systems and water from cooling towers presenting a potential risk (Vincent-Houdek *et al.*, 1993). *Legionella* has been isolated from shower units, nebulisers, humidifiers, cold and hot water circuits, water tanks and calorifiers (Liu *et al.*, 1993). Contamination occurs between different parts of the system, calorifiers operating as an important source (Bartlett *et al.*, 1983). However, the source of infection may sometimes originate outside the hospital premises so this, too, must be included in any epidemiological investigation (Vincent-Houdek *et al.*, 1993).

Simulation experiments suggest that the mode of transmission is via contaminated aerosols from humidifiers and respiratory equipment but not from showers (Woo *et al.*, 1986). If contaminated water becomes airborne in aerosols less than 5 μm in diameter, the bacteria can be inhaled. This leads either to subclinical infection, mild infection not involving the lungs (Pontiac fever) or fulminant pneumonia, which can be fatal. Person-to-person spread has never been reported so patients need not be isolated.

Prevention

The immunocompromised are especially vulnerable so prevention, especially in hospital, is important (Vincent-Houdek *et al.*, 1993). Control measures involve maintaining the hot water temperature at 60 °C and chlorinating incoming water. It is also vital to maintain the system in good working order, closing down redundant parts of the circuit that cannot be maintained at an adequate temperature and monitoring the speed of flow. Water containers and humidifiers should be cleaned and descaled at regular intervals and kept dry if the system is closed down (DoH, 1991). The value of bacteriological sampling in routine prevention is debated (Liu *et al.*, 1993).

Treatment

Treatment involves erythromycin, rifampicin, co-trimoxazole or tetracyclines, together with supportive treatment as required.

Tuberculosis

Tuberculosis is a chronic infection involving the lungs and sometimes other parts of the body that is caused by *Mycobacterium tuberculosis*, the acid-fast bacillus. It is a disease of great antiquity: human remains from the stone age and the time of the Pharaohs show evidence of tuberculosis. An association with overcrowding and poverty was first made in the 1870s, when infection was rife in the UK. Gradual improvements in housing, nutrition and hygiene helped to reduce the incidence, and with the availability of antibiotics, infection became less common. Throughout the 1980s, it was generally considered that the incidence of tuberculosis was declining, but during the 1990s there was a resurgence in the UK, the USA and many other countries, leading the WHO to declare a global health emergency in 1993. The first reversal in the previous trend was recorded in the USA, where resurgence was attributed to an increase in the incidence of HIV and to a relaxation of infection control programmes.

In the UK, the increase is confined to particular groups (Joseph *et al.*, 1992), those at risk including:

- The socially deprived, especially if they are malnourished, the homeless being particularly at risk (Watson, 1993). Most cases are caused by the reactivation of old lesions when health is compromised.

- Those with debilitating illness depressing cell-mediated immunity (Spence *et al.*, 1993), including people with HIV (Charatan, 1991, 1994). This is because damage to the immune system allows dormant infections to reactivate.

- Travellers. In many parts of the world (for example, Africa and Asia), the incidence of tuberculosis is high and travellers may already be infected on their arrival in the UK (Davies and Williams, 1993). Notifications to the CDSC support this view as cases are most common in the South East, Yorkshire and Humberside, which contain the highest proportion of immigrants in the UK.

- Healthcare professionals who have been in contact with infectious patients (Uttley and Pozniak, 1993).

These trends have been confirmed by analysing all new cases of tuberculosis in England and Wales since 1987 (Doherty *et al.*, 1995). Another possible contributory factor could be that some health authorities are no longer routinely offering vaccination, although it is recommended for all children aged between 10 and 14 years (NHSE, 1996).

Transmission

Transmission occurs by inhaling infectious airborne particles released in aerosols. The length of contact between the source and the potential new case increases the risk of transmission because the longer the period of exposure, the greater the risk of inhalation. Mycobacteria have tough, waxy walls, and the host response is primarily cell mediated rather than humoral. The bacilli multiply slowly and when phagocytosed are able to resist destruction by lysosomal enzymes. Instead, they continue to grow within macrophages and escape when the macrophages die, leading to their growth in the extracellular environment. Tuberculosis (primary) infection is possible with and without the full manifestation of the disease (post-primary or secondary infection).

Tuberculosis (primary) infection

Inhaled bacteria set up a single focus of infection in the lung, with involvement of the hilar lymph nodes (the primary complex). There is a local inflammatory reaction followed by healing to leave a calcified lesion visible on chest X-ray. There are usually few symptoms, and recovery is often spontaneous. The individual is not infectious to others and reacts negatively to bacteriological tests although he or she usually has a positive tuberculin skin test (Heaf test) (Figure 14.7). However, at the time of primary infection, bacteria are carried to the regional lymph nodes within the macrophages, gain access to the bloodstream and are carried to extrapulmonary sites. Extrapulmonary manifestations are severe – acute tuberculous bronchopneumonia, miliary tuberculosis, tuberculous meningitis and involvement of the bones, joints or kidneys. Even in the patient who apparently resists primary infection, the bacilli remain dormant for years, any condition compromising cell-mediated immunity reactivating them.

Test method:	Uses a multiple-puncture Heaf gun to inoculate tuberculin purified protein derivative (PPD) into the skin (that is, intradermally)

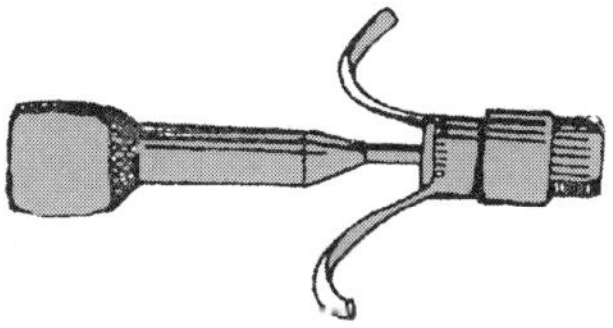

Applications:	Used as a routine screening test, for example prior to BCG immunisation
Test read:	3–7 days
Grades of reaction:	0 faint marks I discrete papules (4 or more) II papules joined (coalesced) to form a ring III raised area of induration IV raised area surrounded by blisters or ulcers

Figure 14.7 Heaf multiple-puncture tuberculin test

Post-primary infection

Post-primary (secondary) infection, the form mainly seen nowadays, occurs either through reactivation of the bacilli within old primary lesions or through reinfection. Pulmonary infection results in the development of one or more lesions near the apex of the lung. These do not usually involve the hilar lymph nodes. The infection is chronic and destructive, resulting in fibrosis, tissue loss and cavity formation. Spontaneous recovery is not a feature of post-primary tuberculosis, and patients may be infectious to others before treatment becomes effective.

Diagnosis

The diagnosis of active tuberculous infection is made by isolation and culture of the bacteria from sputum or gastric washings. Obtaining sputum requires the help of a physiotherapist. In addition, patients have a positive tuberculin skin test and may exhibit clinical signs and symptoms of disease (weight loss, night sweats, low grade pyrexia and malaise), although these are too non-specific to allow a firm diagnosis.

Prevention

Prevention involves:

- Immunisation – Childhood tuberculosis has been controlled through BCG immunisation administered routinely since the 1950s. The present high level of immunity in the general population can be maintained only by ensuring that a comprehensive immunisation programme continues (NHSE, 1996).

■ Mass radiography – This is used in conjunction with the segregation and treatment of known cases, with a follow-up of contacts.

■ Pasteurisation of milk – Pasteurisation has eradicated the risk of bovine tuberculosis in the UK. However, tuberculosis infection within dairy herds is viewed very seriously. Affected cattle are slaughtered and other stringent restrictions are put in place by MAFF, milk, for example being destroyed and the movement of cattle prohibited.

Treatment

See Chapter 4.

Multidrug resistant tuberculosis

Multidrug resistant tuberculosis (MDR-TB) is a new and dangerous development that complicates treatment. It is widespread in Russia.

Viral haemorrhagic fevers

The viral haemorrhagic fevers – Lassa fever, Ebola fever and Marburg disease – are caused by RNA arenaviruses. These are carried by rodents and monkeys in parts of tropical Africa. In 1967, seven animal handlers in the German town of Marburg died after contact with infected laboratory monkeys imported from Uganda, these being the first cases of viral haemorrhagic fever reported in Europe. Occasional cases are reported in people who have been in the bush and in health professionals working abroad. In recent years a number of outbreaks have been reported. For example, in 1995, an outbreak in Zaire killed 245 people.

Early symptoms are non-specific, and many people familiar with the onset of malaria attribute vague feelings of malaise to this infection. However, the disease progresses rapidly, with a decline in blood count, haemorrhage into the internal organs, the appearance of a bleeding rash, seizures and death. Blood splashing is common, and the spillage of infectious secretions can be difficult to contain in primitive field hospitals. The mortality rate is very high, death typically occurring within 10 days of infection.

Transmission

Transmission is by blood and body fluids. The viral haemorrhagic fevers are thought to be highly infectious. The long incubation period of 21 days means that travellers can arrive in the UK apparently healthy, developing symptoms after their arrival. The occasional cases of viral haemorrhagic fever seen in the UK tend to be reported in cities with good links to major airports.

Prevention

Prevention is attained by avoiding exposure to potentially infected wildlife. The most stringent form of isolation is used when caring for infected patients (see Chapter 5). Greater care is now being taken during contact with mammals imported from tropical Africa.

Diagnosis

The diagnosis is made by testing for viruses in the blood.

Treatment

Treatment is not currently available.

Rabies

Rabies causes infection of the brain and spinal cord. It is caused by a rhabodovirus able to infect all warm-blooded animals (Elliott, 1996). Cases have been recorded for more than 2000 years, and the disease has always been much feared because of its dramatic manifestations and because, in untreated cases, it is invariably fatal. The victim develops seizures and hydrophobia, falls into a coma and perishes. In some cases involving the brainstem, the infection follows a less dramatic course but nevertheless ultimately results in paralysis and death. The incubation period varies from 1 to 8 weeks.

Transmission

Transmission is via saliva in a bite from an infected animal. Viruses travel from the site of infection along the peripheral nerves to the brain. Transmission has also been recorded through corneal grafts from infected donors and from handling the tissues of infected animals.

Prevention

Prevention is currently achieved by enforcing quarantine on all imported livestock. Rabies was well established in the British Isles throughout the Middle Ages, and despite legislative measures, cases were reported until 1903. In Europe, however, rabies is endemic in wildlife so there is the potential for its transmission to domestic animals and humans. There are currently fears that it might to return to the UK because of a relaxation in the quarantine laws or via the Channel Tunnel, but these fears must be kept in perspective. In 1996, a woman developed rabies having been bitten by an infected bat that was not believed to have arrived via the transport system.

Vaccination is available for those at risk. Many countries in Europe and other parts of the world operate a mandatory system of vaccination and microchip registration, with documentation for pet animals. Pet animals with the relevant up-to-date documentation (a 'pet passport') including evidence of effective vaccination are allowed to cross frontiers without the need for quarantine (which is expensive and distressing for both pet and owner). At the time of writing the UK is planning the introduction of a similar system.

Diagnosis

Diagnosis is made by clinical examination and a history of contact with an infected animal.

Treatment

A suspect wound should be thoroughly cleansed with soap and water as soon as possible, and the site should be flooded with rabies immunoglobulin. Post-exposure prophylaxis is achieved by administering rabies immunoglobulin and vaccine. Dual treatment is given because the immunoglobulin provides rapid, albeit short-acting, immunity to cover the delay associated with active immunity from the vaccine.

REVISION CHECKLIST: KEY AREAS

❑ Introduction to epidemiology: Epidemiological patterns – the distribution of contagious disease, Factors affecting the incidence of infectious disease, Interpreting epidemiological data, International recommendations

❑ Control of communicable disease in the UK: Notifiable infections

❑ Changing trends of infectious disease: Malaria, Meningitis, Toxoplasmosis, Slow virus infections, Enteric fevers, Cholera, *Helicobacter* infection, Legionnaires' disease, Tuberculosis, Viral haemorrhagic fevers, Rabies

---

Activities – linking knowledge to clinical practice

1. **Select** one 'new' disease and conduct a search of the literature to establish:

(a) when and where it was first documented

(b) how it first presented

(c) the causative organism and how long it took scientists to establish its identity

(d) avenues for its control in both hospital and the community

(e) whether official figures are kept for the number of new cases appearing. If so establish where they are published and obtain the latest figures.

SELF-ASSESSMENT

1. An epidemic is:
   (a) the scientific study of disease ☐
   (b) never present in hospital ☐
   (c) a substantial increase in the number of cases of a condition simultaneously affecting several people ☐
   (d) always present in the population ☐

2. In a prospective epidemiological study, data are collected as new cases appear.
   True? ☐ False? ☐

3. Incidence is defined as the proportion of existing cases of a condition in a given population at a particular point in time.
   True? ☐ False? ☐

4. BSE is caused by:
   (a) a virus ☐
   (b) a prion ☐
   (c) bacteria ☐
   (d) a non-transmissible agent ☐

5. Malaria is caused by *Anopheles,* with *Plasmodium* parasites acting as the vector.
   True? ☐ False? ☐

6. You cannot catch malaria in the UK.
   True? ☐ False? ☐

7. *Neisseria meningitidis* causes:
   (a) a positive Kernig's sign ☐
   (b) turbulent CSF ☐
   (c) headaches ☐
   (d) photophobia ☐

8. Staphylococci have always been the predominant pathogens in hospital.
   True? ☐ False? ☐

9. *Toxoplasma gondii* is transmitted by:
   (a) eating contaminated meat ☐
   (b) handling cat litter ☐
   (c) any contact with cats ☐

10. Cholera is caused by a vibrio.
    True? ☐ False? ☐

11. Typhoid is caused by a vibrio.
    True? ☐ False? ☐

12. Tuberculosis is diagnosed by ....?

13. Legionnaires' disease is transmitted in water via the faecal-oral route.
    True? ☐ False? ☐

References

Bartlett CLR, Kurtz JB, Hutchinson JGP *et al.* (1983) 'Legionella in hospital and hotel water supplies'. *Lancet* **2**: 1315.

Barton S (1994) 'New therapies for the treatment of genital warts'. *Nursing Times* **90**(20): 38–40.

Behrens RH and Roberts JA (1994) 'Is travel prophylaxis worthwhile? Economic appraisal of prophylaxis measures against malaria, hepatitis A and typhoid in travellers'. *British Medical Journal* **309**: 918–22.

British Medical Association (1989) *Infection Control: The British Medical Association Guide.* Edward Arnold, London.

Cartwright K, Reilly S, White D and Stuart J (1992) 'Early treatment with parenteral penicillin in meningococcal disease'. *British Medical Journal* **305**: 143–7.

Charatan F (1991) 'Tuberculosis soars in New York'. *British Medical Journal* **303**: 209–10.

Charatan F (1994) 'New York makes progress in fight against tuberculosis'. *British Medical Journal* **308**: 807–8.

Conlon C (1990) 'Imported malaria'. *Practitioner* **243**: 841–3.

Davies D (1996) 'The causes of meningitis and meningococcal disease'. *Nursing Times* **92**(6): 25–7.

Davies PD and Williams CS (1993) 'Tuberculosis is increasing in England and Wales'. *Tubercle and Lung Disease* **74**: 350–51.

Dawood R (1987) *Travellers' Health*. Oxford University Press, Oxford.

Department of Health (1986a) *Report of the Committee of Inquiry into the Outbreak of Salmonella Food Poisoning at Stanley Royd Hospital*. HMSO, London.

Department of Health (1986b) *Report of the Committee of Inquiry into the Outbreak of Legionnaires' Disease in Stafford in 1985* (Badenoch Report). HMSO, London.

Department of Health (1988) *Report of the Committee of Inquiry into Future Development of the Public Health Function* (Acheson Report). HMSO, London.

Department of Health, Health and Safety Commission (1991) *The Prevention and Control of Legionellosis Including Legionnaires' Disease. Approved Code of Practice*. HMSO, London.

Desmonts G and Couvreur J (1974) 'Congenital toxoplasmosis: a prospective study'. *New England Journal of Medicine* **290**: 1110–16 .

Doherty MJ, Spence DPS and Davies PDO (1995) 'The increase in tuberculosis notifications in England and Wales since 1987'. *Tubercle and Lung Disease* **76**: 196–200.

Donowitz LG (1986) 'Failure of the overgown to prevent nosocomial infection in a paediatric intensive care unit'. *Paediatrics* **77**: 35–8.

Elliott R (1996) 'Menace across the channel'. *Nursing Times* **91**(27): 62–6.

Evans R, Burke JP, Classen D, Gardner RM, Menlove RL (1992) 'Computerised identification of patients at high risk for hospital-acquired infection'. *American Journal of Infection Control* **20**: 4–10.

Farmer RDT, Miller DL and Lawrenson R (1996) *Lecture Notes on Epidemiology and Public Health Medicine* (2nd edn). Blackwell Science, Oxford.

Fraser DW, Tsai T and Orenstein W (1977) 'Legionnaires' disease: description of an epidemic and of pneumonia'. *New England Journal of Medicine* **297**: 1183–97.

Gransden WR (1991) 'Predictors for bacteraemia'. *Journal of Hospital Infection* **18** (Supplement A): 308–16.

Griffiths G (1990) '*Toxoplasma gondii* and toxoplasmosis'. *Nursing Standard* **4**(28): 28–30.

Grist N and Reid D (1991) 'Typhoid immunisation'. *Practice Nurse* **6**: 114–17.

Hohlfeld P, Daffos F and Costa JM (1994) 'Pre-natal diagnosis of congenital toxoplasmosis with a polymerase chain reaction test on amniotic fluid'. *New England Journal of Medicine* **331**: 695–9.

Holmes S (1996) 'Making sense of bovine spongiform encephalopathy'. *Nursing Times* **92**(180): 38–40.

Institute of Food Science and Technology (1996) *Bovine Spongiform Encephalopathy: Position Paper*. IFST, London.

Joseph CA, Watson JM and Fern KJ (1992) 'BCG immunisation in England and Wales: a survey of policy and practice in schoolchildren and neonates'. *British Medical Journal* **305**: 495–8.

Joynson DHM and Payne R (1988) 'Screening for toxoplasma in pregnancy'. *Lancet* **2**: 795–6.

Kornelisse FR, de Groot R and Neijens HJ (1995) 'Bacterial meningitis: mechanisms of disease and therapy'. *European Journal of Paediatrics* **154**: 85–96.

Kreger BE, Craven DE and Carling PC (1989) 'Gram-negative bacteraemia. Reassessment of aetiology, epidemiology and ecology in 612 patients'. *American Journal of Medicine* **68**: 332–3.

Liu WK, Healing DE, Yeomans JT *et al.* (1993) 'Monitoring of hospital water supplies for Legionella'. *Journal of Hospital Infection* **24**: 1–9.

Matthews D (1991) 'Bovine spongiform encephalopathy'. *Journal of the Royal Society of Health* **111**: 3–5.

Moreland SCH (1991) 'Malaria and international air travel'. *Journal of the Royal Society of Health* **2**: 21–3.

Najero-Morrondo J (1991) 'Malaria control: history shows its possible'. *World Health* **5**: 4–5.

National Health Service Executive (1996) *Tuberculosis: Two reports of the Interdepartmental Working Group on Tuberculosis.* Letter (96) 51. NHSE, London.

Pennington Group (1997) *Report on the Circumstances Leading to the 1996 Outbreak of Infection with E. coli 0157 in Central Scotland: the Implications for Food Safety and the Lessons To Be Learnt.* Stationery Office, Edinburgh.

Spence DPS, Hotchkiss J, Williams CSD *et al.* (1993) 'Tuberculosis and poverty'. *British Medical Journal* **307**: 759–61.

Uttley AHC and Pozniak A (1993) 'Resurgence of tuberculosis'. *Journal of Hospital Infection* **23**: 249–53.

Vincent-Houdek M, Muytjens HL, Bongaerts GPA *et al.* (1993) 'Legionella monitoring: continuing story of nosocomial prevention'. *Journal of Hospital Infection* **25**: 117–24.

Watson JM (1993) 'Tuberculosis in Britain today'. *British Medical Journal* **306**: 221–2.

Woo AH, Yu AH and Goetz A (1986) 'Potential in-hospital modes of transmission of *Legionella pneumophila.* Demonstration experiments for dissemination by showers, humidifiers and rinsing of ventilation bag apparatus'. *American Journal of Medicine* **80**: 567–73.

Further reading and information sources

Burnet M and White DO (1972) *The Natural History of Infectious Disease.* Cambridge University Press, Cambridge.

Schaechter M, Medoff G and Schlessinger D (1989) *Mechanisms of Microbial Disease.* Williams & Wilkins, Baltimore.

Webber R (1996) *Communicable Disease Epidemiology and Control.* CAB International, London.

Appendix I Answers to self-assessment questions

CHAPTER 1

1. False

2. False

3. *Proteus, Candida*

4. (a) *Pseudomonas*
   (e) *Salmonella typhi*

5. False

6. True

7. True

8. Virulence is the ability of a pathogen to cause disease

9. False

10. True

CHAPTER 2

1. False

2. (a) Redness
   (b) Heat
   (c) Swelling
   (d) Loss of function
   (e) Pain

3. (a) Phagocytosis – ability of some granulocytic leucocytes to engulf foreign material. Most marked for neutrophils
   (b) Chemotaxis – chemical attraction between cells

   (c) Diapedesis – ability of neutrophils to squeeze between the endothelial cells of capillaries and enter the surrounding tissues

4. True

5. (c) Proteins

6. False

7. False

8. False

9. False

10. (e) None of these answers is correct

CHAPTER 3

1. False

2. Gram stain, wet film, dark ground illumination

3. All bacteria in a colony are derived from the same original cell and are therefore identical

4. In the case of fungi, special culture media incorporating antibiotics are used to inhibit bacterial growth. The cultures are kept for a prolonged period because many fungi are slow growing and diagnosis is based on morphology rather than biochemical or serological tests. Special cultures are used to grow viruses, and in some cases diagnosis is made by detecting antibodies in the patient's blood, or by the particular appearance under the electron microscope. As in the case of bacteria, serology is sometimes used

5. (i) Transport the specimen in a robust, leak-proof container
   (ii) Ensure that the outside of the container is not contaminated
   (iii) Avoid overfilling the container
   (iv) Wash the hands after collecting the specimen
   (v) Label with a biohazard label if appropriate

CHAPTER 4

1. True

2. In ideal circumstances, chemoprophylaxis is restricted to treat patients with a known infection or with a known risk of infection (see Table 4.1)

3. True

4. (b) *Pseudomonas*
   (d) *Klebsiella aerogenes*

5. (b) Cephalosporins
   (c) Penicillins

6. (c) Tetracyclines

7. Superinfection arises when the body's normal commensal flora is suppressed by antibiotics and replaced by drug-resistant organisms

8. Virus infections are difficult to treat because they are not sensitive to antibiotics. Most of the antiviral agents available also have severe side-effects. Viruses are intracellular parasites, which makes it difficult for drugs to attack them. In addition, viral infections are usually well established before symptoms occur

CHAPTER 5

1. (a) Destroy micro-organisms

2. True

3. False

4. (a) Gram-positive bacteria
   (d) *Mycobacterium tuberculosis*

5. (a) Potential harmfulness to users
   (b) Potential harmfulness to patients
   (c) Bactericidal effectiveness
   (d) Potential harmfulness to the environment

6. True

7. (a) Before aseptic procedures

(b) After handling patients

(c) After handling any items that are or could be soiled

(d) Before handling food

8. (b) Hands

9. False

10. False

CHAPTER 6

1. False

2. True

3. True

4. MRSA is difficult to eradicate, and many patients become carriers. Some strains are more readily disseminated than others,

(EMRSA), and treatment is difficult because of antibiotic resistance

5. EMRSA is more readily disseminated than other strains of MRSA

6. False

7. False

CHAPTER 7

1. (a) The presence of 100 000 or more pathogens per ml of urine

2. (b) A collection of micro-organisms and their extracellular products bound to a solid surface

3. True

4. False

5. (a) *Staphylococcus epidermidis*
  (b) *Escherichia coli*
  (f) *Proteus*

6. Complications secondary to urinary infection include encrustation, blockage, leakage and pain

CHAPTER 8

1. (c) A nick from scalpel blade

2. An abscess is defined as a localised collection of purulent material contained within a fibrin membrane

3. True

4. True

5. False

6. (b) Streptococci

7. False

8. False

CHAPTER 9

1. (c) *Bacteroides* spp.

2. The prevalence of lower respiratory tract infection in hospital is 22.9 per cent

3. True

4. True

5. (b) The mouth
   (c) The stomach
   (d) The suction catheter

6. False

7. (a) Patients in congestive cardiac failure
   (b) Those with chronic bronchitis
   (d) Anyone taking corticosteroids for more than a year

8. (c) An antitussive
   (d) Paracetamol dose calculated on body weight

CHAPTER 10

1. False

2. Bacteraemia is defined as the presence of bacteria in the blood

3. Septicaemia is defined as the multiplication of bacteria in the blood

4. True

CHAPTER 11

1. False

2. True

3. (a) Via the faecal-oral route
   (b) By person-to-person spread
   (c) On contaminated fingers
   (d) Via fomites

4. False

5. (a) Protozoal
   (c) Able to survive disinfection of water
   (d) A common hazard for the traveller

6. (c) A Gram-positive sporing rod
   (d) Consuming improperly canned food

7. (a) A harmless commensal in the human gut
   (b) A cause of travellers' diarrhoea
   (c) Spread by food-handlers
   (d) Able to produce enterotoxins causing severe foodborne illness

8. The symptoms and signs of hepatitis A virus infection are anorexia, nausea, vomiting, epigastric pain, jaundice and malaise

9. Microwave ovens are a potential health hazard only if used incorrectly, that is, if the instructions relating to the equipment and to reheating or cooking the food are not followed

CHAPTER 12

1. (a) Semen
   (b) Packed cell transfusions
   (c) Unfixed tissues
   (d) Synovial fluid

2. (a) Hepatitis B
   (b) Hepatitis C
   (c) Delta virus

3. False

4. False

5. (c) HBeAg

6. (a) Hepatitis B virus

7. True

8. False

CHAPTER 13

1. False

2. (b) Chancres

3. False

4. (a) *Neisseria gonorrhoeae*

5. True

6. (d) Podophyllin

7. False

8. (b) Protozoal

9. False

CHAPTER 14

1. (c) A substantial increase in the number of cases of a condition simultaneously affecting several people

2. True

3. False

4. (b) A prion

5. False

6. False

7. (a) A positive Kernig's sign
   (b) Turbulent CSF
   (c) Headaches
   (d) Photophobia

8. False

9. (a) Eating contaminated meat
   (b) Handling cat litter

10. True

11. False

12. Tuberculosis is diagnosed by culturing the bacterium *Mycobacterium tuberculosis*

13. False

Appendix II

Glossary

Abscess A localised collection of purulent material contained within a fibrin membrane.

Acquired immunity Immunity that is stimulated by exposure to a microbial antigen. It results from having the disease or receiving a vaccine containing antigenic substances.

Acute bronchitis Inflammation of the bronchi.

Aerobe A micro-organism able to grow in oxygen. Strict (obligate) aerobes must have oxygen for their growth and survival.

Agar Inert polysaccharide derived from seaweed, solid at room temperature, that is used to solidify culture media.

Agglutination The aggregation or clumping together of cells or particles.

Agranulocyte A leucocyte without granules in its cytoplasm.

Allergic reaction Hypersensitivity to a specific allergen (an antigen that produces allergy), for example pollen, dust, drugs or food. An abnormal immune response occurs that results in the release of chemical mediators such as histamine, prostaglandins and 5-hydroxytryptamine, inflammation and an anaphylactic reaction. There are usually local effects such as bronchospasm, rashes and diarrhoea, or rarely a widespread systemic reaction – anaphylactic shock.

Amoeba A microscopic unicellular protozoon. Some species have evolved as human parasites.

Anaerobe A micro-organism that can grow and flourish without the presence of oxygen. Strict (obligate) anaerobes cannot grow in the presence of oxygen, whereas some facultative microbes can grow with or without oxygen.

Anaphylactic shock A severe hypersensitivity reaction to a foreign protein mediated by mast cells and basophils.

Angiogenesis The formation of new blood capillaries.

Antibiotics Chemicals produced by living organisms, which are able to inhibit the growth of other organisms.

Antibodies (immunoglobulins) Proteins secreted by B lymphocytes that are able to bind to antigens during the immune response. They appear in the blood and tissue fluids of the host in the presence of specific antigens.

Antigenicity The ability of micro-organisms and their products to induce antibody production, a property that is utilised during immunisation.

Antigens Foreign cells or molecules that stimulate the immune system of the host and bind to antibodies or lymphocytes.

Antimicrobial agent Any substance that destroys micro-organisms or inhibits their growth.

Aseptic technique Procedures that exclude pathogenic micro-organisms from a particular environment, for example the use of sterile equipment and non-touch technique.

Atelectasis Collapse of the alveoli.

Attenuation The process by which vaccines are produced that retain microbial antigenicity without pathogenicity; that is, they induce antibody production without causing the disease.

Autoclaving The application of moist heat (steam under pressure) to achieve sterilisation.

Autolysis The self-destruction of an organism through the release of its own enzymes.

Bacillus A genus of Gram-positive micro-organisms. Also a general name for any rod-shaped bacterium.

Bacteraemia The presence of bacteria in the blood.

Bacteria Unicellular micro-organisms, widely distributed within a variety of environments. Some may be pathogenic (disease producing) whereas others perform useful functions, for example producing an environment that is hostile to harmful pathogens in the body.

Bactericidal agent A substance able to kill bacteria.

Bacteriological growth curve A typical sequence of events through which a newly inoculated culture of bacterial cells passes. It encompasses an initial lag phase (without multiplication, as the cells adapt to their new surroundings), a logarithmic phase (of optimal growth), a stationary phase (the total number of cells present remaining static as the rate of multiplication equals the number of cells dying through lack of nutrients) and a final decline phase (the number of cells decreasing as the nutrient supply is expended).

Bacteriophage (phage) A virus that parasitises bacteria.

Bacteriostatic agent A substance able to prevent bacterial replication but unable to kill bacteria.

Bacteriuria The presence of 100 000 or more pathogens per ml of urine.

Barrier nursing *See* Isolation.

Basophil A phagocytic granulocyte present in the blood, which contains heparin and histamine.

B cells B lymphocytes. Part of the humoral immune response, these become plasma cells, which produce antibodies (immunoglobulins).

Binary fission A method of microbial reproduction in which the micro-organism divides into two genetically identical 'daughter' cells.

Biofilm A collection of micro-organisms and their extracellular products bound to a solid surface.

Blood–brain barrier The membranes surrounding the brain and spinal cord allow the passage of some but not all chemical substances. This selective chemical permeability is commonly referred to as the blood–brain barrier.

Body fluids These include blood, all blood products (plasma, packed cells and white cell infusions), cerebrospinal fluid, amniotic fluid, pleural fluid, peritoneal fluid, pericardial fluid, synovial fluid, semen, vaginal fluid, saliva, unfixed tissues and organs, urine and faeces.

Bradykinin A chemical (peptide) mediator of the inflammatory response. It causes vasodilatation, involuntary muscle contraction, increased vessel permeability and pain.

Bronchitis Inflammation of the bronchial mucosa. Acute bronchitis is caused by a variety of viruses and bacteria. Chronic bronchitis is characterised by inflammation, excess mucus production, reduced mucociliary clearance and the eventual impairment of gaseous exchange. The chronic condition is made worse by repeated respiratory infections.

Capsule A mucus layer surrounding the cell wall of some types of bacterium. Helps to prevent desiccation when adverse environmental conditions are encountered.

Carrier An individual harbouring micro-organisms and able to transmit them without manifesting the signs and symptoms of infection.

Cell-mediated immunity Part of the immune response involving the action of T lymphocytes, which release regulatory chemicals and destroy foreign or abnormal cells.

Cellulitis The diffuse inflammation of connective tissue.

Cellulose A polysaccharide (complex carbohydrate) found as a component of plant cell walls.

Cell wall The outer layer that surrounds the cell membrane of certain cell types: some bacteria and all plant cells.

Chancre The primary lesion of syphilis; a hard, painless, highly infectious ulcer.

Chemoprophylaxis The prevention of infection by administering antibiotics before signs and symptoms appear.

Chemotaxis The movement (attraction or repulsion) of cells in response to chemicals, for example, leucocytes are attracted to areas of infection by the release of bacterial substances.

Chemotherapy The use of chemical substances to treat disease in palliation and cure. Covers antimicrobial drugs and drugs used to treat malignancy. In common usage, chemotherapy has come to mean the cytotoxic drugs used in cancer treatment.

Cilia Microscopic 'hair-like' processes found on the surface of some cells, for example respiratory mucosa and uterine tubes. Their ability to beat in a rhythmic way enables mucus to be cleared from the lungs, the process of mucociliary clearance.

Cleaning A procedure to remove vegetative micro-organisms in order to maintain the appearance, structure and effective functioning of the clinical environment and its contents.

Clinical infection Pathogenic invasion eliciting a response from the host (pyrexia and inflammation).

Clinical waste Waste generated by healthcare facilities (both human and animal). Disposal by incineration reduces the risk associated with hazardous waste, be it toxic or infectious.

Coagulase A bacterial enzyme capable of clotting plasma. It is produced by some staphylococci.

Coccus A general name for any spheroidally shaped bacterium, for example *Streptococcus* and *Staphylococcus*.

Cohort A group of individuals sharing a particular characteristic. Infection control in healthcare facilities is assisted by 'cohorting' similarly infected individuals together during outbreaks of infection.

Collagen Strong fibres giving strength to connective tissues such as skin, bone and tendons.

Colonisation The establishment of pathogenic micro-organisms at a particular body site with little or no host response to the pathogen. Colonisation can lead to a large number of micro-organisms, which form a reservoir for infection and cross-infection.

Colony A collection of bacteria growing on a solid culture medium that is large enough to be seen by the naked eye.

Commensal Micro-organisms that live in close association with their host. In their correct location, they do no harm and may even have a beneficial effect.

Communicable An infectious disease, one that is transmitted directly or indirectly from one person or animal to another.

Condylomata lata Flattened, wart-like lesions appearing during the secondary stage of syphilis at anatomical sites that are usually moist.

Conjugation A method by which bacteria exchange genetic material via sex pili. It is of particular importance in Gram-negative bacilli.

Cross-infection An infection acquired from outside the individual. *See* Exogenous.

Croup Laryngeal spasm.

Cystitis Inflammation of the urinary bladder, usually caused by bacteria such as *Escherichia coli*.

Cytokines A generic term used to describe cellular signalling molecules, such as the interferons and interleukins, involved in the modulation of body defences. Cytokines produced by lymphocytes are sometimes called lymphokines.

Decontamination Encompasses cleaning, disinfection and sterilisation.

Dermatophyte Superficial fungal infection of the skin involving the hair and nails.

Diploid Describes a cell containing a full set of paired chromosomes.

Disinfection Process causing the destruction of vegetative micro-organisms but not their spores.

Ectoparasite A parasite that lives upon the surface of its host, for example the flea.

Electron microscopy Using a beam of electrons rather than light to produce images of extremely small particles such as virus particles.

ELISA (enzyme-linked immunosorbent assay) A method that utilises enzyme-labelled antibodies to detect and measure other antibodies and antigens.

Encrustation The deposition of crystalline solids, mainly calcium and magnesium salts, on the surface of a catheter and drainage apparatus.

Endemic disease Disease always present in a given population.

Endocarditis Inflammation of the endocardium (the lining of the heart) and heart valves. Bacterial endocarditis is commonly caused by staphylococci and streptococci.

Endogenous infection Self-infection, the organisms responsible originating from the same individual.

Endotoxin An intracellular toxin contained in the cell wall of some Gram-negative bacteria, the toxin being released only when the bacterial cell is destroyed. The effects may include fever, malaise and inflammation. *Compare* Exotoxin.

Eosinophil A weakly phagocytic granulocyte playing a role in the allergic response and protecting the body against parasites.

Epidemic The same condition simultaneously affecting several people.

Epidemic infection A substantial increase in the number of people becoming carriers or infected with a particular organism.

Epithelialisation The growth of epithelium over the surface of a wound.

Epithelium The surface layer of cells covering the external and internal body surfaces.

Eukaryotic Cells with a true nucleus. The genetic material is enclosed within a nuclear membrane.

Exogenous (cross-infection) Caused by organisms originating from an external source – other patients, staff or the environment.

Exotoxin A toxin released through the bacterial cell wall into the extracellular fluid. These are secreted by Gram-positive bacteria and can have widespread effects. For example, the toxin of *Clostridium botulinum* inhibits the transmission of nerve impulses to cause paralysis.

Facultative Describes a micro-organism that can adapt and survive in different environmental conditions. *See* Anaerobe.

Fibroblast A connective tissue cell producing collagen.

Flagellum A microscopic projection from the surface of some cells, such as spermatozoa and some micro-organisms. It is concerned with cell movement.

Fluorescent antibody technique A method of detecting antibodies by the use of fluorescent dyes. The antibody, when attached to the dye, can be seen by using ultraviolet light with a special fluorescent microscope.

Fomite Any item that has been in contact with an infectious source and is in turn able to transfer infection.

Foodborne infection (invasive intestinal gastroenteritis) An infective condition caused by the activity of bacteria multiplying within the gastrointestinal tract.

Food intoxication Foodborne disease caused by bacterial toxins present in food.

Fungus A diverse group of simple plants that includes mushrooms, moulds and yeasts. Some are human pathogens, but many others are used in the food and pharmaceutical industries.

Gangrene Massive tissue death (necrosis) resulting from loss of the blood supply. Infection may be present in some types.

General paralysis of the insane A manifestation of tertiary syphilis involving the nervous system, characterised by memory loss, incontinence and disintegration of the personality, with a sudden or insidious onset.

Genus A biological subdivision of a family of plants or animals. A genus may contain several related species.

Gram staining A staining method used to identify and classify some bacteria. Gram-positive micro-organisms stain violet and Gram-negative ones pink.

Granulation tissue The outgrowth of new capillaries and connective tissue from the surface of a wound.

Granulocyte A leucocyte containing granules of enzymes within its cytoplasm. Includes basophils, neutrophils and eosinophils.

Gummata The lesions of tertiary syphilis. Obstruction to the blood supply results in necrosis and the formation of chronic ulcers that are probably not infectious.

Haemolysin A chemical produced by many bacteria that causes disruption of the red blood cell membrane.

Hepatitis Inflammation of the liver often caused by viruses, for example hepatitis B virus.

Histamine A chemical mediator released by many tissues and blood cells. Released during inflammation, it causes vasodilation, increased blood flow and increased vessel permeability. It is also implicated in the signs and symptoms of some allergic conditions, for example hay fever.

Hospital acquired infection (HAI) Infection arising from hospital stay or treatment. *See* Nosocomial infection.

Humoral immunity Part of the immune response involving B lymphocytes, plasma cells and the production of antibodies.

Hypersensitivity reaction Extreme sensitivity to an allergen.

Immunisation The administration of antigens to induce a state of immunity.

Immunity A state of resistance to an infectious agent, either intrinsic or acquired.

Immunocompromised patient An individual whose immune system is prevented from responding to pathogens in the normal way, through poor health or the action of drugs, or because he or she is undergoing an invasive procedure.

Immunodeficiency An impairment of humoral or cell-mediated immunity, which may be congenital or acquired. Causes include a failure to produce antibodies, AIDS and chemotherapy.

Immunoglobulins *See* Antibodies.

Immunosuppression The condition in which the activity of the immune system is depressed through treatment (radiotherapy or drugs) or disease.

Incidence The number of new cases of a disease occurring in a population over a specific period of time.

Incubation period The time from contact with an infectious disease until the signs and symptoms appear.

Infection The successful invasion, establishment and growth of micro-organisms within the tissues of a host.

Infectious *See* Communicable.

Inflammation The reaction of the tissues to trauma, characterised by heat, redness, pain and swelling.

Inoculum The material, such as urine or sputum, containing micro-organisms that is used to inoculate culture medium in the laboratory.

Interferons (IFNs) Antiviral proteins produced by T lymphocytes and other cells. They act as cellular signalling chemicals to modulate the immune response by stimulating other immune cells, macrophages, for examples, are activated to become killer cells. *See* Cytokines.

Invasive device/procedure One that bypasses the body's natural defences against infection, for example catheterisation, intubation or incision.

Isolation Various measures used to contain an infectious disease or protect vulnerable individuals. *See* Protective isolation.

Kaposi's sarcoma A malignant neoplasm of reticulo-epithelial cells first appearing as brown or purple lesions, usually on the feet, and spreading to other areas with metastasis to the lymph nodes and viscera. Affects those with HIV disease but is otherwise rare.

Latent infection An infection in which the individual is infected by the micro-organism without the signs of disease being obvious.

Leucocyte Generic name for all white blood cells: neutrophils, eosinophils, basophils, monocytes and lymphocytes.

Leucopoiesis The formation of leucocytes.

Live attenuated vaccine A vaccine produced from living micro-organisms, for example that for MMR (measles, mumps and rubella). The micro-organisms are changed to remove their ability to cause disease while still being able to stimulate antibody production. *See* Attenuation.

Lymphocyte Agranulocytic leucocytes, divided into T and B cells.

Lymphokines Chemicals released by T cells. They control all the cells of the immune system by activating or suppressing other cells involved in the immune response.

Lysozyme A bactericidal enzyme found in many body fluids, for example tears, saliva and nasal secretions.

Macrophage Large phagocytic cells that play an important scavenging role in the inflammatory response.

Malaise A general (non-specific) feeling of illness or discomfort.

Mast cell The term given to basophils once they have entered the tissues.

Memory cell Cells derived from B and T lymphocytes, which persist in the body. They 'remember' a specific antigen and are able to respond quickly if that antigen is encountered again.

Meningitis Inflammation of the meninges (the three membranes covering the brain and spinal cord). Meningitis may be bacterial or viral.

Methicillin-resistant *Staphylococcus aureus* (MRSA) A strain of *Staphylococcus aureus* that is resistant to most antimicrobial agents, including methicillin and flucloxacillin.

Microbe *See* Micro-organism.

Micro-organism An organism, usually too small to be seen without a microscope, for example bacteria, viruses, fungi and protozoa.

Monocyte A type of phagocytic leucocyte. It moves into the tissues from the blood to become a macrophage.

Mycelium Filaments produced by moulds (a type of fungus). It is these filaments that can be seen on mouldy food.

Myocarditis Inflammation of the myocardium, the muscle layer of the heart.

Natural killer (NK) cell A type of lymphocyte able to destroy virus infected cells and those showing malignant change.

Necrosis The localised death of tissue in response to injury, poor blood supply or disease.

Neutrophil A phagocytic granulocyte playing a key role in the inflammatory response.

Non-specific urethritis Non-gonococcal urethritis.

Normal flora The micro-organisms that normally colonise the body.

Nosocomial infection Infection not present or incubating at the time of hospital admission.

Obligate Of a micro-organism, requiring specific environmental conditions for its survival. *See* Aerobe and Anaerobe.

Opportunistic infection Infection caused by organisms that do not usually exhibit pathogenic properties but which become pathogenic in patients who are seriously ill or undergoing invasive treatment.

Opsonisation The process by which bacteria are marked as foreign cells, rendering them more susceptible to phagocytosis.

Otitis media Inflammation of the middle ear.

Pandemic The simultaneous occurrence of a large number of infections of the same kind.

Parasite An organism that lives in or on another living organism (the host). It confers no benefit upon the host, which it exploits for its physical needs.

Parenteral Literally meaning 'outside the alimentary tract'. Applies to therapy such as fluids, nutrients or drugs given via a route other than the alimentary tract, for example by injection.

Parenteral transmission Literally, the delivery of a substance by any route other than via the alimentary tract. Usually now taken to mean transmission via blood.

Pathogen An agent able to cause disease.

Pathogenicity The capacity of micro-organisms to cause disease.

Pericarditis Inflammation of the pericardium (the membrane covering of the heart). This can be caused by bacteria or viruses.

Peritonitis Inflammation of the peritoneum (the membrane lining the abdominal cavity and covering some of the organs). It may be caused by bacterial infection or chemical irritation.

Petri dish A plastic dish that, when filled with agar, is used to grow bacteria in the laboratory.

pH The hydrogen ion concentration. A method of expressing acidity (hydrogen ions) or alkalinity (hydroxyl ions). It utilises a logarithmic scale with a range from 0 to 14 (pH 0 representing the greatest concentration of hydrogen ions, pH 7 neutrality, the number of hydrogen and hydroxyl ions being equal, and pH 14 the greatest concentration of hydroxyl ions).

Phage *See* Bacteriophage.

Phagocyte A leucocyte that is capable of phagocytosis, for example a neutrophil, monocyte or macrophage.

Phagocytosis The cellular engulfment of bacteria and particulate matter.

Phlebitis Inflammation of the vein. Usually caused by chemical or mechanical irritation but may become complicated by infection.

Plasma cells Transient immune cells derived from B lymphocytes. They secrete specific antibodies.

Plasmid Extrachromosomal DNA present in the cytoplasm of some bacteria.

Pleomorphism A state in which the size and shape of bacterial cells become highly variable, sometimes ceasing to display the typical morphological characteristics of the species and thus making identification difficult.

Pneumonia Inflammation of the lung. In bronchopneumonia, the affected tissue is distributed widely around the bronchi. In lobar pneumonia, the area of consolidation is localised. Nosocomial pneumonia is hospital-acquired infection of the lower respiratory tract developing at least 72 hours after admission.

Polymorphonuclear leucocyte A leucocyte containing a many-lobed nucleus. This can be a neutrophil, an eosinophil or a basophil.

Prevalence The total number of cases of a disease present in a population at a single point in time.

Primary intention The type of healing that occurs in clean surgical wounds where the skin edges are in apposition.

Primary response The immune response that results from the first contact with an antigen. There is an initial lag phase of 2–3 weeks before antibody production reaches a protective level.

Prion A virus-like infectious agent that consists of protein but no nucleic acids. Prions are responsible for the transmission of such diseases as Creutzfeldt–Jakob disease, bovine spongiform encephalopathy and scrapie in sheep.

Prokaryotic Describing a cell that lacks a true nucleus and nuclear membrane, the genetic material lying within the cytoplasm.

Prophylaxis Measures taken to prevent disease, for example immunisation and perioperative antimicrobial drug therapy.

Protective isolation Special measures taken to protect immunocompromised individuals from infection.

Protozoa Microscopic unicellular animals. Many are harmless, but others are responsible for human diseases including malaria, toxoplasmosis and cryptosporidiosis, which affects immunocompromised individuals.

Pseudomembranous colitis A serious, sometimes life-threatening condition in which large areas of the intestinal epithelium undergo necrosis. Most cases develop after patients have received broad-spectrum antibiotics, which suppress the normal intestinal flora.

Puerperal sepsis A local infection, which results from childbirth, arising in the genital tract leading to septicaemia.

Pus Matter resulting from infection. It consists of bacterial cells, leucocytes, cell debris and tissue fluid.

Pyelonephritis Ascending urinary tract infection spreading outwards from the pelvis of the kidney to its cortex. In some cases, the source of infection is the blood rather than the lower urinary tract.

Reservoir of infection A source of micro-organisms, for example a human carrier of *Salmonella typhi*.

Reverse transcriptase A viral enzyme that catalyses the synthesis of nucleic acids.

Rickettsia A group of micro-organisms that have the characteristics of both bacteria and viruses. They cause diseases such as typhus and Rocky Mountain spotted fever.

Risk assessment A method of identifying and assessing a particular risk or hazard. Subsequent management seeks to minimise the potential risk by the use of specific precautions, for example handwashing protocols.

Saprophyte A free-living micro-organism obtaining nourishment from decaying animals and plant tissue.

Screening A preventative measure employed to identify potential or incipient disease.

Secondary intention The type of healing that occurs in a wound where there is tissue loss, for example a pressure sore. Here, the wound heals from the base.

Secondary response The immune response occurring when B lymphocytes encounter an antigen on a second or subsequent occasion. The memory cells produce antibodies very quickly (without a lag phase).

Septicaemia Multiplication of bacteria in the blood.

Seroconversion The secretion of specific antibodies following exposure to an antigen.

Serology The study of blood sera with particular emphasis on the reactions concerned with immunological function and diagnosis.

Serotyping A method of classifying microbial strains based on their antigenic characteristics. The surface antigens are identified in the laboratory by using the specific antibodies.

Serum The plasma component of coagulated blood with all the cellular elements removed.

Sharp Any item able to cut or penetrate skin or mucous membranes (needles, razors, lancets, scalpel blades, microscope slides, ampoules, wires and stitch-cutters).

Slough Necrotic tissue that detaches from healthy tissue following infection.

Source of infection The site from which a micro-organism responsible for an infection has emanated.

Species Smaller subdivisions within a genus.

Spirochaetes An order of slender, spiral-shaped bacteria. Genera included in the order are *Treponema*, *Leptospira* and *Borrelia*.

Spore A bacterial adaptation to unfavourable environmental conditions. Cells survive as their metabolism slows, and they become surrounded by a thick capsule. When favourable conditions return, the spore is able to germinate.

Sterilisation The destruction of all micro-organisms and their spores.

Stevens–Johnson syndrome An adverse, potentially fatal reaction to co-trimoxazole characterised by a bullous rash, fever and ulceration of the mouth.

Strain Micro-organisms of the same species that have different physical and chemical features.

Subclinical infection The presence of infection without any obvious signs or symptoms of the disease.

Surveillance The process of monitoring the occurrence of diseases, for example notifiable infectious diseases, within a population.

Tabes dorsalis A manifestation of tertiary syphilis involving the posterior columns of the spinal cord and the associated sensory nerve roots, resulting in disordered gait and a loss of sense of position in the legs (locomotor ataxia).

T cells T lymphocytes that facilitate cell-mediated immunity. They differentiate into active T cells that destroy foreign cells carrying specific antigens and regulate the immune response.

Titre The measurement of antibody concentration, for example in the blood.

Toxin A poisonous substance, usually of microbial origin.

Toxoid A microbial toxin that has been modified to retain antigenicity without pathogenicity. It is used to produce immunity against specific diseases, for example tetanus. *See* Attenuation.

Transduction The transfer of genetic material from one bacterium to another by a bacteriophage.

Transformation The transfer of genetic material from one bacterium to another through the cell wall into the cytoplasm.

Universal precautions Precautions taken routinely during contact with blood or body fluids, for example wearing gloves and a plastic apron, and decontaminating the hands after removing the gloves.

Vaccine An extract prepared from inactivated or weakened organisms that is used to induce a state of immunity to the pathogen in the recipient.

Vibrio A genus of comma-shaped bacteria. *Vibrio cholerae* causes cholera.

Virulence The ability of a micro-organism to cause infection.

Virus A micro-organism containing either DNA or RNA. They can only replicate inside a living host cell. Visualisation is only possible using electron microscopy.

White blood cell *See* Leucocyte.

Yeast A simple, single-celled fungus, for example *Candida albicans*.

Ziehl–Neelsen stain A staining technique used in the identification of acid-fast bacilli such as *Mycobacterium tuberculosis*.

Zoonoses Diseases transmitted from animals to humans, for example anthrax and rabies.

Index